...mporary Perspectives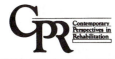
...abilitation

...**. Wolf, PhD, FAPTA**
...**n-Chief**

The Biomechanics
of the Foot and Ankle

The Biomechanics of the Foot and Ankle

Edition 2

Robert A. Donatelli, PhD, PT, OCS
Instructor, Division of Physical Therapy
Department of Rehabilitative Medicine
Emory University School of Medicine
and
National Director of Sports Rehabilitation
Physiotherapy Associates
Atlanta, Georgia

F. A. DAVIS COMPANY • Philadelphia

F. A. Davis Company
1915 Arch Street
Philadelphia, PA 19103

Printed in the United States of America

Last digit indicates print number: 10 9 8 7 6 5 4 3 2 1

Publisher: Jean-François Vilain
Developmental Editor: Crystal S. McNichol
Production Editor: Marianne Fithian
Cover Designer: Louis J. Forgione

As new scientific information becomes available through basic and clinical research, recommended treatments and drug therapies undergo changes. The author and publisher have done everything possible to make this book accurate, up to date, and in accord with accepted standards at the time of publication. The author, editors, and publisher are not responsible for errors or omissions or for consequences from application of the book, and make no warranty, expressed or implied, in regard to the contents of the book. Any practice described in this book should be applied by the reader in accordance with professional standards of care used in regard to the unique circumstances that may apply in each situation. The reader is advised always to check product information (package inserts) for changes and new information regarding dose and contraindications before administering any drug. Caution is especially urged when using new or infrequently ordered drugs.

Library of Congress Cataloging-in-Publication Data

The biomechanics of the foot and ankle / [edited by] Robert A. Donatelli;
  editor-in chief, Steven L. Wolf.—Ed. 2.
    p. cm.—(Contemporary perspectives in rehabilitation)
  Includes bibliographical references and index.
  ISBN 0-8036-0031-3 (alk. paper)
    1. Foot—Abnormalities. 2. Ankle—Abnormalities. 3. Foot—
Abnormalities—Patients—Rehabilitation. 4. Ankle—Abnormalities—
Patients—Rehabilitation. 5. Foot—Mechanical properties.
6. Ankle—Mechanical properties. I. Donatelli, Robert. II. Wolf,
Steven L. III. Series: Contemporary perspectives in rehabilitation
(Unnumbered).
    [DNLM: 1. Foot—physiology. 2. Ankle Joint—physiology.
3. Biomechanics. 4. Foot Diseases—therapy. 5. Gait. WE 880 B615
1995]
RD781.B53 1996
617.5'85—dc20
DNLM/DLC
for Library of Congress
    95-24075

Dedication to the Second Edition

I would like to dedicate this book to my mother, Rose Donatelli. Her love and support has sustained me through the rough times in association with my demanding schedule.

Dedication to the First Edition

I would like to dedicate this book to my best friend, Scot Irwin. His love and support have enabled and motivated me to pursue my interest in the area of foot and ankle biomechanics. His friendship has encouraged me to persevere through the good times and hard times in our practice.

Foreword

Soon after the first edition of *The Biomechanics of the Foot and Ankle* appeared in 1990 it became apparent that many courses in orthopedics for students and clinicians had found a suitable text in which the anatomy, pathomechanics, and treatment of the foot and ankle could be studied. Over the next 5 years the obvious challenge posed by the success of the first edition was how to configure an even better book. The decision was made to maintain the three-section format of the first edition. The original chapters on normal anatomy and biomechanics and abnormal biomechanics conceived by Donatelli to be all-inclusive could only be improved by updating references and findings relevant to this subject matter. The same could be said for the chapter by Corradi-Scalise and Ling on normal development of gait. Consequently, aside from some logical changes in formatting, these contributions are retained and newer material added wherever appropriate.

During the past 5 years we did not remain dormant and merely rest on the laurels of the first edition. Bob Donatelli and F. A. Davis Company actively sought constructive criticism about the volume, including soliciting input on how the text could be improved. We deduced that Section I on "Biomechanics of the Foot and Ankle" needed a comprehensive treatise on gait. Subsequently, we were fortunate to recruit Leslie Russek to write such a chapter. This task proved substantial, because Russek had to contain her enthusiasm to write a tome by condensing material often covered in volumes so that it read in a clear, yet challenging matter. We believe that she has succeeded in producing a magnificently condensed synopsis of multiple issues about ambulation including determinants of gait, temporal and spatial characteristics, kinematics, neural control mechanisms, muscle activation patterns, kinetics, and several other important considerations. At the same time, her writing style confronts the analytic skills of the reader.

Section II, "Biomechanical Evaluation" retains some original contributions and brings new issues to the foreground. Luke Bordelon's clinical assessment of the foot retains its unique perspective, but references are updated. The same can be said of the presentation by Vito and Kalish on radiographic evaluation but now scanning and imaging techniques and their interpretation are added. Mike Wooden has updated his chapter on functional orthotics. Bruce Greenfield has been joined by Marie Johanson to contemporize information on overuse syndromes, including a discussion on tissue degeneration with overuse. The original presentation by Nathan Schwartz on the diabetic foot has been reformatted and expanded with Jennifer Bottomley co-authoring the chapter. New information on pathomechanics of the diabetic foot, treatment suggestions, and general considerations of such issues as nutrition, exercise, drug therapy, and patient education have been added.

Section III, "Treatment Approaches to Restore Normal Movement" has been expanded to meet the needs of readers. The original chapter on biomechanical orthotics by Donatelli and Wooden provides updated references and expands the section on laboratory orthotics. Karen Davis and Jeff Cooper have joined forces with John Garbalosa to augment John's original contribution on physical therapy treatment of foot and ankle pathologies through the inclusion of two case study learning formats and two other cases addressing specific sports injuries. Greenfield and Bennett have composed a comprehensive chapter on application of closed kinetic chain rehabilitation in treating lower extremity problems. This new chapter addresses theory and justifies exercise progression in an exceptionally comprehensive manner. Last, Paul Speigl joins Karen Seale to present surgical interventions for foot and ankle problems. Added to the original offering is a detailed presentation on arthritis.

Throughout the text the original problem-solving format is kept to meet the continuing requests of students and clinicians not to abandon this valuable instructional mode. By following our convictions as well as adhering to the requests of our readers, we believe that the second edition of *The Biomechanics of the Foot and Ankle* is superior to its first born. It offers compelling information that will strengthen support to justify therapeutic interventions for this often unappreciated anatomical area.

Steven L. Wolf, PhD, FAPTA
Series Editor

Preface

The first edition of *The Biomechanics of the Foot and Ankle* was influenced by an almost explosive proliferation of physical therapists fabricating and prescribing foot and ankle orthotics. Physical therapy management of foot and ankle disorders has become a subspecialty within the physical therapy orthopedic specialty. More and more articles are being published by physical therapists on foot mechanics and orthotics intervention.

The second edition of the book has deliberated on the concept of the foot as an important part of the lower kinetic chain. Two new chapters have been added, Chapter 4, "Closed Kinetic Chain and Gait" by Leslie Russek and Chapter 12, "The Application of Kinetic Chain Rehabilitation in the Lower Extremities," by Bruce Greenfield and J. Gregory Bennett. The addition of the chapter by Russek, in particular, establishes the knowledge base needed for the understanding of the lower kinetic chain during ambulation. Combined with the chapters 1 and 2 by Donatelli, "Normal Anatomy of Biomechanics" and "Abnormal Biomechanics," and Chapter 3, "Normal Development of Gait" by Deborah Corradi-Scalise, the first section has evolved as a detailed functional analysis of the lower extremity.

In Section II, "Biomechanical Evaluation," Chapter 6, "Biomechanical Radiographic Evaluation," by George Vito and Stanley Kalish, contains new information on advances in radiology of the foot and ankle. Chapter 7, "Biomechanical Evaluation for Functional Orthotics," by Michael J. Wooden, has been reinforced by the addition of new information based on research establishing the reliability of evaluation methods described in the chapter. Chapter 8, "Evaluation of Overuse Syndromes," and Chapter 9, "The Diabetic Foot," have been strengthened by the contributions of two new authors, Marie Johanson and Jennifer M. Bottomley, respectively. Johanson increased the understanding of overuse injuries of the lower kinetic chain, and Bottomley added the physical therapist's perspective. Both authors emphasized the conservative management of overuse syndromes and diabetes by developing patient cases. The clinicians faced with the problems of evaluation of these complete pathologies will be enlightened by the information added to these chapters.

As mentioned previously, Section III now contains a new chapter by Greenfield and Bennett. In addition, all the existing chapters have been significantly revised. Chapter 10, "Biochemical Orthotics," has been updated to reflect the wealth of new research on the effectiveness of foot orthotic intervention. In Chapter 11, "Physical Therapy," Karen E. Davis, Jeff Cooper, and John C. Garbalosa have added four new cases on foot and ankle problems in the professional and recreational athlete. Finally, Chapter 13, "Surgical Intervention," by Paul V. Spiegl and Karen S. Seale now contains new information on the surgical management of foot and ankle disorders.

Any rehabilitation professional entrusted with the care and treatment of mechanical abnormalities of the foot and ankle as it relates to the lower kinetic chain will benefit from this book. We hope that its contents, like those of its predecessors in the *Contemporary Perspectives in Rehabilitation* series will hold true to the philosophy of the series—comprehensive, clinically relevant presentations that are well documented, contemporary, and personally challenging to the student and clinician alike.

Robert A. Donatelli, PhD, PT, OCS

Acknowledgments

Love and thanks to my staff at Physiotherapy Associates in Jonesboro, Georgia: Zita, Tammie, John, Ronnie, Karen, Paula, Bobbie and Carolyn, their support and professionalism has enabled me to peruse my educational endeavors. A special thanks to my soul mate, Judy D. I appreciate Steve Wolf for his support through the development of the second edition; and to Jean François Vilain and his colleagues at F. A. Davis.

Contributors

Ian J. Alexander, MD
Department of Orthopedic Surgery
The Cleveland Clinic Foundation
Cleveland, Ohio

J. Gregory Bennett, MS, PT
Dominion Physical Therapy
NOVA Health System
Fairfax, Virginia

R. Luke Bordelon, MD
Clinical Assistant Professor
   of Orthopedics
Louisiana State University
School of Medicine
New Orleans, Louisiana

Jennifer M. Bottomley, MS, PT
Outpatient Rehabilitation Coordinator
Hillhaven Corp.
Lexington, Massachusetts
Core Faculty
Harvard Medical School Division
   on Aging
Cambridge, Massachusetts

K. R. Campbell, PhD
Department of Musculoskeletal
   Research
The Cleveland Clinic Foundation
Cleveland, Ohio

Jeff Cooper, MS, ATC
Head Athletic Trainer
Philadelphia Phillies
Philadelphia, Pennsylvania
and
Consultant to Physiotherapy Associates
Atlanta, Georgia

Deborah Corradi-Scalise, MA, PT
Department of Physical Therapy
Hebrew Academy for Special Children
Woodmere, New York
Private Practice
Baldwin Harbor, New York

Karen E. Davis, MPT, ATC
Physiotherapy Associates
Atlanta, Georgia

Robert A. Donatelli, PhD, PT, OCS
Instructor, Division of Physical Therapy
Emory University School of Medicine
and
National Director of Sports
   Rehabilitation
Physiotherapy Associates
Atlanta, Georgia

John C. Garbalosa, MMSC, PT
Center for Locomotion Studies
Pennsylvania State University
University Park, Pennsylvania

Bruce Greenfield, MSc, PT, OCS
Instructor, Division of Physical Therapy
Department of Rehabilitative Medicine
Emory University School of Medicine
Atlanta, Georgia

Marie Johanson, MS, PT, OCS
Clinic Director
Physiotherapy Associates
Atlanta, Georgia

Wen Ling, PhD, PT
Assistant Professor
Department of Physical Therapy
New York University
New York, New York

Stanley Kalish, DPM
Associate Professor, Department of
    Surgery
New York College of Podiatric Medicine
Attending Podiatrist, HCA/Doctor's
    Hospital
Tucker, Georgia
Staff Podiatrist
Henry General Hospital
Atlanta, Georgia

Leslie N. Russek, PhD, PT
Research Physical Therapist
Physiotherapy Associates
Glen Burnie, Maryland

Nathan Schwartz, DPM
Assistant Clinical Professor
Emory University
Atlanta, Georgia
Private Practice
Windy Hill City
Marietta, Georgia

Karen S. Seale, MD
Assistant Professor and Head of Foot
    and Ankle Surgery Section
Department of Orthopedic Surgery
University of Arkansas
Little Rock, Arkansas

Paul V. Spiegl, MD
Private Practice
Orthopedic Surgery
Atlanta, Georgia

George Vito, DPM
HCA/Doctors Hospital
Tucker, Georgia

Michael J. Wooden, MS, PT, OCS
National Director of Clinical Research
Clinic Director
Physiotherapy Associates
Lilburn, Georgia
Instructor, Division of Physical Therapy
Department of Rehabilitation Medicine
Emory University School of Medicine
Atlanta, Georgia

Contents

Biomechanics of the Foot and Ankle

CHAPTER 1

Normal Anatomy and Biomechanics

Robert A. Donatelli, PhD, PT, OCS

The study of normal mechanics in the musculoskeletal system is the analysis of forces and their effects on anatomic structures, such as bones, muscles, tendons, and ligaments.[1] The study of forces acting on the musculoskeletal structures can be divided between the examination of bodies at rest (static) and bodies in motion (dynamic).[1] Kinetics is the study of the relationship between the forces and the resulting movement of the musculoskeletal structures.[1] This chapter focuses on descriptions of movements and forces acting on the functional joints of the normal human foot and ankle. Because the prenatal and postnatal development of the human foot are important in the establishment of an organ of locomotion, the development of the functional joints of the foot and ankle is briefly discussed. Consideration of the ligaments, tendons, and muscles and their influences on movement is also included. A glossary of key terms appears at the end of this chapter.

What is a normal foot? Four of Cailliet's[2] criteria for normalcy are absence of pain, normal muscle balance, central heel, and straight and mobile toes. Adequate distribution of weight-bearing forces on the foot while standing and during the stance phase of gait is also an important criterion of normalcy.

The foot is the terminal joint in the lower kinetic chain that opposes external resistance. Proper arthrokinematics within the foot and ankle influence the ability of the lower limb to attenuate the forces of weight bearing. The lower extremity should distribute and dissipate compressive, tensile, shearing, and rotatory forces during the stance phase of gait. Inadequate distribution of these forces can lead to abnormal movement, which, in turn, produces excessive stress and results in the breakdown of connective tissue and muscle. The normal mechanics of the foot and ankle are the combined effects of muscle, tendon, ligament, and bone function. The coordinated and unified effect of these tissues within the foot, ankle, and lower extremity results in the most efficient force attenuation.

The foot, for the purposes of this chapter, can be divided into three sections: the rearfoot, midfoot, and forefoot. The rearfoot converts the torque of the lower limb. The transverse rotations of the lower extremity are converted into sagittal, horizontal, and frontal plane movements. The rearfoot also influences the function and movement of the midfoot and forefoot. The midfoot transmits movement from the rearfoot to the forefoot and promotes stability. The movements and function of the midfoot depend on the mechanics of the rearfoot. The forefoot adapts to the ground as the terrain changes, adjusting to the uneven surface. The forefoot accommodation depends on the normal mechanics of the rearfoot.

The bones of the foot are shown in Figures 1–1 and 1–2.

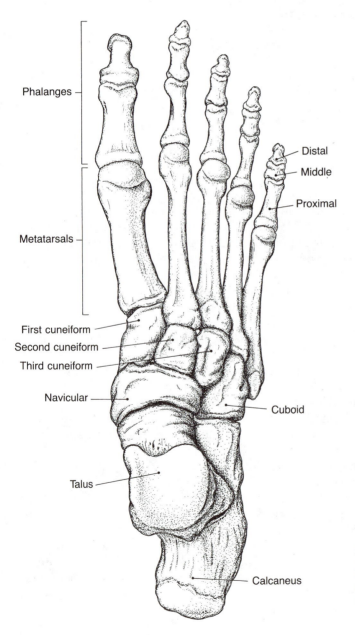

FIGURE 1–1. Dorsal view of the bones of the foot. (From Rothstein, JM, et al: The Rehabilitation Specialist's Handbook. FA Davis, Philadelphia, 1991, p 40, with permission.)

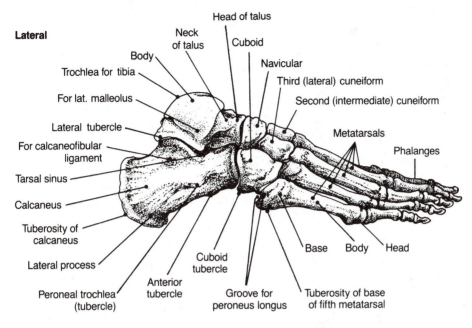

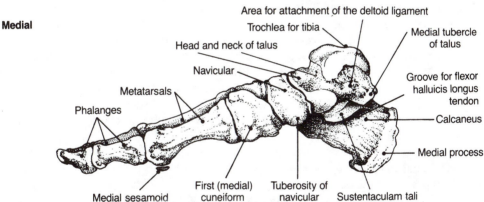

FIGURE 1–2. Lateral (*top*) and medial (*bottom*) views of the bones of the foot. (From Rothstein, JM, et al: The Rehabilitation Specialist's Handbook. FA Davis, Philadelphia, 1991, p 39, with permission.)

DEVELOPMENT OF THE HUMAN FOOT FOR LOCOMOTION

Early Development

REARFOOT

The rearfoot is made up of the talus and the calcaneus. The importance of the calcaneus and the talus is apparent from their early development within the fetus and from the evolutionary changes that have enhanced their function. The calcaneus is the first of the tarsal bones to begin ossification (Table 1–1). The ossification center appears between the 5th and 6th fetal month. The talus is the second tarsal bone to ossify, at

TABLE 1–1 Ossification Schedule of the Bones of the Foot and Ankle

Bone	Ossification Period
Tibia (distal epiphysis)	6–10 mo gestation to 18 y
Fibula (distal epiphysis)	11–18 mo to 17 y
Talus	8 mo gestation to 17–18 y
Calcaneus	5–6 mo gestation to 16 y (women) or 20 y (men)
Navicular	Boys, 3 y to 17–18 y
	Girls, 2 y to 17–18 y
Cuboid	Birth–21 days to 17–18 y
Cuneiforms	Lateral, 4–20 mo to 17–18 y
	Medial, 2 y to 17–18 y
	Intermediate, 3 y to 17–18 y
Metatarsals	1–12 wk gestation to 16–18 y
	2 or 3–9 wk gestation to 16–18 y
	4 or 5–10 wk gestation to 16–18 y
Phalanges	Proximal, 1–2.2 y to 13–16 y
	Distal, 2.5–4.7 y to 11.5–14.7 y
	Intermediate, 15 wk gestation to 18 y

about the 8th fetal month.[3] The talus and calcaneus have exhibited evolutionary changes associated with the development of the foot into the body's primary weight-bearing, balancing, and propulsive organ.[4] The calcaneus has become quite large (for additional propulsive leverage) and has developed a sturdy tuberosity for increased weight bearing.[4] The talus articulates with the calcaneus on facets parallel to the ground for additional balance and adaptation. The articulations of the talus in humans differ from those of other primates, in which the articular facets are steeply sloped.[4]

The calcaneus of the fetus at 3 months represents an average of 25.3% of the total foot length; in adults it is 35%.[5] The posterior segment of the calcaneus grows faster than the anterior segment, contributing to the mechanical efficiency of the triceps surae. The talar body increases more rapidly in height than in length, contributing to the development of the talocrural joint.

The foot develops in a supinated position. Correction of fetal supination is accomplished by changes in the rearfoot. As lateral rotation of the talar head and neck occurs, the forefoot varus is reduced. The lack of this rotation is the major cause of forefoot varus.[6,7] Another characteristic of fetal supination is a varus calcaneus (inverted position). Three months after birth, the varus angle of the calcaneus is 36.8°, compared with a varus angle of 3.6° in adults.[5] Finally, an adducted position of the forefoot is corrected by changes in the position of the talus and calcaneus. The talar neck–calcaneal angle decreases from 42° at birth to 23° in the adult. The talar trochlear and calcaneal angle reduces from 9° at birth to 1° in the adult (Fig. 1–3).

MIDFOOT

The midfoot is made up of the navicular and cuboid bones. The midtarsal joint is the major articulation of the midfoot formed by the approximation of these two bones, which articulate with the calcaneus and the talus, respectively. Ossification of the cuboid bone takes place from birth to 21 days of age.[3] The navicular is one of the last of the tarsal bones to ossify, which it does between the 2nd and 5th years.

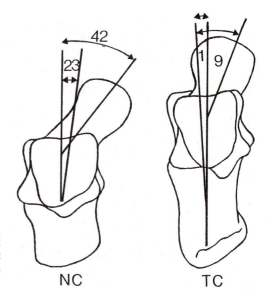

FIGURE 1–3. Talar trochlear and calcaneal angle. Calcaneal angle (NC) is 42° in the infant and 23° in the adult. Trochlear-calcaneal angle (TC) is 9° in infants and 1° in adults.

FOREFOOT

The forefoot includes the cuneiforms, metatarsals, and phalanges. In the fetus, the first metatarsal grows faster than the second. After birth, the first and second metatarsals grow at the same rate. The first metatarsal is shorter and thicker than the second. The intermetarsal angle between the first and second metatarsal bones decreases from 32° at age 2 months, to 8.9° at age 9 months, and 6.2° in the adult.[5] The primary ossification centers of the metatarsals appear between the 8th and 10th weeks of life.

The hallux is the most prominent of the phalanges. Ossification of the medial and lateral sesamoids of the great toe takes place between the ages of 12 and 14 years. By the age of 2 years, the ossification centers of the medial cuneiform and the proximal phalanges have appeared. Between the ages of 2 and 3 years, the ossification centers of the middle cuneiform and middle phalanges appear.

Development During Childhood

The infant foot appears excessively pronated because the medial arch is occupied by a fat pad.[8] The infant foot is very supple. The total range of motion of the subtalar joint is 50°. The ankle joint or talocrural joint exhibits a combined dorsiflexion and plantar flexion range of 20° to 50°.[9]

From the age of 5 to 10 years in girls and 5 to 12 years in boys, the foot grows 0.9 cm per year. At the age of 10 and 12 years, respectively, the foot is at 90% of the adult size. At the age of 14 and 16 years, respectively, the foot is at the adult size.[8]

By 6 to 8 years of age, the bones of the foot assume adult shape.[8] The adult pattern of gait develops between 3 and 5 years of age, slightly ahead of the bones of the foot.[3]

Early in the developmental stages, the rearfoot largely influences the midfoot and forefoot's form and function. Lack of lateral rotation of the talar head, inadequate reduction in the talar-calcaneal angles, and insufficient changes in the varus angle of the calcaneus can produce deformities of the forefoot and rearfoot. Abnormal pronation and supination in the adult may be attributed to the imperfect development of the foot within the fetus. The evolutionary changes in the development of the foot are secondary to alterations in function. The foot has become the primary organ of weight bearing, balance, and propulsion.

FUNCTIONAL ANATOMY AND MECHANICS OF THE ADULT FOOT

The functional joints of the foot and ankle are the ankle (talocrural), the subtalar, the midtarsal (transverse tarsal), the tarsometatarsal (TMT), and the metatarsophalangeal (MTP) joints.

The rearfoot, midfoot, and forefoot function as a unit during the stance phase of gait. Alterations in any one of these structures influence the function of the entire foot and ankle during the stance phase. The interdependency and interrelationships of the rearfoot, midfoot, and forefoot are established by muscle and connective tissue structures. Movement of one joint influences movement of other joints in the foot and ankle. Furthermore, the soft tissue structures establish an interdependency of the foot and ankle to the entire lower limb. Therefore, alterations in the mechanics of the foot and ankle can influence the function of the lower limb.

This section discusses the principles of movement, the specific movements of the joints of the foot and ankle, and their combined function during the stance phase of gait. Periarticular stability and muscle function are reviewed.

Principles of Motion

Motion can be divided into two components, translation and rotation.[11] Translation, movement of an object in a straight line, occurs when the line of force passes through the center of the object. Rotation is movement of an object in an arc around a fixed axis. It occurs when the line of force does not pass through the center of the object. The greater the distance between the line of force and the center of the object or center of mass, the greater the rate of rotation.[11] Rotational movement is always perpendicular to the axis of rotation. For example, when a door swings open, the movement of rotation occurs around and perpendicular to the fixed axis of the hinge. Movement is also described according to the body plane in which it occurs (the plane of motion). The primary planes of motion in the foot and ankle are the frontal, sagittal, and transverse planes. The frontal plane movements are inversion and eversion. The sagittal plane movements are dorsiflexion and plantar flexion. The transverse plane movements are adduction and abduction.

The joints of the foot and ankle function as hinges.[10,13] Motion must occur perpendicular to the axis. If not, partial dislocation or impingement may occur.[14] A true hinge joint provides 1° of freedom, or motion, in one plane.[14,15] The interphalangeal (IP) joints of the toes provide 1° of freedom, or movement, in one body plane. The MTP joints have two independent axes of motion. Each axis provides 1° of freedom, therefore giving the joints 2° of freedom. The midtarsal, subtalar, and talocrural joints

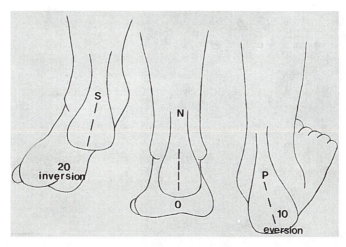

FIGURE 1–4. Open kinetic chain pronation and supination. (P = pronation; S = supination; N = neutral.)

and the first and fifth rays all provide movement in the three cardinal body planes. As described by Root et al,[14] the fifth ray is the fifth metatarsal, and the first ray is the first metatarsal and the first cuneiform.

TRIPLANAR MOVEMENT OF THE FOOT AND ANKLE

The ankle, subtalar, and midtarsal joints and the first and fifth rays have axes of motion that are oblique to the body planes. The axes of motion are at an angle to three body planes.[14] The movement remains perpendicular to the axis, whereas the plane of movement occurs at an angle to all three body planes. If movement occurs in all three body planes simultaneously, it is referred to as triplanar motion.[14] The triplanar movements of the foot and ankle are supination and pronation.[14] The three body plane motions in pronation are abduction (transverse plane), dorsiflexion (sagittal plane), and eversion (frontal plane).[14,15] Conversely, supination is a combined movement of adduction, plantar flexion, and inversion (Fig. 1–4).[14,15] The amount of movement occurring in each body plane depends on the position of the axis. For example, if the axis lies close to the frontal plane, more motion occurs in dorsiflexion and plantar flexion. If the axis of motion is closer to the sagittal plane, more motion occurs in adduction and abduction than in dorsiflexion and plantar flexion. Motion at the subtalar joint represents the purest triplanar movement. The oblique axis of the subtalar joint is equidistant from the planes of movement;[10,14] therefore, the amounts of sagittal, transverse, and frontal planar motion are equal during movement at the subtalar joint.

Rearfoot Stability and Mechanics

ANKLE (TALOCRURAL) JOINT MECHANICS

The tibiotalar, fibulotalar, and tibiofibular joints are three articulations that make up the ankle, or talocrural, joint (Fig. 1–5). The superior surface of the talus bone is wedge shaped and is referred to as the trochlea.[10,11] It may be as much as 6 mm wider

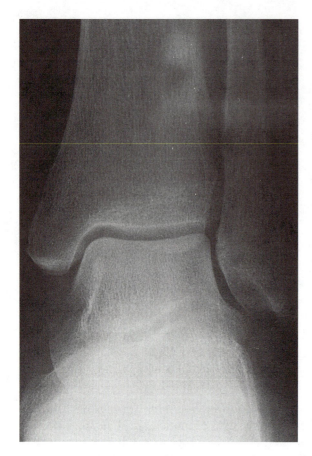

FIGURE 1–5. Ankle joint radiograph (horizontal view) of tibiofibula, tibiotalar, and fibulotalar.

anteriorly than it is posteriorly.[10] Dorsiflexion is the close-packed position of the talocrural joint. In the close-packed position, there is maximum congruency of the trochlea of the talus with the distal fibula and tibia. The "mortise" is another term used to describe the ankle joint. The mortise is formed by the distal end of the tibia, its medial malleolus, and the lateral malleolus of the fibula.[19]

Hicks[13] and Barnett and Napier[16] identify two axes of ankle joint motion. The dorsiflexion axis is oriented in a downward and lateral direction, and the plantar flexion axis is downward and medial. In the frontal plane, the axis of the ankle joint is observed as slightly distal to the medial and lateral malleoli, in a downward and lateral direction. The oblique anteroposterior inclination of the ankle axis as measured in the transverse plane is called "tibial torsion" or "malleolar torsion."[10] In the normal adult foot, the external tibial torsion is 23° (Fig. 1–6).[10]

Singh et al[20] describe an axis of rotation of the talocrural joint. A single constant axis of rotation was determined to be distal to the tips of the malleoli. The axis of rotation for the talocrural joint is offset in two planes. The transverse and frontal planes demonstrate an offset rotation axis of approximately 20°. This offset produces conjoint movements of both varus-valgus and inversion and eversion with flexion and extension. The study by Singh et al further verifies that the talocrural joint is a triplane joint capable of assisting in torque conversion by the rearfoot. Measurement of the ankle

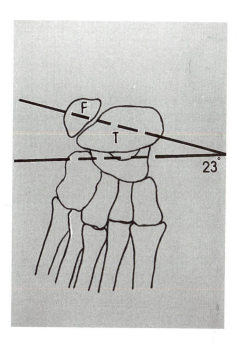

FIGURE 1–6. Malleolar torsion measured by the position of the distal ends of the malleoli, using a goniometer. (F = fibula; T = tibia.)

motion using an axis parallel to the floor and perpendicular to the long axis of the foot does not mimic normal motion at the ankle joint.

The triplanar movements of supination and pronation occur at the joints of the ankle because of the obliquity of the axes to the body planes. The trochlea, the dome of the talus, is cone shaped with a medial apex.[5] The cone shape of the trochlea describes two arcs of motion. The small anteromedial arc corresponds to dorsiflexion, and the larger posterolateral arc corresponds to plantar flexion.[5] The arc of movement during dorsiflexion allows the talus to move into abduction or external rotation, and the plantar flexion arc describes medial rotation or adduction.[5]

From full plantar flexion to dorsiflexion, 1.5 mm of lateral excursion of the fibula and 2.5° of lateral rotation was measured.[5] Throughout the dorsiflexion and plantar flexion range of motion, the malleoli of the fibula and tibia hug the talus for all positions of the joint.[10] Close and Inman[17] measured 1 mm of tibial and fibular malleoli separation during dorsiflexion of the ankle. The dorsiflexion movement was studied during normal walking during weight bearing. The normal range of motion of the ankle joint is 20° of dorsiflexion and 50° of plantar flexion.[18] The most clinically tested movements of the ankle joint are dorsiflexion and plantar flexion;[5] however, the ankle joint is classified as a triplanar joint.[14]

The *closed kinetic chain* ankle movement is influenced by the obliquity of the axis from the tips of the fibular and tibial malleoli. From initial contact to weight acceptance, medial rotation of the lower limb is accompanied by ankle joint plantar flexion and a toe-in position of the foot.[10] During midstance, anterior excursion of the tibia on the talus is initiated as the foot is fixed against the ground.[10] The anterior movement of the tibia on the talus in the closed kinetic chain may be referred to as *closed kinetic chain dorsiflexion*. At heel-off, plantar flexion results in lateral rotation of the leg.

The maximum amount of rotation of the tibia around the oblique axis of the ankle joint is 11°. The average amount of tibial rotation is 19°.[10] The subtalar joint must assist the ankle in accommodating the transverse rotations of the lower limb. The greater the obliquity of the ankle joint axis, the more triplanar movement is available. There is a 1:1 relationship between subtalar adduction and tibial internal rotation.[10]

ANKLE (TALOCRURAL) JOINT STABILITY

Stormont et al[19] determined that stability of the weight-bearing ankle depends on several factors, including the congruity of articular surfaces, the orientation of ligaments, and the position of the ankle at the time of stress. McCullough and Burge[21] added muscle action to the dynamic stability of the weight-bearing ankle.

During loading of the ankle, or weight bearing, 100% of inversion and eversion ankle joint stability was accounted for by the joint articular surface; however, in the unloaded or non–weight-bearing position, none of the stability was contributed by the articular surface. The three lateral collateral ligaments accounted for 87% of resistance to inversion in the unloaded position. The most important stabilizer was the calcaneofibular ligament (Fig. 1–7). The anterior talofibular ligament was the second most significant stabilizer, resisting inversion of the ankle in the non–weight-bearing position.[19] The deltoid ligament afforded 83% of the ankle joint stability during eversion in the unloaded condition.[19]

Internal and external rotation of the foot on the leg were generally more stable during weight bearing.[19] The primary stabilizers for internal rotation included the anterior talofibular ligament and the deltoid ligament. External rotation was stabilized by the calcaneofibular ligament. The posterior talofibular ligament was the pri-

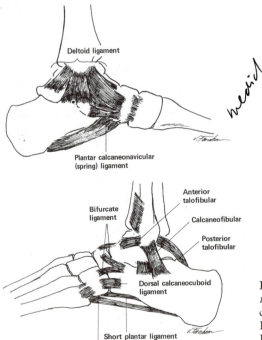

FIGURE 1–7. Medial (*top*) and lateral (*bottom*) ligaments of the posterior ankle/foot complex. (From Norkin, CC and Levangie, PK: Joint Structure and Function, ed 2, FA Davis, Philadelphia, 1992, p 385, with permission.

mary stabilizer during plantar flexion.[19] Abnormal talar rotation is prevented by the distal tibiofibular ligaments and the anterior two thirds of the deltoid ligament.[21]

Harper[22] has shown that the excursions of the talus are limited by the medial and lateral structures of the ankle. Tilting of the talus secondary to a valgus stress, anterior excursions, and lateral tilting were the three movements examined in the study. The lateral supporting structures of the joints of the ankle were the major restraint against anterior talar excursion.

Talar tilt is limited in plantar flexion by the anterior talofibular ligament, in neutral position by the anterior talofibular ligament, and in dorsiflexion by the calcaneofibular ligament plus the posterior talofibular ligament.[23] The anterior talofibular ligament undergoes an increasing strain of 3.3% from 10° of dorsiflexion to 30° of plantar flexion. The calcaneofibular ligament was isometric in the neutral position throughout the flexion arc.[23] The anterior talofibular and calcaneofibular ligaments are synergistic, so that when one is relaxed, the other is strained.[23]

Clinically a positive anterior drawer sign (anterior position of the talus relative to the tibia) and talar tilt can be demonstrated roentgenographically (Fig. 1–8), indicating torn lateral collateral ligaments. The deltoid ligament is the primary restraint to a valgus stress. It is an important factor in preventing rearfoot valgus deformities. Over-

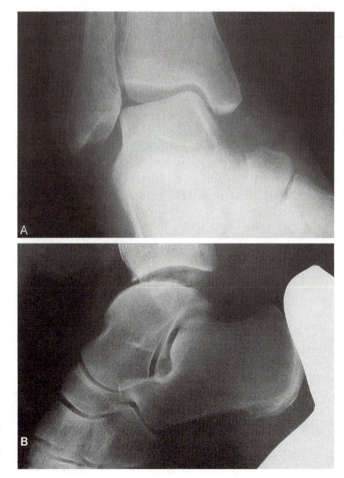

FIGURE 1–8. (*A*) Talar tilt (1.8B) of 23° and (*B*) positive anterior drawer sign, indicating torn collateral ligaments.

stretching of this structure can produce flatfoot. The lateral malleolus of the fibula is the primary restraining structure to lateral talar shifts.[22] The lateral malleolus is a key structure requiring reduction and stabilization in the management of ankle fractures.

The final consideration regarding the ankle joint is its weight-bearing capability. Frankel and Nordin[24] reported 11 to 13 cm[2] of weight-bearing surface in each ankle. (Each ankle carries 49.3% of the body weight, if the feet represent 1.4% of the total body weight.[11]) The weight bearing is shared by the tibiotalar and fibulotalar joints.[11] Lambert[25] demonstrated that one sixth of the 49.3% of body weight is carried by the fibula. Because of the large surface area, the load transmission across the ankle joint is less than that across either the hip joint or the knee joint.[11,24] The talocrural joint is an efficient weight-bearing structure.

From heel strike to footflat, the compressive forces increase within the ankle joint to approximately three times body weight. At heel-off, articular compressive forces reach 4.5 to 5.5 times body weight, secondary to the large plantar flexion movement of the Achilles tendon.[23] Tangential "fore and aft" or shear forces were also calculated in the normal gait cycle, reaching mean peak value of 36% body weight from push-off to heel-off.[23]

SUBTALAR JOINT MECHANICS

The talus and calcaneus are the bones that make up the subtalar joint. The subtalar joint is one of the most important joints of the lower extremity and is responsible for the conversion of the rotatory forces of the lower extremity. The mechanics of the subtalar joint dictate the movements of the midtarsal joint and forefoot.

Movement between the talus and calcaneus occurs around an oblique axis. The axis of the subtalar joint extends anteromedially from the neck of the talus to the posterolateral portion of the calcaneus.[10] The average inclination of the axis is 42° from the horizontal and 23° from the midline (Fig. 1–9).

The movement is perpendicular to the axis. Because the axis of the subtalar joint is oblique to three body planes, the motion is triplanar—dorsiflexion, abduction, and eversion for pronation and plantar flexion; adduction and inversion for supination.

Subtalar joint supination and pronation are measured clinically by the amount of

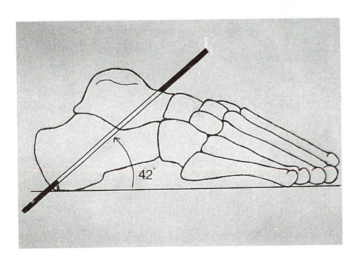

FIGURE 1–9. Subtalar joint axis of motion 42° from the horizontal.

calcaneal inversion and eversion. Root et al[14] describe an inversion to eversion ratio of 2:3 to 1:3, 20° of inversion and 10° of eversion. The midposition of the subtalar joint is subtalar joint neutral. To allow the necessary amount of supination and pronation during the stance phase, the subtalar joint should function as closely as possible to the neutral position (Fig. 1–10). For example, if the calcaneus is everted 10° at heel strike, excessive pronation of the subtalar joint after heel strike follows. If the subtalar joint is maximally pronated directly after heel strike, torque conversion and shock absorption are significantly reduced.

Bones and soft tissue structures limit the amount of calcaneal eversion and inversion. Inversion is limited by the cervical ligament, calcaneofibular ligament, the peroneus longus and brevis, and the sustentaculum tali striking the talar tubercle.[5] Eversion of the calcaneus is limited by the cervical ligament, lateral process of the talus striking the sinus tarsi surface of the calcaneus, tibiocalcaneal portion of the deltoid ligament, medial talocalcaneal ligament, posterior tibialis tendon and muscle, and the flexor digitorus longus tendon muscle.

In the closed kinetic chain, an important function of the subtalar joint is to act as a torque converter of the lower leg. The transverse plane rotations of the lower kinetic chain are attenuated at the subtalar joint. In addition, the transverse plane movements of the lower limb depend on the oblique subtalar joint axis.[10] For example, movement of the leg on a fixed foot produces medial and lateral displacement of the lower leg that is accompanied by transverse rotation at the subtalar joint.[10] Figure 1–11 shows how transverse rotation of the lower leg is converted at the subtalar joint. Pronation of the subtalar joint produces internal rotation of the tibia, evidenced by the increased space between the tibia and fibula (Fig. 1–11B). Supination of the subtalar joint produces external rotation of the tibia (Fig. 1–11D). The space between the fibula and tibia is reduced; the tibia is superimposed over the fibula.

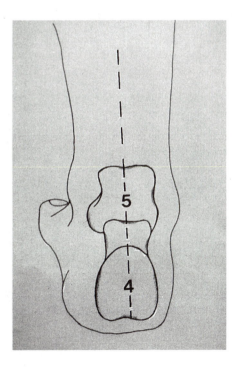

FIGURE 1–10. Neutral position of subtalar joint.

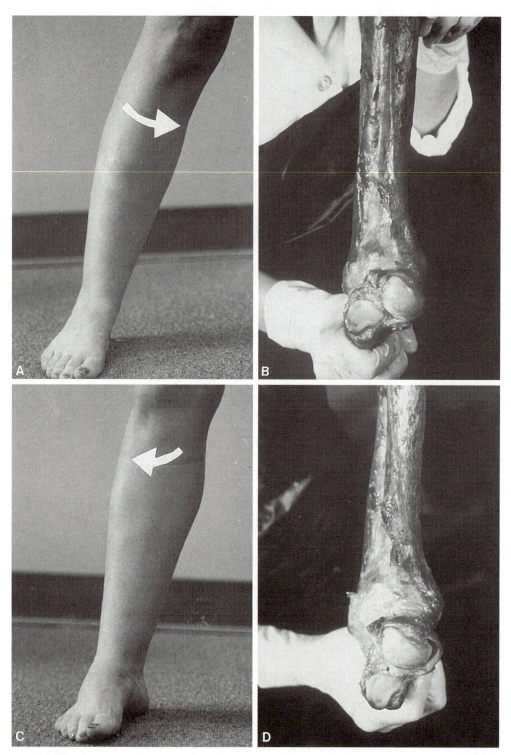

FIGURE 1–11. Transverse rotation of subtalar joint pronation and internal rotation of the tibia. Medial displacement of the tibia (*A*) normal leg; (*B*) dissection. Transverse rotation of the subtalar joint supination and external rotation of the tibia. Lateral displacement of the tibia (*C*) normal leg; (*D*) dissection.

During normal ambulation, the transverse rotations of the lower limb are transmitted to the foot. Sarrafian[5] describes the anterior tibiotalar ligament as contributing to transmission of internal rotation of the tibia to the talus and the posterior talotibial ligament as contributing the transmission of external rotation of the tibia to the talus.

Tibial rotation is clearly demonstrated during the stance phase of walking.[10] The tibia has been found to rotate an average of 19°. The foot does not rotate by moving from a toe-in to a toe-out position during ambulation. Therefore, a mechanism must exist to permit the rotations of the lower limb to occur without movement of the foot. At the beginning of the stance phase, as the tibia rotates internally, the talus plantar flexes and adducts. The talus converts the transverse plane rotations of the tibia into sagittal and transverse plane movements of the talus. The calcaneus simultaneously rolls into eversion to complete the torque conversion. This movement of the talus and calcaneus is closed kinetic chain pronation (Fig. 1–12). During the end of the stance phase, the tibia rotates externally, pushing the talus into dorsiflexion and abduction. Simultaneously the calcaneus inverts to complete the torque conversion. This is closed kinetic chain supination (Fig. 1–13).

The combined closed kinetic chain movement of the rearfoot is important for torque conversion and shock absorption. The obliquity of the ankle joint and subtalar joint axes allows the foot to accommodate for the transverse plane rotations of the lower limb. Talar movement is coordinated at the ankle and subtalar joint. The conical shape of the trochlea and the oblique axis of the ankle joint allow plantar flexion and adduction of the talus immediately after heel strike. As the foot makes contact with the ground, movement occurs around the subtalar joint axis. Subtalar joint closed kinetic chain pronation results in plantar flexion and adduction of the talus. In addition, the calcaneus everts to complete the triplanar movement. Therefore, immediately after heel strike, the knee flexes, the tibia internally rotates, the ankle plantar

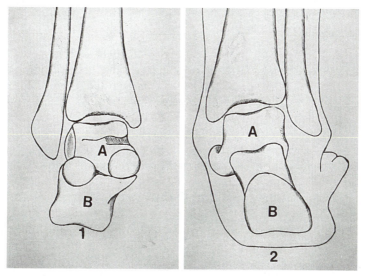

FIGURE 1–12. Anterior (1) and posterior (2) views of closed kinetic chain pronation. (A = talus; B = calcaneus.)

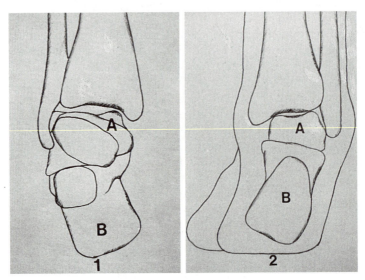

FIGURE 1–13. Anterior (1) and posterior (2) views of closed kinetic chain supination. (A = talus; B = calcaneus.)

flexes, and the subtalar joint pronates as the sequence of events is controlled by the eccentric action of muscle and the tensile strength of ligaments.

As the foot reaches midstance, a reversal occurs at the subtalar joint. In early midstance, the subtalar joint stops pronating and begins to reverse its movement. The tibia moves anterior to the talus. The neutral position of the subtalar joint is reached at midstance. The tibia continues to move anterior to the talus until late midstance. Supination begins during late midstance as the tibia continues to move anterior to the talus. The talus is abducted and dorsiflexed as the tibia externally rotates.

SUBTALAR JOINT STABILITY

The subtalar joint is made up of two articular areas. The posterior articulation consists of the convex calcaneus and the concave talus. The anterior articulations include medial, central, and lateral facets between the talus and calcaneus.[5,26] In a study by Viladot et al[26] of 100 calcanei, three different anterior calcaneal facets of the subtalar joint were identified: an ovoid form, a bean-shaped structure with a narrow medial aspect, and two separate articular surfaces.[26] The calcaneus forms an important part of the anteromedial subtalar joint. The sustentaculum tali is the anteromedial aspect of the calcaneus that supports the head and neck of the talus.[10]

Harris and Beath[28] have reported variations in the anteromedial projection of the calcaneus. They classified the support of the anteromedial calcaneus as weak, moderate, or strong. The degree of support depends on how far distally the anteromedial aspect of the calcaneus extends. Excessive plantar flexion and adduction of the talus, components of abnormal pronation of the subtalar joint, are increased by the lack of anteromedial support of the calcaneus. The talus literally falls off the calcaneus in a medial and anterior direction, as a result of weight-bearing forces and poor osseous support. Furthermore, the sustentaculum tali forms a fulcrum around which the tibialis posterior, flexor hallucis longus, and flexor digitorum longus tendons pass. The contraction of their muscles gives the hindfoot dynamic stability.[26]

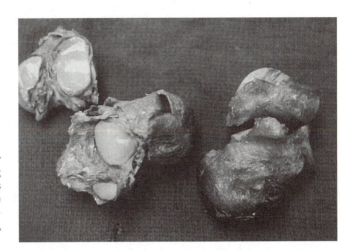

FIGURE 1–14. (*Left*) Axilla or interosseous ligament dividing the anterior and posterior facets of the subtalar joint. (*Right*) Talus and calcaneus in the normal anatomical relationship, talus superior to calcaneus.

The ligaments of the subtalar joint are important to joint stability. A review of the literature indicates confusion in the description and nomenclature of the subtalar joint ligaments. They can be divided into superficial and deep structures. The superficial ligaments include the lateral and posterior talocalcaneal ligaments. The deep ligamentous structures form a wall that divides the subtalar joint. The deep ligaments include the interosseous, cervical, and axial ligaments.[26] Gray[29] separates the cervical ligament from the interosseous ligament. Viladot et al[26] describe the cervical ligament as a portion of the interosseous structure that prevents inversion and eversion.

The ligament in the tarsal canal is the most important ligament formation. The tarsal canal separates the middle and posterior facets of the articulation between the talus and the calcaneus. The ligament of the canal is sometimes referred to as the cruciate ligament of the tarsus, or the axial ligament.[26] Formed mainly by collagen fibers, the axial ligament is thick and strong. It divides the anterior and posterior subtalar joint and is mainly responsible for limiting eversion.[27] Figure 1–14 (*left*) shows a dissection of the axial ligament, which divides the subtalar joint, the inferior surface of the talus, and the superior surface of the calcaneus. Figure 1–14 (*right*) shows the normal relationship of the talus and calcaneus. Overstretching of the axial ligament can result in an acquired heel valgus deformity. Conversely, severe limitations in passive calcaneal eversion may be secondary to lack of extensibility of the axial ligament.

Hellman et al[30] determined that the major articular area of the subtalar joint complex is the posterior facet of the talus. The ligament responsible for posterior facet congruence is the calcaneofibular ligament. Maximum tightness of the calcaneofibular ligament was obtained by dorsiflexion and supination.[30] Subtalar joint stability was described by intact bony surfaces held together by the interosseous ligament and the calcaneofibular ligament.

Midfoot Stability and Mechanics

The midtarsal, transverse tarsal, and Chopart's joint are synonymous with the articulations of the calcaneocuboid and the talonavicular joints. The talonavicular articulation resembles the articulation of the acetabulum and the head of the femur. Sarrafian[5] describes the articulation of the head of the talus, the navicular, and the anteromedial calcaneal portion as the "acetabulum pedis." The concave portion of the acetabulum pedis is formed by osseous and ligamentous structures. The floor of the acetabulum pedis is formed by the navicular bone. The convex surface of the head of the talus bone is analogous to the head of the femur.

The calcaneocuboid joint is a saddle, or sellar, joint. As in all saddle joints, the convex and concave joint surfaces are at right angles to each other.[29] The convex joint surface of the calcaneocuboid joint is transverse (or within the horizontal plane), and the concave joint surface is vertical (or perpendicular to the horizontal plane).[5] If the convex and concave joint surfaces are a perfect match, only rotation is allowed to occur.[5] The rotational movement between the calcaneus and cuboid is described as pivotal.[31]

Rotational movements of the midtarsal joint allow the forefoot to twist on the rearfoot. The navicular and cuboid move as a unit with the anterior part of the foot. There is minor relative movement between the navicular and the cuboid.[5,31,32] Therefore, the forefoot, or anterior unit, is capable of moving on the calcaneus and talus by movement of the midtarsal joint.

Manter[31] and Elftman[32] describe two axes of motion at the midtarsal joint (Fig. 1–15). The first axis is longitudinal (extending lengthwise through the foot) and slopes upward and mediad.[14,31,32] Inversion and eversion are the movements occurring around the longitudinal axis.[14,31,32] Clinically, inversion and eversion of the midtarsal joint can be observed in the normal rise and drop of the medial arch of the foot in the weight-bearing position.[31,32]

Manter[31] describes a "screwlike" action of the cuboid and navicular bones rather than a rotation around the longitudinal axis. The "screwlike" action of the cuboid and navicular occurs during closed kinetic chain inversion and eversion. Eversion turns

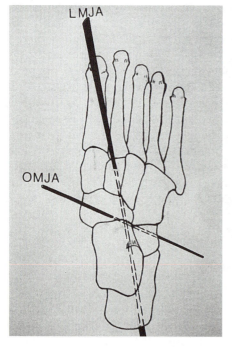

FIGURE 1–15. Midtarsal joint axes. (LMJA = longitudinal midtarsal joint axis; OMJA = oblique midtarsal joint axis.)

the navicular in a medial direction and displaces it distally.[31] The forward movement of the navicular releases the head of the talus, allowing it to move anteriorly. Forward displacement of the talus is opposed by plantar muscles and ligaments.[31] The forward displacement of the talus and navicular is brought about by pronation of the subtalar joint.[31] The rotational movements of the talus and of the navicular are in opposite directions. For example, observing the right foot from behind, pronation turns the navicular counterclockwise with respect to the calcaneus, and the talus undergoes clockwise rotation.[31]

A rotation also occurs at the calcaneocuboid articulation. During the push-off phase of gait, the pivotal movement of the calcaneus and cuboid allows the cuboid to become fixed. A stable cuboid acts as a fulcrum for the peroneus longus muscle. The peroneus longus pulls around the cuboid, plantar flexing the first ray in the push-off phase of gait. The pivotal movement of the cuboid and calcaneus is accomplished by supination of the subtalar joint.

The second axis of the midtarsal joint is oblique or transverse. Several authors describe the transverse axis of the midtarsal joint as being inclined 52° from the horizontal and 57° from the frontal plane.[14,31-35] Movement at the transverse axis is a combination of dorsiflexion and abduction and plantar flexion and adduction. Increased motion along the transverse axis occurs with abnormal pronation. In severe cases of flatfoot, the forefoot is dorsiflexed and abducted on the rearfoot.[31] The dorsiflexion component may be compensatory to ankle joint equinus. The increased abduction results from anteromedial displacement of the navicular and talus with rearfoot pronation. Therefore, every degree of subtalar joint pronation produces an increase in midtarsal joint instability.[36]

Rearfoot and Midfoot Closed Kinetic Chain Function

The ankle, subtalar, and midtarsal joints depend on each other during the stance phase of gait. Immediately after heel strike, the ankle plantar flexes, causing internal rotation and adduction of the tibia and talus. The subtalar joint pronates, producing forward displacement of the talus and the navicular. The calcaneus everts, allowing maximum range of motion of the midtarsal joint. The articular surfaces of the navicular and cuboid are more parallel to each other, producing a supple forefoot. During midstance, the tibia advances over the talus in closed kinetic chain dorsiflexion. External rotation of the tibia and abduction of the talus accompanies closed kinetic chain dorsiflexion. During push-off, the subtalar joint supinates, producing a pivotal movement of the cuboid and calcaneus, stabilizing the cuboid. A fixed cuboid acts as a fulcrum for the peroneus longus muscle, facilitating plantar flexion of the first ray or first metatarsal in push-off.

TRIPLANAR MOVEMENTS

The normal mechanics of the rearfoot and midfoot depend on the obliquity of the axes of motion. Because there are wide variances in the direction of the axis of the ankle, subtalar, and midtarsal joints, greater range of motion in one cardinal plane and restricted movement in another may be possible from patient to patient.[33,35]

Predominance of motion in one cardinal plane is referred to as *planar dominance.*

Variance in the direction of the axis for the ankle, subtalar, and midtarsal joints alters the triplanar motion and determines the planar dominance. For example, if the subtalar joint axis of motion is inclined 68° from the horizontal instead of 42°, movement of the subtalar joint is increased in the transverse plane and limited in the frontal plane. An individual with these variances has difficulty compensating for frontal plane deformities intrinsic to the foot, such as forefoot varus.

Conversely the more parallel the subtalar axis is to the sagittal plane, the greater the amount of inversion and eversion. Patients demonstrating greater ranges of inversion and eversion should be able to compensate successfully for frontal plane deformities and respond better to functional orthoses. Patients who demonstrate reduced ranges of inversion and eversion are less capable of compensating for frontal plane deformities.

The obliquity of the ankle joint determines how much torque conversion is necessary at the subtalar joint. If the axis of the ankle joint is horizontal, it cannot function as a triplanar joint. Thus, the movement of the tibia cannot be resolved about the axis of the ankle joint and must take place at the subtalar axis.[37]

Inman[10] reports a heel lift can be therapeutic and clinically useful for determining the obliquity of the ankle joint axis. In patients with an oblique ankle joint axis, the use of a heel lift increases both plantar flexion and the toe-in position of the foot directly after heel strike. The toe-in position facilitates supination of the foot, reducing the stress of excessive pronation.

The primary planar dominance of the ankle, subtalar, and midtarsal joints determines the primary planar compensation.[35] The clinical significance of planar dominance becomes evident when selecting a surgical procedure or in determining the foot orthoses prescription. For example, orthotic control of excessive transverse plane motion is difficult. The functional foot orthoses are designed to control frontal plane movement of the forefoot and rearfoot. Controlling a foot with excessive frontal plane movement is easier than controlling one with excessive transverse plane movement. Off-the-shelf arch supports may be somewhat helpful to reducing the symptoms in those patients demonstrating excessive frontal plane movement.[35]

As we become more sophisticated in our understanding of foot function, assessment of the foot's biomechanics will take on added significance. Bordelon[38] describes normal ranges for the cardinal body plane movements of the foot and ankle. Passive motion of the foot in the transverse plane demonstrates 30° of adduction and 15° of abduction. Passive forefoot motion in the frontal plane demonstrates 25° of varus and valgus, or inversion and eversion, respectively. Passive motion of the heel in the frontal plane is 10° of eversion and 20° of inversion. Finally, ankle joint sagittal plane movement is 50° of plantar flexion and 20° of dorsiflexion. The evaluation of planar dominance can begin with these cardinal plane ranges (Table 1–2).

Forefoot Stability and Mechanics

The normal movement and stability of the forefoot depend on stable metatarsals and good mobility of the MTP and IP joints. The metatarsal heads tolerate the vertical forces of weight bearing, whereas the toes stabilize the forefoot dynamically. The forefoot extends from the TMT joints, or Lisfranc's joint, distally. The tarsometatarsal joints allow flexion and extension of the metatarsal bones and a certain degree of supination and pronation of the marginal rays. Sarrafian[5] describes the supination

TABLE 1–2 Passive Range of Motion
of the Foot and Ankle

Transverse Plane Movement

30° of forefoot adduction
15° of forefoot abduction

Frontal Plane Movement

25° of forefoot inversion (varus)
25° of forefoot eversion (valgus)
10° of rearfoot eversion
20° of rearfoot inversion

Sagittal Plane Movement

50° of plantar flexion
20° of dorsiflexion

and pronation of the first and fifth rays as longitudinal axial rotations. The combination of the sagittal motions and the axial rotations of the first and fifth rays results in a supination and pronation twist of the forefoot, as defined by Hicks.[13] A supination twist is a result of first ray extension (dorsiflexed) and fifth ray flexion (plantar flexed) (Fig. 1–16). A pronation twist is a result of first ray flexion (plantar flexed) and fifth ray extension (dorsiflexed) (Fig. 1–16).[5,13]

In a standing position, a high medial arch is produced by external rotation of the tibia, supination of the subtalar and midtarsal joints, and pronation twist of the forefoot. Conversely a low medial arch is produced by internal rotation of the tibia,

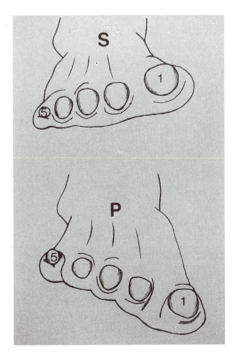

FIGURE 1–16. Forefoot supination twist (S); forefoot pronation twist (P).

pronation of the subtalar and midtarsal joints, and a supination twist of the fore-foot.[5,13] The forefoot pronation and supination twist depends on the coordinated movement of the midtarsal and subtalar joints. The actual twisting movement of the forefoot results from the reciprocal movement of the first and fifth metatarsals.

METATARSALS

Hicks[13,39] describes the metatarsals as beams supporting the longitudinal arches. The beams are tied together by a "tie rod" or plantar aponeurosis. On weight bearing, the metatarsals and calcaneus are forced apart, and tension develops within the tie rod.

Perry[40] describes the plantar fascia, or the aponeurosis, and the intrinsic musculature as the force transmitters from one end of the arch to the other. As the MTP joints are dorsiflexed in push-off, a "windlass effect" tightens the tie rod (Fig. 1–17).[39–41] The plantar fascia is a broad, dense band of longitudinally arranged collagen fibers.[41] Collagen fibers are designed to resist tensile forces. As increased loads are applied, the plantar fascia becomes progressively stiffer or more able to resist deformation.[42] Hence, tension at one end of the tie rod is transmitted to the other end, pulling the ends closer together.

The plantar aponeurosis has three components, central, lateral, and medial.[5] The central component originates from the posteromedial calcaneal tuberosity. The lateral or peroneal component originates from the lateral margin of the medial calcaneal tubercle and is connected with the origin of the abductor digiti minimi muscle. Finally, the medial or tibial component fibers originate distally and medially and are continuous with the abductor hallucis muscle.[5] As noted previously, the plantar aponeu-

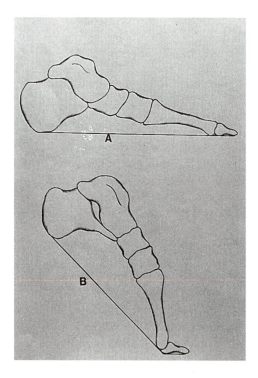

FIGURE 1–17. The windlass effect. (*A*) Plantar aponeurosis slack position. (*B*) Tightening of the plantar aponeurosis in push-off.

rosis originates predominantly from the medial aspect of the calcaneus. Therefore, tension of the tissue promotes inversion of the calcaneus and supination of the subtalar joint. Thus, the windlass mechanism is important in establishing a rigid lever for push-off.

Numerous authors have demonstrated that the longitudinal arches are not supported by muscle.[44–47] Lapidus[48] was one of the first to describe the concept of the foot functioning as a truss. A truss is a triangular structure with two beams connected by a tie rod. The vertical forces transmitted to the foot in weightbearing are attenuated by the truss mechanism. Therefore, intrinsic and extrinsic muscles are not used in static arch support.[4] Mann and Inman[49] reports activity of the intrinsic muscles, abductor hallucis brevis, flexor hallucis brevis, flexor digitorum brevis, and abductor digiti minimi in stabilizing the transverse tarsal joint during the stance phase of gait. In normal feet, the onset of intrinsic muscle activity is initiated at approximately midstance, or after 35% of stance phase. In contrast, the onset of intrinsic muscle activity in flat-footed subjects was within the first 25% of the stance phase.[49,50] A fallen or flattened arch cannot be raised by exercises.[44]

Huang et al[51] reported that the highest relative contribution to medial arch stability was provided by the plantar fascia, followed by plantar ligaments and the spring ligament. The plantar fascia was a major factor in maintenance of the medial longitudinal arch.

The transverse arch is formed by the cuneiforms and the cuboid (Fig. 1–18).[5] Support of the forefoot is by means of the heads of the metatarsals. The metatarsals are held together by ligament and muscle. The six elements that prevent splaying the forefoot include Lisfranc's ligament, the transverse metatarsal ligament, the interosseous muscles, the peroneus longus muscle, the plantar extension of the posterior tibial tendon, and the adductor hallucis muscle (Fig. 1–19).[52]

Cavanagh[53] reported that in a symptom-free population, the static peak pressures in the forefoot were 2.5 times lower than the peak pressures under the heel. Thus, about 60% of the weight-bearing load is carried by the rearfoot, 8% by the midfoot, and 28% by the heads of the metatarsals. These peak pressures during standing are approximately 30% of those produced during walking and 16% of those during running.[53] The second and third metatarsal heads bear the greatest forefoot pressures.[54]

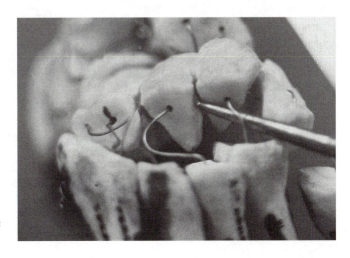

FIGURE 1–18. Transverse arch cuboid and cuneiforms.

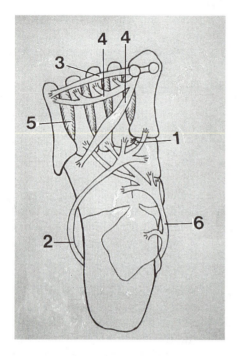

FIGURE 1–19. Structures within the forefoot to prevent "splaying." (1) Lisfranc's ligament; (2) peroneus longus tendon; (3) transverse metatarsal ligament; (4) adductor hallucis; (5) interosseous muscle; (6) posterior tibialis tendon.

The fact that the first ray does not bear the greatest pressure in standing indicates that it has a more dynamic function during push-off. Earlier studies by Stokes et al[55] indicated that the forces under the first metatarsal during walking were found to be the highest. Hutton and Dhannedran[56] reported that the first ray is the largest and strongest of all. The first metatarsal bone is twice as wide as the second metatarsal and four times as strong.[56] Furthermore, the peroneus longus, posterior tibialis, and anterior tibialis muscles attach to the first ray and function to stabilize it dynamically in the propulsive phase of gait. The head of the first metatarsal has a large joint surface and sesamoid bones to give the flexor hallucis longus a mechanical advantage, minimizing joint forces.[55] Finally, the inclination angle of the first metatarsal to the horizontal is greater than that of the other metatarsals, reducing the shearing and bending forces of weight bearing.[55]

TOES

The function of the toes is important to the biomechanics of the forefoot. During walking, the toes help to stabilize the longitudinal arch and maintain floor contact until the final phase of push-off.[50] Approximately 40% of the body weight is borne by the toes in the final stages of foot contact.[55] During the stance phase of gait, the greatest load is through the first MTP joint.[50] Weight-bearing forces to the toes are attenuated by the tension in the toe flexor tendons and tendon sheaths.[55] During standing, the peak pressure to the toes is minimal.[51]

Dorsiflexion of the toes, especially the first MTP joint, is important to the windlass mechanism. MTP joint movement occurs in two cardinal body planes. The sagittal plane movement of the MTP joint is flexion and extension, and the transverse plane movement is abduction and adduction. Sixty degrees to 70° of dorsiflexion is necessary for tension to develop within the aponeurosis. The instant center of rotation of the first MTP joint is within the head of the metatarsal. Hallux valgus and hallux rigidus deformities, which are subluxations of the first MTP joint, alter the instant center of rotation of the MTP joint. Often with these deformities the center of rotation falls outside the head of the first metatarsal.[57] The mobility of the sesamoid bones is important to the normal mechanics of the first MTP joint. Displacement of the medial and lateral sesamoids during dorsiflexion of the MTP joint was measured to be 10 to 12 mm.[57] Hallux valgus deformities demonstrate significantly less sesamoid displacement than normal joints.[57] Hallux valgus produces lateral subluxation of the sesamoid bones and the flexor hallucis longus muscle. The altered position of the sesamoid bones transforms the flexor hallucis longus and brevis from flexors to adductors, contributing to the severe loss of plantar flexion.[57]

The sesamoid bones are the attachment sites for several important soft tissue structures. Flexor hallucis brevis, oblique head and transverse component of the adductor hallucis, flexor hallucis longus fibrous tunnel, and the deep transverse metatarsal ligament all insert into the borders of the medial and lateral sesamoid bones.[5] The sesamoid bones maintain proper alignment of the flexor hallucis longus tendon and are also responsible for absorbing vertical pressures in push-off. Figure 1–20 shows the first MTP joint with the sesamoid bones in place. The flexor hallucis longus passes between the sesamoids.

The last four toes are attachment sites for the extensor digitorum tendon, the flexor digitorum tendon, the dorsal and plantar interossei, and the lumbrical muscles.[53] The interosseous and lumbrical muscles dynamically stabilize the toes on the floor in the tiptoe position.[52] Failure of the lumbrical and interosseous muscles to function accounts for toe deformities such as claw toes.[52]

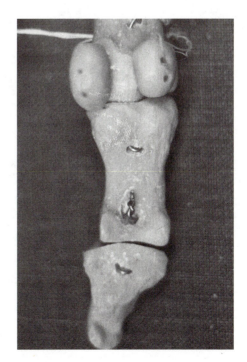

FIGURE 1–20. Sesamoids of the first metatarsophalangeal joint that houses the flexor mechanism of the flexor hallucis longus tendon.

Summary of Closed Kinetic Chain Function

The triplanar joints of the foot include the talocrural, subtalar, midtarsal, first ray, and fifth ray. Pronation and supination are the triplanar movements of the foot. Pronation occurs directly after heel strike, for shock absorption, adjustment to the terrain, and torque conversion. Supination occurs during the push-off phase of gait. Supination of the subtalar joint allows the foot to function as a rigid lever for propulsion. A rigid foot during the propulsive phase allows muscle pulleys to be established. The pulleys established by the tarsal bones change the direction of pull of the muscle, increasing the efficiency of muscle function. Table 1–3 summarizes the closed kinetic chain movements of the foot and ankle.

TABLE 1–3 Closed Kinetic Chain Mechanics of the Foot and Ankle

---

Heel Contact to Weight Acceptance

Rearfoot
  Talocrural plantar flexion
  Subtalar joint pronation
  Tibial internal rotation
  Talar adduction and plantar flexion
  Calcaneal eversion
Midfoot
  Midtarsal pronation
  Unlocking of cuboid/navicular
  Forward displacement (clockwise rotation) of talus
  Counterclockwise rotation of navicular
Forefoot
  Supination twist-dorsiflexion of the first ray

Early Midstance/Midstance/Late Midstance

Rearfoot
  Early—Talocrural: anterior movement of the tibia over the talus; subtalar reversal of pronation
  Midstance—Closed kinetic chain dorsiflexion; subtalar: neutral position
  Late—Continued anterior movement of tibia over talus; subtalar: supination abduction and
    dorsiflexion of talus
Midfoot
  Midtarsal reversal of pronation
Forefoot
  Full weight bearing of the metatarsal heads

Push-off and Propulsion

Rearfoot
  Talocrural: tibial external rotation
  Subtalar: supination
Midfoot
  Midtarsal supination-cuboid/navicular and rigid-talus counterclockwise rotation-navicular
    clockwise rotation
Forefoot
  Pronation twist-first ray plantar flexion
  Sesamoids weight bearing

MUSCLE FUNCTION AND NORMAL MECHANICS

During walking, muscle is used to initiate movement, stabilize osseous structures, and decelerate movement.[12] Electromyographic studies are commonly used to analyze the function of muscle during the gait cycle. The combined knowledge of electromyographic activity and foot function during the gait cycle is necessary to give the clinician a complete picture of muscle function. This section describes the functions of the major muscles of the foot and ankle during the different phases of the gait cycle (Table 1–4).

The anterior tibialis is an important muscle during the swing phase. Directly after toe-off, early swing, and midswing, the anterior tibialis assists dorsiflexion of the foot

TABLE 1–4 Muscle Function During the Stance Phase of Gait

Muscle	Action
Heel Contact to Weight Acceptance	
Anterior tibialis	*Eccentric*—control pronation of subtalar joint
Extensor hallucis longus Extensor digitorum	*Eccentric*—decelerate plantar flexion and posterior shear of tibia on talus
Posterior tibialis	*Eccentric*—decelerate pronation of subtalar joint and internal rotation of tibia
Soleus Gastrocnemius	
Midstance	
Posterior tibialis Soleus Flexor hallucis longus Flexor digitorum longus	*Eccentric*—decelerate forward movement of tibia
Posterior tibialis Soleus Gastrocnemius	*Concentric*—supinate subtalar and midtarsal joints
Push-off and Propulsion	
Peroneus longus Abductor hallucis	*Concentric*—plantar flex first ray
Peroneus brevis	*Antagonistic*—to supinators of subtalar and midtarsal joints
Flexor digitorum longus	*Concentric*—stabilize toes against ground
Extensor hallucis longus and brevis	*Concentric*—stabilize first metatarsophalangeal joint
Abductor hallucis Abductor digiti quinti Flexor hallucis brevis Flexor digitorum brevis Extensor digitorum brevis Interossei, lumbricals	*Concentric*—stabilize midtarsal and forefoot, raise medial arch of foot in push-off

for clearance of the ground. Just before heel strike, slight supination of the foot is accomplished by the accelerating or concentric action of the anterior tibialis muscle.[19] Directly after heel strike, the anterior tibialis and the toe extensors (extensor digitorum longus and extensor hallucis longus) demonstrate maximal electrical activity.[4,12] The decelerating function of these muscles resists plantar flexion of the foot at heel strike and controls pronation of the forefoot during the contact period.[19] The anterior tibialis at heel strike and immediately afterward decelerates the tibia, resisting a posterior shear force.

Immediately after heel strike, there is no activity of the pronators. As previously noted, pronation is a controlled passive movement. As the forefoot makes contact with the ground, the posterior tibialis, soleus, and gastrocnemius muscles further decelerate pronation of the subtalar joint and internal rotation of the lower extremity.[19,58]

During midstance, the soleus, posterior tibialis, flexor hallucis longus, and flexor digitorum longus muscles reduce the forward momentum of the tibia.[19] The activity of the posterior tibialis, soleus, and gastrocnemius maintains stability of the midtarsal joint by accelerating subtalar joint supination during the midstance and early propulsive phases of gait.[19] External rotation of the lower leg is initiated by swing-through of the contralateral limb and the action of the gastrocnemius rotating the femur externally.[19,59]

As the foot prepares for push-off, supination of the subtalar joint is initiated to establish a rigid lever and pulleys for extrinsic muscles. For example, at heel-off the peroneus longus plantar flexes the first ray. The plantar flexion of the first metatarsal is facilitated by the cuboid pulley. The cuboid changes the direction of pull of the peroneus longus, increasing efficiency of plantar flexion of the first ray. The abductor hallucis muscle also plantar flexes the first metatarsal during propulsion.[19] The peroneus brevis is active in the early propulsive phase as an antagonist to the muscles that supinate the subtalar and midtarsal joints.[19]

The extensor digitorum longus assists the lumbricals in stabilizing the IP joints during propulsion. The flexor digitorum longus stabilizes the toes against the ground during push-off.[19] The extensor hallucis longus and flexor hallucis longus and brevis stabilize the first MTP joint during propulsion.

The intrinsic muscles include the abductor hallucis, abductor digiti quinti, flexor hallucis brevis, flexor digitorum brevis, extensor digitorum brevis, interossei, and lumbricals. Several authors have reported that the intrinsic muscles of the foot play a dynamic role in stabilization of the midtarsal joint and forefoot during the push-off phase.[4,49]

SUMMARY

The normal biomechanics of the foot and ankle can be divided into static and dynamic components. The static components include the bones, joint surface congruity, ligaments, and fascia. The dynamic components include the kinetics of the tarsal bones and muscle function.

The combined effects of the static and dynamic structures of the foot and ankle are responsible for force attenuation within the foot and lower limb. The windlass effect of the plantar aponeurosis, the tensile strength of the plantar ligaments, the beam effect of the metatarsals, and the joint congruity of the tarsal and metatarsal bones encompass the static mechanisms for force attenuation.

The triplanar movements of the foot and ankle and the interrelationship of muscle function are the dynamic components of force attenuation. Pronation is initiated at heel strike and is controlled by an eccentric action of muscle and the restraining characteristics of connective tissue. Pronation allows the foot to absorb compressive forces, adjust to uneven terrain, and maintain equilibrium. Supination establishes a rigid lever for push-off and creates pulley systems for several extrinsic foot muscles. Pronation occurs directly after heel strike and reaches its maximum at footflat. Resupination occurs during earlier midstance, allowing the foot to pass through a neutral position at midstance. Supination begins during late midstance and continues until toe-off.

Understanding the functional biomechanics of the foot and ankle has profound implications for clinical applications. The inability of the lower limb to convert transverse rotation at the subtalar joint could have detrimental effects on other joints in the chain, such as the knee, midtarsal joint, and forefoot. It is imperative for the clinician treating lower extremity dysfunction to have an understanding of the normal biomechanics of the foot and ankle. Furthermore, the clinician must understand the interdependency of the foot and ankle and the normal function of the lower kinetic chain.

GLOSSARY

Adduction/Abduction: Movements of the foot and ankle in the transverse plane.

Closed kinetic chain: A series of joints in which the terminal joint is the first joint to meet with resistance during movement.

Closed kinetic chain dorsiflexion: Anterior movement of the tibia on the talus.

Dorsiflexion/Plantar flexion: Movements of the foot and ankle in the sagittal plane.

Inversion/Eversion: Movements of the foot and ankle in the frontal plane.

Kinetic chain: A series of joints interconnected by soft tissue and muscle in which movement of one joint will influence the movements of others in the chain.

Neutral position of the subtalar joint: The position one third of the way through the total range of motion of the subtalar joint from the fully everted position to full inversion. Midposition of the subtalar joint range of motion, zero pronation, and zero supination.

Open kinetic chain: A series of joints in which the terminal joint is non–weight bearing.

Open kinetic chain pronation: Dorsiflexion, abduction, and eversion.

Open kinetic chain supination: Plantar flexion, adduction, and inversion.

Pronation/Supination: The triplanar movements of the foot and ankle.

Subtalar joint closed kinetic chain pronation: Talar adduction and plantar flexion and calcaneal eversion.

Subtalar joint closed kinetic chain supination: Talar abduction and dorsiflexion and calcaneal inversion.

Triplanar joints of the foot and ankle: Talocrural, subtalar, midtarsal, first ray, and fifth ray.

Triplanar movements: Movement in three body planes simultaneously around an oblique axis. The movement is perpendicular to the axis.

REFERENCES

1. Smidt, GL: Biomechanics and physical therapy, a perspective. Phys Ther 64:1807, 1984.
2. Cailliet, R: Foot and Ankle Pain. FA Davis, Philadelphia, 1968.
3. Tachdjian, MO: The Child's Foot. WB Saunders, Philadelphia, 1985.
4. Conroy, GC and Rose, MD: The evolution of the primate foot from the earliest primates to the Miocene hominids. Foot Ankle 3:342, 1983.
5. Sarrafian, SK: Anatomy of the Foot and Ankle. JB Lippincott, Philadelphia, 1983.
6. Brown, LP and Yavorsky, P: Locomotor biomechanics and pathomechanics: A review. J Orthop Sports Phys Ther 9:3, 1987.
7. Hlavac H: Compensated forefoot varus. J Am Podiatr Med Assoc 60:229, 1970.
8. Jaffe, WL and Laitman, JT: The evolution and anatomy of the human foot. In Jahss, MH (ed): Disorders of the Foot, Vol 1. WB Saunders, Philadelphia, 1982, p 1.
9. McCrea, JD: Pediatric Orthopaedics of the Lower Extremity. Futura, Mt. Kisco, NY, 1985.
10. Inman, VT: The Joints of the Ankle. Williams & Wilkins, Baltimore, 1976.
11. Kotwick, JE: Biomechanics of the foot and ankle. Clin Sports Med 1:19, 1982.
12. Inman, VT, Rolston, HJ, and Todd, F: Human Walking. Williams & Wilkins, Baltimore, 1981.
13. Hicks, JH: The mechanics of the foot. 1. The joints. J Anat 87:345, 1953.
14. Root, ML, Orien, WP, and Weed, JN: Clinical Biomechanics. Vol 11: Normal and Abnormal Function of the Foot. Clinical Biomechanics, Los Angeles, 1977.
15. Gross, CM: Gray's Anatomy. Lea & Febiger, Philadelphia, 1968.
16. Barnett, CH and Napier, JR: The axis of rotation at the ankle joint in man: Its influence upon the form of the talus and the mobility of the fibula. J Anat 86:1, 1952.
17. Close, JR and Inman, VT: The action of the ankle joint. Prosthetic Devices Research Project, Institute of Engineering Research, University of California, Berkeley. Series 11, Issue 22:5 The Project Berkeley, University of California, Berkeley, 1952.
18. Morris, JM: Biomechanics of the foot and ankle. Clin Orthop 22:10, 1977.
19. Stormont, DM, et al: Stability of the loaded ankle. Am J Sports Med 13:295, 1985.
20. Singh, AK, et al: Kinematics of the ankle: A hinge axis model. Foot Ankle 13:439, 1992.
21. McCullough, CL and Burge, PD: Rotatory stability of the load-bearing ankle. J Bone Joint Surg 62B:460, 1980.
22. Harper, MC: Deltoid ligament: An anatomical evaluation of function. Foot Ankle 8:19, 1987.
23. Stiehl, JB: Biomechanics of the ankle joint. In Stiehl, JB (ed): Inman's Joints of the Ankle, ed 2. Williams & Wilkins, Baltimore, 1991, p 39.
24. Frankel, VH and Nordin, M: Basic Biomechanics of the Skeletal System. Lea & Febiger, Philadelphia, 1980.
25. Lambert, KL: The weight-bearing function of the fibula. A strain gauge study. J Bone Joint Surg 53A:567, 1971.
26. Viladot, A, et al: The subtalar joint: Embryology and morphology. Foot Ankle 5:54, 1984.
27. Kapandji, IA: The Physiology of the Joints, Vol II, The Lower Limb. Churchill Livingstone, London, 1970.
28. Harris, R and Beath, T: Hypermobile flat-foot with short tendoachilles. J Bone Joint Surg 30A:116, 1948.
29. Warwick, R and Williams, P (eds): Gray's Anatomy, British ed 35. Philadelphia, WB Saunders, 1973.
30. Hellman, AE, et al: An anatomic study of subtalar instability. Foot Ankle 10:224, 1990.
31. Manter, JT: Movements of the subtalar joint and transverse tarsal joints. Anat Rec 80:397, 1941.
32. Elftman, H: The transverse tarsal joint and its control. Clin Orthop 16:41, 1960.
33. Phillips, RD, et al: Clinical measurement of the axis of the subtalar joint. J Am Podiatr Med Assoc 75:119, 1985.
34. Subotnick, SI: Biomechanics of the subtalar joint and midtarsal joints. J Am Podiatr Med Assoc 65:756, 1975.
35. Green, DR and Carol, A: Planal dominance. J Am Podiatr Assoc 74:98, 1984.
36. Phillips, RD and Phillips, RL: Quantitative analysis of the locking position of the midtarsal joint. J Am Podiatr Med Assoc 73:518, 1983.
37. Wright, DG, et al: Action of the subtalar and ankle-joint complex during the stance phase of walking. J Bone Joint Surg 46A:361, 1964.
38. Bordelon, LR: Surgical and Conservative Foot Care. Charles B. Slack, Thorofare, NJ, 1988.
39. Hicks, JH: The mechanics of the foot. II. The plantar aponeurosis. J Anat 88:25, 1954.
40. Perry, J: Anatomy and biomechanics of the hindfoot. Clin Orthop 177:9, 1983.
41. Mann, RA: Surgical implications of biomechanics of the foot and ankle. Clin Orthop 146:111, 1980.
42. Wright, DG and Rennels, DC: A study of the elastic properties of plantar fascia. J Bone Joint Surg 46A:482, 1964.
43. Sarrafian, SK: Functional characteristics of the foot and plantar aponeurosis under tibiotalar loading. Foot Ankle 8:4, 1987.

44. Jones, RL: The human foot. An experimental study of its mechanics, and the role of its muscles and ligaments in the support of the arch. Am J Anat 68:1, 1941.
45. Basmajian, JV and Stecko, G: The role of muscles in arch support of the foot. J Bone Joint Surg 45A:1184, 1963.
46. Smith, JW: Muscular control of the arches of the foot in standing: An electromyographic assessment. J Anat 88:152, 1954.
47. Hicks, JH: The mechanics of the foot. IV. The action of muscles on the foot in standing. Acta Anat 27:180, 1956.
48. Lapidus, PW: Kinesiology and mechanical anatomy of the tarsal joints. Clin Orthop 30:20, 1963.
49. Mann, RA and Inman, VT: Phasic activity of intrinsic muscles of the foot. J Bone Joint Surg 46A:469, 1964.
50. Mann, RA and Hagy, JL: The function of the toes in walking, jogging and running. Clin Orthop 142:24, 1979.
51. Huang, CK, et al: Biomechanical evaluation of the longitudinal arch stability. Foot Ankle 14:353, 1993.
52. Viladot, A: The metatarsals. In Jahss, MH (ed): Disorders of the Foot, Vol 1. Philadelphia, WB Saunders, 1982, p 659.
53. Cavanagh, PR: Pressure distribution under symptom-free feet during barefoot standing. Foot Ankle 7:262, 1987.
54. Gieve, DW and Rashi, T: Pressures under normal feet in standing and walking as measured by foil pedobarography. Ann Rheum Dis 43:816, 1984.
55. Stokes, IAF, et al: Forces acting on the metatarsals during normal walking. J Anat 129:579, 1979.
56. Hutton, WC and Dhaneddran M: The mechanics of normal and hallux valgus feet: A quantitative study. Clin Orthop 157:7, 1981.
57. Shereff, ML, et al: Kinematics of the first metatarsophalangeal joint. J Bone Joint Surg 68A:392, 1986.
58. Sutherland, DH, et al: The role of the ankle plantar flexors in normal walking. J Bone Joint Surg 62A:354, 1980.
59. Mann, RA: Biomechanics of running. In Mack, RP (ed): Symposium on the Foot and Leg in Running Sports. St. Louis, CV Mosby, 1982, p 1.

CHAPTER 2

Abnormal Biomechanics

Robert A. Donatelli, PhD, PT, OCS

This chapter discusses the cause, classification, and mechanics of abnormal pronation and supination. Abnormal pronation and supination within the joints of the foot and ankle are nothing more than hypermobilities and hypomobilities, respectively. For example, a flexible flatfoot (abnormal pronation) describes a hypermobile unit unable to produce an effective push-off during the gait cycle. The lack of efficient propulsion is perpetuated by abnormal mechanics of the rearfoot. The poor mechanics of the subtalar joint may result in first ray (first metatarsal/first cuneiform articulation) hypermobility. The term "first ray insufficiency syndrome" is often used to describe this hypermobility. The insufficiency or hypermobility of the first ray refers to dorsiflexion of the first ray that is unable to bear weight effectively during propulsion. As a result of faulty mechanics, the foot is unable to establish an effective lever for push-off. In addition, the abnormal mechanics reduce the ability of the foot to attenuate the excessive forces of weight bearing. Soft tissue breakdown may occur, causing changes in muscle function and osteologic remodeling. These changes can produce a rigid deformity. The foot becomes unable to function as a shock absorber or mobile adapter to the changing ground surfaces. Thus, a hypermobile foot may become hypomobile as a result of pathologic changes within the soft tissue structures.

ABNORMAL PRONATION

There are many terms to describe abnormal pronation. Flatfoot, pes planus, pes valgoplanus, pronated foot, calcaneovalgus foot, valgus foot, and talipes calcaneovalgus are several of the terms found in the literature that describe or identify abnormal pronation.[1-6] In this text, the term "abnormal pronation" is used to describe the flatfoot deformities noted, and the terms are interchangeable.

The literature classifies the cause of abnormal pronation into three basic categories: congenital, acquired, and secondary to neuromuscular diseases. A discussion of flatfoot associated with neuromuscular disease, however, is beyond the scope of this chapter. The term "congenital" means "to be born with" or "to have been present at birth."[7] Congenital flatfoot can result from genetic factors or malposition of the fetus in the uterus. Congenital deformities can be further classified as rigid or flexible. The most common rigid flatfoot deformities with possible genetic cause include convex pes valgus (congenital vertical talus), tarsal coalition, and congenital metatarsus varus.[5,6] The most common congenital flexible flatfoot deformity is talipes calcaneovalgus.[5,6]

Acquired flatfoot can result from abnormalities that are intrinsic or extrinsic (or both) to the foot and ankle. Intrinsic causes of acquired flatfoot include trauma, ligament laxity, bony abnormalities of the subtalar joint, forefoot varus, forefoot supinatus, rearfoot varus, and ankle joint equinus. Extrinsic factors causing abnormal pronation include rotational deformities of the lower extremity and leg length discrepancies.

Abnormal pronation, or flatfoot, can be a deformity present at birth or an acquired deformity that develops after weight bearing begins. Acquired flatfoot may result from compensation at the subtalar joint. This compensation is an attempt to modify an intrinsic or extrinsic foot abnormality.

Congenital Deformities

RIGID DEFORMITIES

Convex pes Valgus

Convex pes valgus, or congenital vertical talus, is a dislocation of the talocalcaneonavicular joint that the fetus develops in the uterus within the first trimester of pregnancy.[5,8–10] The cause is uncertain, and the deformity may occur either in isolation or in association with central nervous system abnormalities, such as spina bifida and arthrogryposis.[8–10] Convex pes valgus may also occur as an isolated primary deformity of unknown cause.[5]

The most striking characteristic of the convex pes valgus deformity visible on x-ray is plantar rotation of the talus toward a more vertical position (Fig. 2–1). The vertical position of the talus, however, is commonly observed in other flatfoot deformities, such as talipes calcaneovalgus. Thus, the distinguishing feature in convex pes valgus is the position of the navicular, which is completely dislocated, articulating with the dorsal surface of the neck of the talus.[9–12] In talipes calcaneovalgus, there is a sag at the talonavicular articulation, and joint congruity is compromised, without complete dislocation. During the first 3 years of life, the navicular bone cannot be accurately visualized roentgenographically.[5,10] Therefore, the clinician must be aware of other differential characteristics, such as a valgus and equinus (plantar flexed) position of the hindfoot. A dorsiflexion force to the foot causes bending at the midtarsal joint, producing a convexity along the foot's plantar aspect. To compensate for the limited dorsiflexion at the ankle joint, the forefoot abducts and tilts upward at the midtarsal joint, creating a "rocker-bottom" appearance to the plantar aspect (Fig. 2–2).[9,12]

Tarsal Coalitions

Tarsal coalition may be either a complete or incomplete fusion of the talus, calcaneus, cuboid, navicular, and cuneiforms.[5,13–18] The joint fusion may be fibrous, cartilaginous, or osseous and can occur during the development of the fetus.[13] Stormont

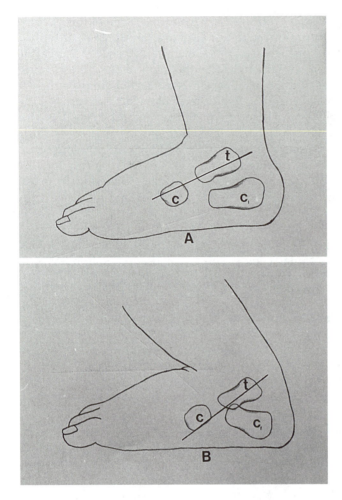

FIGURE 2–1. (*A*) Normal weight bearing. Bisecting line passes through the talus and cuboid. (*B*) Abnormal pronation-talipes calcaneovalgus. Bisecting line passes below the cuboid, indicting a plantar flexed talus that is common in the congenital flatfoot. (c = cuboid; t = talus; c_1 = calcaneus.)

and Peterson[14] found the most common tarsal coalition to be the calcaneonavicular, followed by the talocalcaneal. The cause of tarsal coalitions strongly suggests an hereditary component.[14–16,19–21] Tarsal coalition was observed in 18 cases of rigid equinovarus deformity.[19]

Subtalar joint motion becomes progressively more limited with ossification of the coalition. The fusion can occur at the anterior, middle, or posterior facets of the sub-talar joint. Limitations at the subtalar joint may be difficult for the clinician to determine. Limited mobility of the calcaneus may be concealed by movement at the mid-tarsal joint and tilting of the talus in the mortise or ankle joint.[18] The examiner must grasp the calcaneus firmly and attempt to move it into both eversion and inversion to determine subtalar joint restrictions. Figure 2–3 demonstrates the range of motion of the adult subtalar joint. The calcaneus is forced into a valgus position when talo-calcaneal, calcaneonavicular, or talonavicular coalition occurs.[13] This position causes a breakdown of the midtarsal area, and the arch flattens.

Rigid Metatarsal Deformities

The nomenclature for metatarsal deformities is confusing. Most of the literature describes metatarsus varus and metatarsus adductus synonymously. For the purpos-

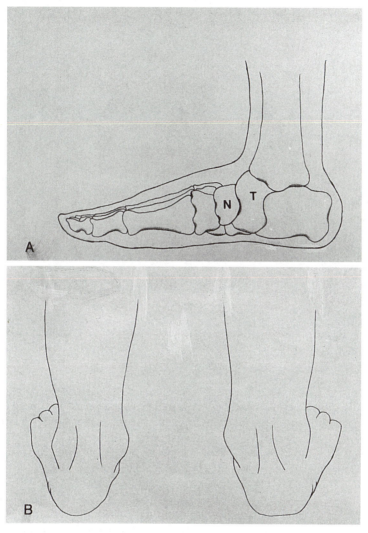

FIGURE 2–2. Rocker bottom foot. (*A*) Navicular (N) articulating with the dorsal aspect of the talus (T) (midtarsal joint line). (*B*) Forefoot is abducted and dorsiflexed at the midtarsal joint; talus is in the vertical position.

es of this chapter, however, the forefoot deformities are divided into rigid and flexible categories. The rigid metatarsal deformity metatarsus varus, as described by Kite,[22] is a medial subluxation of the tarsometatarsal joints.[22] The hindfoot is in a slightly valgus or neutral position, with the navicular lateral to the head of the talus.[5,22] The term "metatarsus adductovarus" is used to refer to the combination of adduction and inversion of the forefoot and is discussed in the next section.

Congenital rigid metatarsal deformities do not present as flatfoot deformity at birth. In fact, the literature describes metatarsus varus as a "third of clubfoot."[22–24] Kite[22] observed 300 cases of congenital metatarsus varus. In 94% of these, the deformity was present at birth. The average age at which the metatarsus varus deformity was recognized was 2.8 months.[22] According to Kite,[22] because most congenital defor-

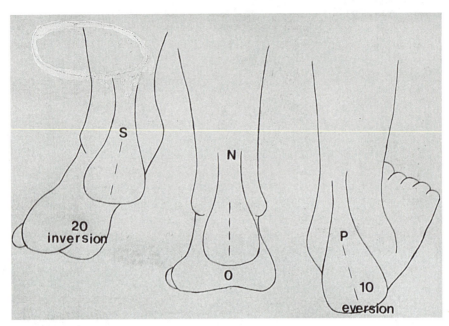

FIGURE 2–3. Range of motion of the subtalar joint is measured by calcaneal inversion and eversion 20/10. Zero is the perpendicular or neutral position of the subtalar joint.

mities are fully developed at birth, metatarsus varus is a congenital muscle imbalance, which increases with the lapse of time after birth, similar to the deformities associated with poliomyelitis. The cause of rigid metatarsus deformities has both genetic and environmental factors.[5] Abnormal pronation secondary to metatarsus adductovarus deformities develops after weight bearing in an attempt to compensate for the deformity.

There are several clinical signs to assist in the diagnosis of a rigid metatarsal deformity. The forefoot cannot be abducted past the midline position (Fig. 2–4). In severe cases, the forefoot cannot passively be reduced from the in-toe position. The clinician must be careful to abduct the forefoot against the resistance of the rearfoot. If the forefoot is abducted against the resistance of the leg, abduction of the foot could occur as a result of external rotation of the leg. Normal dorsiflexion range of motion at the ankle joint is present. Observation of the foot demonstrates a prominent lateral aspect of the foot in the area of the cuboid and the fifth metatarsal.[6,22]

FLEXIBLE DEFORMITIES

Talipes Calcaneovalgus

The most common congenital flexible flatfoot deformity is talipes calcaneovalgus, which occurs in approximately 1 in 1000 births.[5,6,25,26] There is a high correlation between the presence of calcaneovalgus in the newborn and the later development of flatfoot in the older child.[5,15,27]

Tachdjian[5] reports that the cause of talipes calcaneovalgus is a malposition of the fetus in the uterus. As the fetus develops, the posture is determined by the develop-

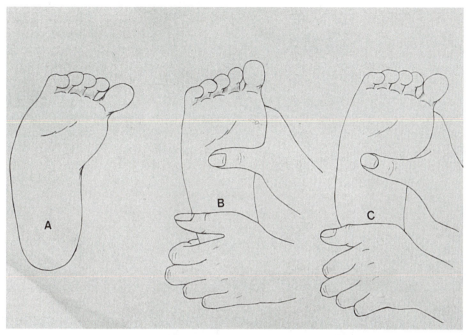

FIGURE 2–4. Range of motion of the forefoot. (*A*) Metatarsus adductus position of the forefoot. (*B*) Passive reduction of the metatarsus adductus deformity to the midline. (*C*) Metatarsus varus. Rigid forefoot deformity unable to abduct the forefoot to the midline.

ment of neuromuscular function. The limbs assume various postures as different muscle groups become active. Between 12 and 26 weeks of fetal development, the feet are dorsiflexed and everted. If such a position persists beyond this stage of development, the feet could be excessively pronated at birth, either unilaterally or bilaterally.[5]

The appearance of the foot in talipes calcaneovalgus is one of dorsiflexion and eversion. The dorsal surface of the foot is in contact with the anterolateral surface of the lower limb (Fig. 2–5). The calcaneus is in a valgus position, and the talus is plantar flexed.[25,26,28,29] The plantar flexed talus can be observed on radiograph and is not to be confused with the convex pes valgus deformity. The latter, as previously mentioned, is associated with central nervous system deformities. In convex pes valgus, a dislocated navicular bone is the distinguishing characteristic.

An important clinical observation of talipes calcaneovalgus is the limitation of plantar flexion at the ankle joint. The plantar flexion range is usually limited to 90° or less. Any attempt to move the foot into plantar flexion beyond 90° is met with resistance of the soft tissue. Furthermore, during the neonate's first 4 to 6 months, stroking of the plantar aspect of the foot produces a dorsiflexion and eversion movement.[6]

Ferciot[26] explains that in talipes calcaneovalgus, there is a tendency for the entire lower limb to be positioned in external rotation, and this positioning occurs during fetal development. He believes there is a delay in the development of the limb bud, with incomplete rotation and a positional stretching of the Achilles tendon. Thus, the feet are held in a position of dorsiflexion and eversion before birth.[26] Rosegger and Steinwendner[30] report that pes calcaneovalgus is attributed to prenatal lie of the fetus.

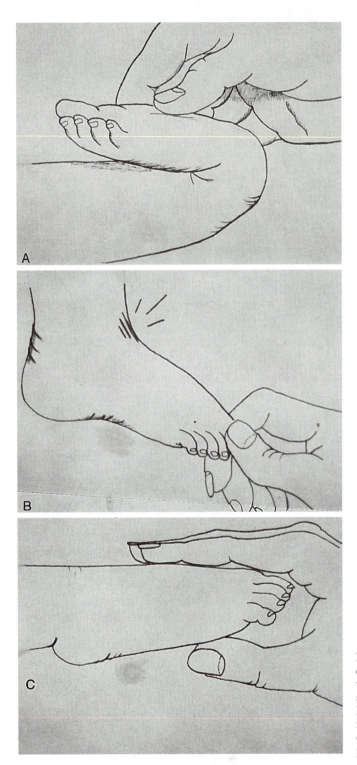

FIGURE 2–5. (*A*) Passive dorsiflexion of the foot. Contact of the forefoot on the anterior aspect of the lower leg. Typical sign found in talipes calcaneovalgus. (*B*) Limited plantar flexion. (*C*) Normal plantar flexion.

According to McCarthy,[31] pes planus or flatfoot becomes a medical problem only when symptoms develop. The mere absence of a well-formed medial arch does not imply pathology. Many apparently flatfeet demonstrate congruent joints, and the extremity function is normal. The development of the foot bones is most often determined at the moment of fertilization by the genes of the patients.[31] Intrauterine development and the genetic factors place the fetus in jeopardy of calcaneovalgus deformities.[31,32]

The cause of flatfoot deformity was suggested to be shoe-wearing in early childhood.[33] A survey of 2300 children between the ages of 4 and 13 years indicated that the incidence of flatfeet among children who used footwear was 8.6% compared with 2.8% in those who did not ($P < .001$). Flatfoot was common in those children who wore closed-toe shoes and less common in children who wore sandals or slippers or were unshod.

Flexible Metatarsal Deformities

For the purposes of this chapter, the flexible metatarsal deformities include those deformities present at birth that are secondary to malposition of the fetus in the uterus. McCrea[6] has the most operative classification system of deformities. His system of classification describes the deformity within the body planes. There are four metatarsal deformities: metatarsus adductus, metatarsus varus, metatarsus adductovarus, and forefoot adductus.[6] Metatarsus adductus is a transverse plane deformity, with adduction of all five metatarsals at the tarsometatarsal joint (Fig. 2–6). Metatarsal varus is a frontal plane deformity of subluxation at the tarsometatarsal joint, with all

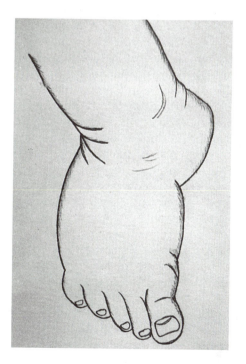

FIGURE 2–6. Metatarsus adductus. Transverse plane deformity with subluxation at the tarsometatarsal joint.

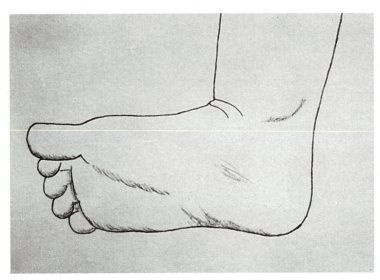

FIGURE 2–7. Metatarsus varus. Frontal plane deformity with subluxation at the tarsometatarsal joint.

of the metatarsals inverted and little or no adduction present (Fig. 2–7). Metatarsus adductovarus is a combination of the frontal and the transverse plane deformities, with adduction and inversion occurring simultaneously at the tarsometatarsal joint (Fig. 2–8). Metatarsus adductovarus is the most common deformity. Forefoot adductus is a single or combined deformity occurring at the midtarsal joint (Fig. 2–9).

Clinical examination of the metatarsus adductus deformities usually reveals a convex lateral border and a concave medial border (Fig. 2–10). Passive movement of the forefoot should reduce the deformity, allowing the forefoot to return to the midline. There are no limitations of the ankle joint into dorsiflexion or plantar flexion, and the calcaneus is in a perpendicular or slightly varus position.[6]

At birth, a metatarsus adductus deformity does not present with the characteristics of flatfoot. According to McCrea,[6] the metatarsus adductus deformities may develop into metatarsal in-toeing abnormalities if they are present when the child begins to weight bear. In-toeing may cause impaired ambulation in the young child. Often, because of the toe-in position, the child is unable to run without tripping and demonstrates an awkward gait. The body's center of gravity is shifted to the lateral aspect of the foot. Normally the weight-bearing stress line is through the central portion of the foot.[6] If the metatarsus adductus deformity is not corrected, foot mechanics are altered with weight bearing. Abnormal pronation develops as a compensation for the forefoot deformity. The rearfoot and the midfoot collapse, which results in abduction of the forefoot, adduction and plantar flexion of the talus, and eversion of the calcaneus.[34,35] The alterations in the foot mechanics allow the center of gravity of the body to shift from a lateral to a more medial position, producing a more stable and less awkward gait. Therefore, metatarsus adductus deformities do not represent true congenital flatfoot. The abnormal pronation develops as a compensation for the deformity after weight bearing.

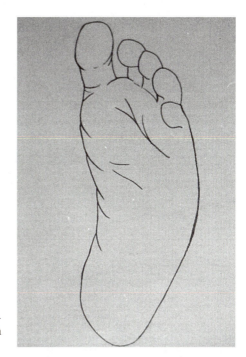

FIGURE 2–8. Metatarsus adductovarus. Combined transverse and frontal plane deformity with subluxation at the tarsometatarsal joint.

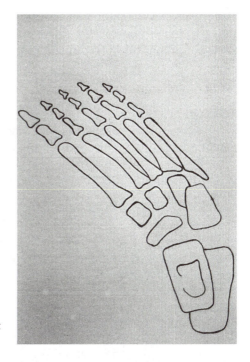

FIGURE 2–9. Forefoot adductus. Subluxation at the midtarsal joint.

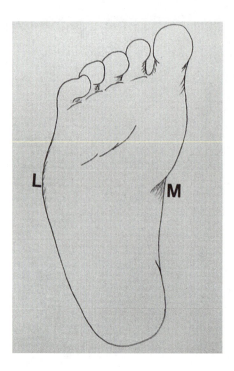

FIGURE 2–10. Concavity of the medial border (M) and convexity of the lateral border (L) of the foot give the appearance of an infant ("C" shaped) foot in metatarsus adductus deformity.

Acquired Deformities

The acquired flatfoot deformity can develop after birth as a result of trauma, ligament laxity, or bony abnormality of the subtalar joint. Acquired flatfoot can also be a compensation for an abnormality that is intrinsic or extrinsic to the foot.[27,34–36]

INTRINSIC DEFORMITIES

Traumatic Flatfoot

Trauma to the tibialis posterior tendon is often described as a cause of acquired adult flatfoot.[37,38] The tibialis posterior is a strong supinator of the foot and produces adduction, inversion, and plantar flexion of the ankle.[34] The muscle-tendon unit of the tibialis posterior is an important stabilizer of the rearfoot, preventing valgus (eversion) deformities.[43]

The primary function of the posterior tibialis is adduction of the midtarsal joint.[42] The tibialis posterior muscle functions early during the stance phase of gait by eccentrically controlling subtalar joint eversion. At the midstance phase of gait, the lesser tarsus is stabilized by the tibialis posterior muscle. During the propulsive phase of gait, the tibialis posterior muscle functions to accelerate subtalar joint supination and assists in heel lift.[42]

The secondary insertions of the tibialis posterior muscle suggest a ligamentous function that provides stability to the rearfoot and midfoot area. The posterior insertion of the tibialis posterior tendon inserts at the sustentaculum tali reinforcing the talonavicular joint. The distal insertion of the tibialis posterior tendon is to the midtarsus area, blending with the short plantar ligament. The distal and posterior inser-

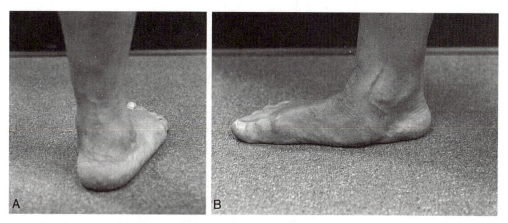

FIGURE 2–11. (*A*) "Too many toes" sign on the right, resulting from a ruptured tibialis posterior tendon. (*B*) Five toes are visible from the posterior aspect of the foot.

tions of the tibialis posterior tendon do not appear to glide.[42] In addition, the tibialis posterior tendon insertions blend with the peroneus longus tendon, long plantar ligament, and talonavicular ligament.

Elongation of the tibialis posterior tendon decreases the resting length of the muscle and adversely affects the contractile force it can exert. Pathologic changes in the tibialis posterior tendon and sheath are accompanied by changes in the talonavicular ligaments, resulting in midfoot abduction and midtarsal joint subluxation progresses.[42] Rupture of the tendon imposes an excessive stress to the hindfoot static structures (ligaments and bone) designed to maintain good alignment. The movement of the calcaneus into the valgus position causes collapse of the talocalcaneal articulation. The calcaneus can be described as subluxing under the talus. The talus moves medially as the calcaneus moves laterally. An important clinical sign in posterior tibialis rupture is the "too many toes sign"; that is, four or five toes can be visualized by an observer from the posterior aspect of the foot when the patient stands (Fig. 2–11). In addition, inability of the patient to rise up onto the toes in the weight-bearing position is an indication of tibialis posterior weakness.

Ligament Laxity

Ligament laxity is an important consideration in the development of a flatfoot deformity. Ligamentous support is important in maintaining the medial arch.[43–45] If sufficient tensile strength is present within the long and short plantar ligaments, the spring ligament, and the plantar fasciae, good joint congruity and alignment are established. A certain amount of ligament laxity is present in the normal child's foot. Young children have a greater range of joint motion than most adults. As the child matures, the margins of increased ranges of joint motion diminish by about half by early adolescence.[6] A child just beginning to walk demonstrates significant medial and lateral instability of the foot.[6] The appearance of flatfoot at this early age may be attributed to ligament laxity. If the tensile strength of the ligaments does not increase as the child matures, a position of pronation is maintained. As the child becomes older and gains weight, stress increases on the ligamentous and muscular structures. The increase in weight-bearing forces may produce microtrauma to the weak ligamentous and muscular structures, eventually producing soft tissue destruction and increased possibility of joint collapse. Prolonged pronation in childhood can produce a structurally irreparable adult flatfoot.[46]

Bony Abnormality of Subtalar Joint

Harris and Beath[47] have reported the significance of the bony architecture in maintaining proper joint congruity between the talus and calcaneus.[47] Bony abnormalities between the articular facets of the talus and calcaneus may be significant factors in the development of flatfoot. The stability and congruity of the subtalar joint depend on ligamentous, muscular, and bony support. The articular surfaces of the subtalar joint are composed of three facets: anteromedial, anterolateral, and posterior. The anteromedial facet is the most important of the three for support of the head and neck of the talus. The anterior medial facet of the subtalar joint is formed by the anterior aspect of the calcaneus and a bony prominence along the anteromedial aspect of the calcaneus called the sustentaculum tali. In the stance phase of gait, from heel strike to footflat, the vertical body weight is shifted to the medial aspect of the foot as the tibia rotates internally.[34] Pronation at the subtalar joint includes plantar flexion and adduction of the talus as the calcaneus moves into eversion. The anteromedial facet and the posterior facet are important articulations for normal pronation. If the anteromedial facet does not provide good support to the head and neck of the talus, the forces at heel strike could push the talus into excessive plantar flexion and adduction, one component of abnormal pronation (Fig. 2–12).

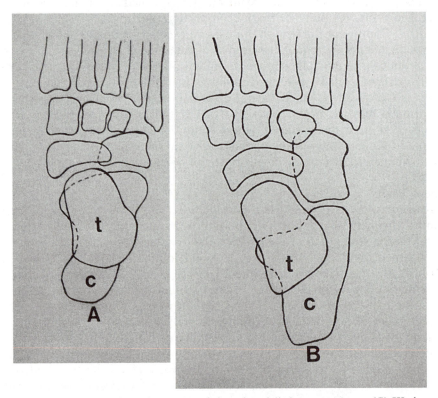

FIGURE 2–12. Anterior calcaneal support of the talus. (*A*) Strong support. (*B*) Weak support, which predisposes the foot in weight bearing to abnormal pronation. (t = talus; c = calcaneus.)

The manner in which the head of the talus is supported by the anterior aspect of the calcaneus can be classified as strong, mild, or weak.[47] Strong support is indicated by a talar head that is placed solidly on the calcaneus with total joint congruity. This strong osseous support to the talar head permits full weight bearing without changing the talocalcaneal position. Mild osseous support is demonstrated when the head of the talus is partially sustained by the anterior aspect of the calcaneus. Weak osseous support results when the head of the talus is without anterior medial calcaneal contact, with only the sustentaculum tali to support the head. When the osseous support is weak, the head and neck of the talus project over the anteromedial end of the calcaneus. The lack of support may produce excessive medial and plantar movement of the talus during the pronation phase, causing the calcaneus to tilt into eversion. The excessive movements of the talus and calcaneus are important components in the development of abnormal pronation and acquired flatfoot deformity.

Compensatory Pronation Caused by Intrinsic Deformities

The four most common intrinsic abnormalities resulting in compensated abnormal pronation are forefoot varus, forefoot supinatus, subtalar varus, and ankle joint equinus.[27,34] The compensation for the deformity usually occurs at the subtalar joint. When the subtalar joint compensates for the deformity by pronating, the compensatory pronation occurs in addition to the normal amount of pronation necessary for ambulation. This compensatory pronation occurs every time the foot is placed on the ground. Furthermore, compensatory pronation may occur at the wrong time. For example, pronation may occur during the supination phase of stance. Root et al[34] report that pronation is most destructive to the foot when it occurs in the push-off phase of gait.

Maximum pronation is normally reached after approximately 25% of the stance phase is completed.[48] Compensatory pronation usually continues past 50% of the stance phase. The foot never supinates.

Compensatory pronation may be excessive, persistent, and untimely during the stance phase, resulting in destruction of the soft tissue and in foot pathology. Because the subtalar joint is triplanar, it has the ability to move in three body planes: frontal, sagittal, and transverse.[34] The ability of the subtalar joint to move in three planes allows it to compensate for deformities in the body planes.[34,35,49]

Compensated Forefoot Varus. Forefoot varus is the most common intrinsic deformity that results in abnormal compensatory pronation.[34,50-53] Root et al[34] define forefoot varus as an inversion of the forefoot on the rearfoot, with the subtalar joint held in neutral (Fig. 2–13).[34] Forefoot varus is a frontal plane deformity that is compensated, in weight bearing, by eversion of the calcaneus (Fig. 2–14). The compensatory movement of the calcaneus into eversion is accompanied by talar adduction and plantar flexion.[25]

Compensation for forefoot varus deformity occurs at the subtalar joint. This compensation can be measured by the amount of calcaneal eversion in the standing position. For example, 8° of forefoot varus should result in 8° of calcaneal eversion. The eversion range of motion of the subtalar joint determines the amount of compensation movement available. For example, if the eversion range of the calcaneus is measured at 10°, the subtalar joint is capable of compensating for a forefoot deformity of up to 10°. If the forefoot varus is greater than 10°, additional compensation must be accomplished elsewhere. A forefoot varus deformity may be totally compensated, partially compensated, or uncompensated at the subtalar joint.

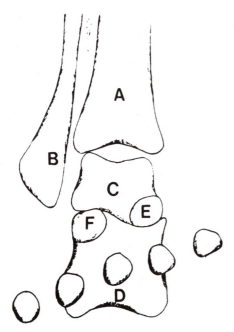

FIGURE 2–13. Forefoot varus. Inversion of the forefoot on the rearfoot with the subtalar joint in neutral. (A = tibia; B = fibula; C = talus; D = calcaneus; E = talonavicular articulation; F = calcaneal-cuboid articulation.)

A forefoot varus deformity alone is not destructive to the foot; however, the method of compensation is detrimental to the normal mechanics of the foot. The subtalar joint must pronate to compensate for the forefoot deformity. In addition, normal pronation must occur to assist the lower kinetic chain to attenuate weight-bearing forces, such as torque conversion, anterior shear, and compression. The combination of normal pronation and compensatory pronation is excessive and may be destructive to the foot and ankle. Many clinicians have observed that compensation for forefoot varus is a clinically significant factor in the development of mechanical pain and dysfunction within the foot, lower third of the leg, and knee.[52,54–56]

McCrea[6] explains that forefoot varus results from prolonged abnormal pronation rather than from a primary cause or result of a flatfoot deformity. As the foot continues to function from a collapsed position of pronation, the forefoot eventually assumes a varus attitude in conjunction with the everted position of the calcaneus. A functional shortening of the muscles attaching to the dorsal medial aspect of the foot maintains this varus position of the forefoot.[6]

DiGiovanni and Smith[57] define forefoot varus as a sagittal plane deformity of the first ray. The dorsal hypermobility of the first ray results from abnormal pronation and is also referred to as "first ray insufficiency."[16] The dorsiflexed hypermobile first ray results from inability of the peroneus longus to stabilize the first ray. The cuboid pulley allows the peroneus longus to plantar flex and abduct the first ray, producing a stable structure from which to push off.[34] The peroneus longus pulley system is reinforced by locking up the midtarsal joint during supination of the subtalar joint.[34,57–59] The cuboid becomes a rigid structure around which the peroneus longus functions. Abnormal pronation reduces the ability of the foot to return to supination. Thus, the midtarsal joint, specifically the cuboid, is in a poor position. The poor position of the cuboid creates an inefficient pulley for the peroneus longus muscle, causing instability of the first ray (Fig. 2–15).[34]

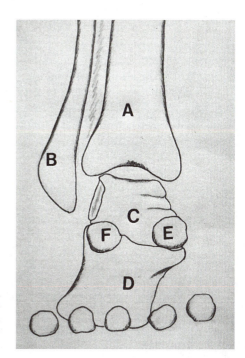

FIGURE 2–14. Compensated forefoot varus in weight bearing. (A = tibia; B = fibula; C = talus; D = calcaneus; E = talonavicular articulation; F = calcaneal-cuboid articulation.)

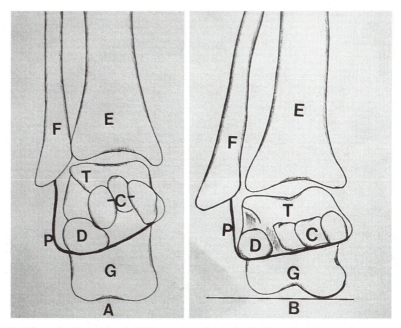

FIGURE 2–15. Cuboid pulley. (*A*) Normal pulley of cuboid. (*B*) Abnormal pronation cuboid pulley is less effective. (E = tibia; F = fibula; P = peroneus longus tendon; D = cuboid; C = cuneiforms; G = calcaneus; T = talus.)

Partially Compensated or Uncompensated Forefoot Varus. Inability of the subtalar joint to pronate, offsetting a forefoot varus deformity, may result in partial or complete compensation at the joints distal to the subtalar joint. Compensations may occur within the joints of the midtarsal or the first ray, or both.

During the stance phase of gait, an uncompensated or partially compensated forefoot varus may manifest itself by an increase in the abduction of the foot from the midline. The abduction of the forefoot occurs around the transverse axis of the midtarsal joint. It is accompanied by eversion. Abduction and eversion are pronation movements occurring at the midtarsal joint. Pronation of the midtarsal joint is in addition to subtalar compensatory pronation or else replaces it.

Jahss[16] refers to talonavicular and navicular cuneiform sag as a collapse of the medial arch. Excessive movement of these joints may occur when the subtalar joint is limited and unable to produce enough compensatory pronation. The excessive mobility of the midfoot and forefoot may cause subluxation of the talonavicular and navicular-cuneiform articulations. These subluxations produce soft tissue trauma and medial arch pain.

Forefoot Supinatus. Forefoot supinatus is difficult to distinguish from forefoot varus. Forefoot supinatus is a soft tissue deformity that occurs around the longitudinal axis of the midtarsal joint.[34] The forefoot is held in a supinated position secondary to contracture or spasm of the anterior tibialis muscle. In contrast, forefoot varus results from failure of the head and neck of the talus to derotate fully from the infantile position.[34]

Forefoot supinatus and forefoot varus are compensated at the subtalar joint during the stance phase of gait. The compensation is the same for both deformities—the subtalar joint pronates if complete compensation occurs to increase weight bearing of the first ray. Another method of compensation for forefoot varus and forefoot supinatus is plantar flexion of the first ray.[34] In the non–weight-bearing position, the first ray is hypermobile and plantar flexed. During the gait cycle, plantar flexion of the first ray is an attempt to correct an uncompensated forefoot varus. This compensation causes instability of the forefoot and rearfoot in the propulsive phase of gait.

Rearfoot Varus. Another intrinsic frontal plane deformity resulting in compensatory pronation is rearfoot varus, not to be confused with the calcaneal varus position as a compensation for forefoot valgus (see Abnormal Supination, later). The rearfoot varus deformity can be described as a varus neutral heel. If the subtalar joint functions from the varus neutral position, the heel contacts the ground in an inverted position. As the heel hits the ground, the rearfoot must be stable. The calcaneus moves from the varus position to a vertical position. The movement of the heel from varus to vertical is a relative eversion or pronation of the subtalar joint. This positioning becomes detrimental to the foot if, in addition to normal pronation, compensatory pronation must also occur.

To protect the ankle from trauma, the subtalar joint must pronate at heel strike. The calcaneal eversion distributes the weight medially, permitting the subtalar joint to function as a shock absorber and to adjust to changing terrain. The inability to pronate causes instability with minimal changes in the contour of the walking or running surface, leaving the patient more vulnerable to ankle sprains.

Many patients demonstrate restricted calcaneal eversion. Patients who complain of repeated ankle sprains may have limited eversion of the calcaneus beyond the vertical position (Fig. 2–16). Limited calcaneal eversion is another example of a rearfoot

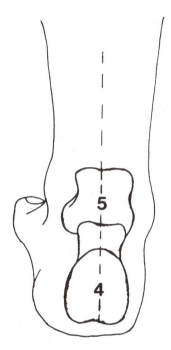

FIGURE 2–16. In the neutral or vertical position of the subtalar joint, a vertical line would bisect both the talus (5) and calcaneus (4).

varus deformity. Limited eversion produces instability of the ankle from heel strike to footflat.

Ankle Joint Equinus. Ankle joint equinus is an intrinsic sagittal plane deformity that causes compensatory pronation.[34,47,53,60–63] Root et al[34] define ankle joint equinus as the lack of dorsiflexion of the ankle with the subtalar joint in neutral position. The most common cause of ankle joint equinus is limited flexibility of the gastrocnemius and soleus muscle groups.[60,61] Harris and Beath[47] reported a congenital shortening of the gastrocnemius and soleus muscles. Sgarlato[64] was the first to distinguish between the soleus or the gastrocnemius as the limiting agent of dorsiflexion of the ankle joint.[64] He demonstrated that a shortened soleus muscle can be distinguished from a shortened gastrocnemius by flexing the knee and passively dorsiflexing the ankle. A shortened soleus prevents 10° of dorsiflexion at the ankle joint with the knee flexed. The gastrocnemius equinus limits dorsiflexion with the knee extended. A combined limitation in dorsiflexion of the gastrocnemius and soleus muscle groups produces restrictions with the knee extended and flexed.[64] The subtalar joint is held in the neutral position in this test.

Anopol[62] describes the foot as a two-lever arm mechanism. The short arm of the lever is the length of the Achilles tendon from insertion on the calcaneus to the center of the ankle joint. The long arm runs from the center of the ankle joint to the metatarsophalangeal joint. The short lever arm of the Achilles tendon can manage twice the force of the long lever arm. For example, every time a person weighing 100 kg takes a step, 100 kg of force is placed on the ball of the foot, and 200 kg is exerted on the calf muscles.[62] If the calf muscles (gastrocnemius and soleus) become tight, dorsiflexion of the ankle joint is limited, increasing the pull of the gastrocnemius. The increased force of the muscle pull may cause the calcaneus to move into eversion to

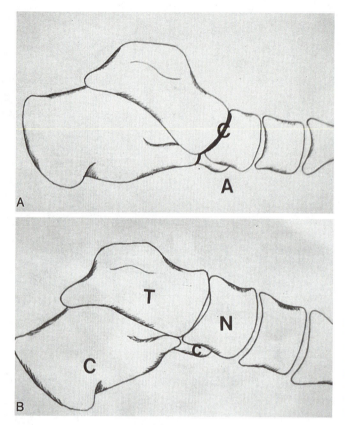

FIGURE 2–17. (*A*) Abnormal pronation of subtalar joint in weight bearing. Movement of the talus anterior to the calcaneus causes an anterior break in the Cyma (C) line. (*B*) Normal subtalar joint in weight bearing. Cyma line (or midtarsal joint line) is "S" shaped.

place the lateral aspect of the tendon on slack. Therefore, a tight Achilles tendon may be the cause of excessive pronation of the subtalar joint.

Furthermore, limited dorsiflexion of the ankle joint during the stance phase produces an inability of the tibia to move anterior to the talus from footflat to midstance. This limitation may also be compensated for by pronation of the subtalar joint. A common finding in a flatfoot is the change in the alignment of the midtarsal joint line (Fig. 2–17). The lateral weight-bearing radiograph of a normal foot demonstrates a line forming an S, called the Cyma line. This anatomic line passes between the talus and the navicular bones and the cuboid and calcaneus (midtarsal joint line). Excessive pronation of the subtalar joint causes an anterior break in the Cyma line. The anterior movement of the talus that occurs during pronation of the subtalar joint may compensate for the lack of anterior movement of the tibia.

EXTRINSIC DEFORMITIES

Rotational deformities and leg length discrepancies (LLDs) are the two most common extrinsic abnormalities of the lower extremities causing compensatory pronation.

Rotational Deformities

The rotational deformities of the lower extremity can be divided into deformities of the thigh and the lower leg. Rotational deformities of the thigh include femoral anteversion, retroversion, antetorsion, and retrotorsion. The lower leg deformities include internal and external tibial torsion.

The limb buds orginate in a laterally rotated, abducted, and flexed position relative to the pelvis.[65] Early in development, the limb first rotates medially to bring the great toe to the medial side of the foot and to rotate the knee and leg into an anterior position.[65,66] The normal rotational process may be altered by genetic or environmental factors.[66]

Cause. Considerable confusion exists in the literature regarding the terminology of rotational deformities of the thigh or femur. "Femoral version" and "torsion" are often used synonymously when discussing rotational deformities. Femoral torsion, also called the "angle of declination," is defined (for the purposes of this chapter) as a twist in the femur bone. Femoral version is defined as an altered relationship between the femoral head and neck and the acetabulum.[6] Femoral version may be caused by contractures of the soft tissue structures around the hip. The soft tissue contractures can be precipitated by intrauterine positioning of the lower extremity.[6,66] Malposition in the uterus is also the most common cause of torsional deformities of the femur and tibia.[66] Sitting and sleeping postures may perpetuate or delay resolution of femoral torsion or version deformities of the femur or tibia.[66,67] Rotational variations of the femur and tibia have a genetic factor. Evaluation of the parents' rotational profiles can often predict a child's rotational variations.[66] The cause of excessive external tibial torsion can be iatrogenic.[66] The management of clubfoot deformities using long leg cases or Denis Browne splints may create a lateral rotational deformity of the tibia.

Femoral torsion and version and tibial torsion may be caused by soft tissue deformities, malposition in the uterus, sitting postures, sleeping postures, and genetic and iatrogenic factors.

Rotational Deformities of the Thigh. The femoral antetorsion angle is used to describe the relationship of anterior rotation of the proximal head and neck of the femur to the condyles of the distal femur (Fig. 2–18).[66,68] If the femur were placed on the table top with the posterior aspect of the condyles in contact with the table, the head and neck of the femur would be elevated away from the table anteriorly. Therefore, the axis of the head and neck would form an angle with the transcondylar axis of the femur. The angle of declination, or anteversion, is 30° to 40° at birth and between 8° and 15° in the adult.[6]

Excessive femoral anteversion or medial femoral torsion can produce an in-toeing gait.[6,66,68] Patients who have significant femoral anteversion or medial femoral torsion deformity have hip internal rotation of 60° to 90° and external rotation of less than 25°.[68] The foot progression angle can help to determine the degree of in-toeing or out-toeing during gait. The foot progression angle can be defined as the angle between the axis of the foot and the line of progression.[66] In-toeing is expressed as a negative value, and out-toeing is a positive value. Normally the foot progression angle should be between +8° and +12°, or that of an out-toe foot position.[68] Excessive femoral retroversion or lateral femoral torsion deformities are rare (Fig. 2–19).[68] These deformities would cause excessive out-toeing or a foot progression angle of +15° or more.

Clinically, to distinguish between hip anteversion and medial femoral torsion deformities, it is important to evaluate the range of motion of the hip in four positions. Test the patient in a supine posture, with the hip and knee extended; the knee flexed and hip extended; the hip flexed 90° and knees extended; and the hip and knee

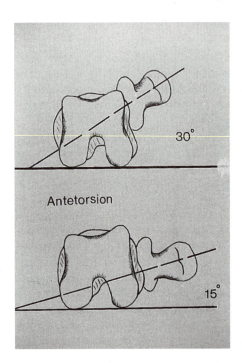

FIGURE 2–18. Antetorsion of 30° (*top*) is abnormal; 15° is normal (*bottom*).

flexed. If the findings are consistent in all four positions, there is probably osseous torsion.[69] If there is an inconsistency in rotational values from one position to another, however, one must suspect soft tissue contractures. Roentgenographic procedures such as fluoroscopy, axial scans, and computed tomography are also used to determine the degree of femoral torsion deformities.[68]

Compensations throughout the lower extremity may occur if femoral anteversion or medial femoral torsion deformities persist beyond the age of 4 or 5 years.[68] In the case of femoral anteversion or medial femoral torsion, the child develops an awkward gait. Excessive compensatory external tibial torsion (greater than 22°) may develop to reduce clumsiness and occasional stumbling in the child with an excessive in-toe gait. Extreme external tibial torsion increases the stress to the medial aspect of the foot.[65] Increased medial force to the subtalar joint produces calcaneal valgus, plantar flexion, and adduction of the talus (abnormal compensatory pronation).[70] Abnormal foot pronation may precipitate patellar malalignment and knee pain. Furthermore, hip and buttock pain may result from strain to the external rotators in an attempt to walk straight.

Five percent to 15% of femoral rotational deformities in children are not spontaneously corrected by skeletal maturity.[6,68] The child who continues to demonstrate excessive femoral torsion at the age of 8 rarely demonstrates significant spontaneous torsion changes, even with conservative management.[68]

Rotational Deformities of the Lower Leg. Tibial torsion is the transverse plane abnormality that occurs in the lower leg. It results from the axial relationship of the foot to the thigh, which is due to rotation or twisting of the tibia along its longitudinal axis.[66] "Malleolar torsion" is a term coined by Root as the preferred term for tibial torsion.[34] Malleolar torsion presents as an excessive anterior or posterior displace-

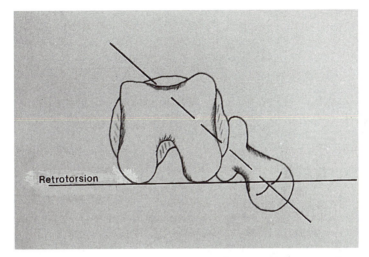

FIGURE 2-19. Retrotorsion is rare and can result in out-toeing.

ment of the medial malleolus relative to the lateral malleolus. The normal adult external torsion angle is approximately 20° (Fig. 2–20).[71]

Internal tibial (malleolar) torsion is present when the angle of malleolar torsion is less than zero. Internal torsion deformity of the tibia is usually associated with congenital metatarsus adductus, clubfoot, and developmental genu varum (bow legs).[67] Hutter and Scott[71] advocate conservative treatment of internal tibial torsion deformities if they are still present at age 3. Correction of tibial torsion is possible during the growth period by application of a night splint, which produces a rotational stress in a direction opposite to that of the deformity (Fig. 2–21). Spontaneous correction of torsion deformities after age 8 is rare. Internal tibial torsion is the most common cause of in-toeing.[66] Metatarsus adductus is also associated with internal tibial torsion and in-toeing.[66]

Abnormal external tibial torsion, as previously noted, is usually a result of a compensation for in-toeing. When external tibial torsion is greater than 20°, pronation at the subtalar joint is clinically evident.[34]

Leg Length Discrepancies

Most authors in the podiatric and osteopathic literature divide LLDs into structural and functional leg length differences.[72–74] Structural LLDs are true anatomic differences in the length of the tibia or femur, or both. Functional LLDs are either the shortening or lengthening of a limb, secondary to joint contracture or muscle imbalances.[73]

Structural LLD may be caused by uneven development of the lower extremity in utero, fractures, epiphyseal irritation with lengthening, sacral or innominate deformity, or unilateral coxa vara.[75] Functional LLD may be secondary to a tight unilateral psoas muscle, unequal lumbar muscle spasms, hip fascia tightness, shortening or ligamentous laxity, or pronated feet.[75] Botte[72] describes how muscle imbalances may produce a functional LLD. Ipsilateral hip flexor tightness, secondary to muscle guarding or spasm, may cause ipsilateral limb shortening. In the case of the functional LLD, a change in position of the tight muscle may reduce the LLD. The clinician can safe-

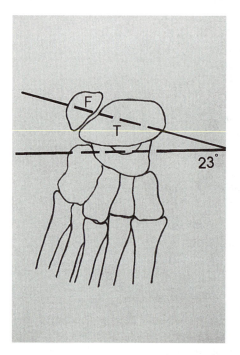

FIGURE 2–20. External torsion of the tibia (or external malleolar torsion) of 23° is within normal limits.

ly assume that if a LLD is suspected, regardless of the cause, there is always an associated asymmetry to be found. At some point(s) between the head and the foot, the body attempts to compensate for an unbalanced lower kinetic chain.

In relationship to the foot and ankle, the most important biomechanical compensation for LLD is at the subtalar joint.[72–74] On the long limb side, the subtalar joint pronates in an attempt to reduce the vertical height of the leg, whereas on the short limb side, the subtalar joint supinates in an attempt to increase the length of the leg (Figs. 2–22 and 2–23). The inclination angle of the calcaneus is increased in the

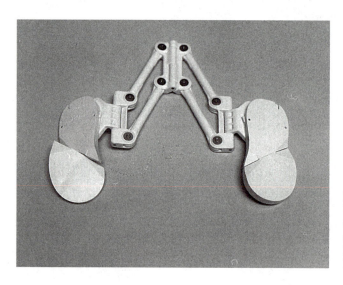

FIGURE 2–21. Derotation brace by Langer Biomechanics Group CRS counter-rotation system. (Courtesy of Langer Biomechanics Group, Deer Park, NY.)

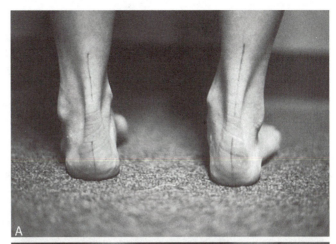

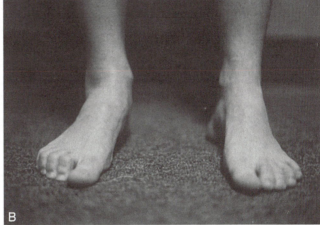

FIGURE 2–22. Posterior (*A*) and anterior (*B*) views of the foot in LLD. The right subtalar joint is pronated, reducing the length of the long leg. The left subtalar joint is supinated to increase the length of the short leg.

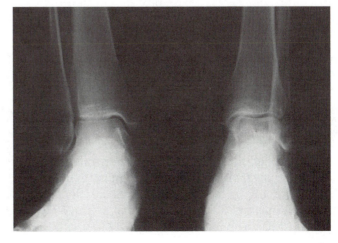

FIGURE 2–23. Anterior radiograph of the patient in Figure 2–22. Note the tibia and fibula relationship. In the right ankle, the tibia is internally rotated and the talus is adducted. In the left ankle, the tibia is externally rotated. The syndesmosis space is open and visible on the right, and reduced on the left.

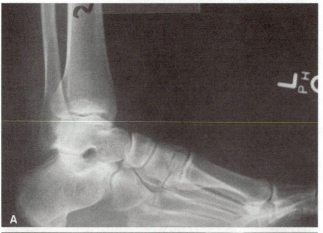

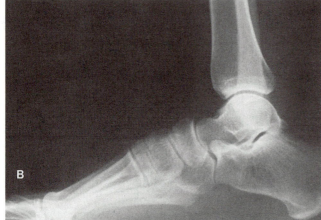

FIGURE 2–24. (*A*) Weight-bearing radiograph of the shorter foot in LLD. Note the increased inclination angle of the calcaneus on the supinated foot. (*B*) Weight-bearing radiograph of the longer foot in LLD. Note the decreased inclination angle of the calcaneus on the pronated foot.

supinated foot and decreased in the pronated foot (Fig. 2–24). Plantar flexion, adduction, and subsequent calcaneal eversion actively shorten the long leg by reducing the vertical height of the subtalar and talocrural areas (Fig. 2–25). The subtalar joint on the contralateral lower extremity may reciprocally supinate, "thereby increasing the calcaneal inclination, in an effort to lengthen the shorter limb and balance the pelvis."[74]

These changes in the kinetic chain may not cause any problem for the sedentary individual, but an athlete or runner may suffer from the effects of an abnormal gait cycle. Blustian and D'Amico[74] observed that the longer leg maintains a prolonged stance phase. As the cadence increases, double support diminishes, subjecting the longer leg to greater stress for longer periods.[74] More complaints of pain and dysfunction are likely to be present on the side with the longer leg and pronated subtalar joint.

Compensations for a LLD do not follow consistent patterns, and the clinician should be aware of various patterns that may exist.[76] Accommodation to a short leg may have any of the following compensation patterns: pelvic tilt, sacral tilt, pelvic side shift, pelvic rotation, and lumbar scoliosis.[75]

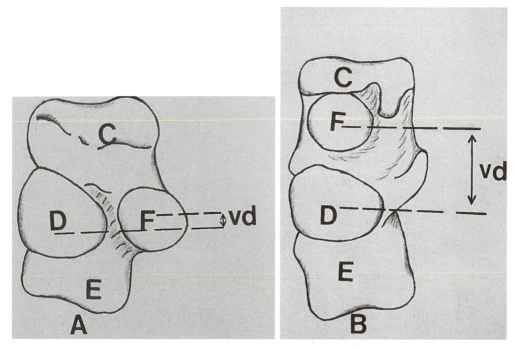

FIGURE 2–25. (*A*) Pronation of the subtalar joint (anterior view). Reduced vertical distance (vd) reduces the height of the rearfoot. (*B*) Supination of the subtalar joint (anterior view). Increased vertical distance increases the height of the rearfoot.

SUMMARY

Congenital or acquired abnormal pronation (Table 2–1) changes the alignment of the calcaneus, talus, cuboid, and navicular bones. The change in alignment produces poor articular congruity and alters the arthrokinematics of the ankle, subtalar, and midtarsal joints. The excessive arthrokinematic movements produce excessive forces within the foot and ankle and throughout the lower kinetic chain. The tibia, talus, and calcaneus move simultaneously, as the foot pronates. The talus and tibia are rotated medially, and the calcaneus rolls laterally into eversion. In abnormal pronation, the calcaneus has been described as subluxing under the talus. Such arthrokinematics are abnormal because they are excessive and persistent throughout the stance phase. Normal pronation compensation is a temporary condition of the subtalar joint.[34] Normal compensation might occur in response to a change in the terrain.

Changes in the mechanics of the rearfoot and midfoot produce certain anatomic changes typical of flatfoot. These can be observed in the weight-bearing or (in severe cases) in the non–weight-bearing position. The changes include everted position of the calcaneus, medial bulging of the navicular tuberosity, abduction of the forefoot on the rearfoot, and a reduction in the height of the medial arch.[34,77] As a result of the excessive pronation, the soft tissue structures are traumatized over a long period of time, resulting in breakdown and pathology.

TABLE 2–1 Abnormal Pronation

I. *Congenital Abnormal Pronation*

    A. Rigid deformities
        1. Vertical talus–convex pes valgus
        2. Tarsal coalitions
        3. Rigid metatarsal deformity
    B. Flexible deformities
        1. Talipes calcaneovalgus
        2. Flexible metatarsal deformities

II. *Acquired Abnormal Pronation*

    A. Intrinsic deformities
        1. Traumatic
        2. Ligament laxity
        3. Bony abnormalities of subtalar joint
        4. Compensatory pronation for intrinsic deformities
            a. Compensated forefoot varus
            b. Partially compensated or uncompensated forefoot varus
            c. Forefoot supinatus
            d. Rearfoot varus
            e. Ankle joint equinus
    B. Extrinsic deformities
        1. Rotational deformities of the lower extremity
        2. Leg length discrepancy

ABNORMAL SUPINATION

Abnormal supination is the inability of the foot to pronate effectively during the stance phase of gait. This is commonly referred to as the high-arched foot, or pes cavus. Abnormal supination is a hypomobility of the joints of the foot and ankle that may result from muscle imbalances and soft tissue contractures. Abnormal supination usually is associated with a rigid structure that is unable to function as an efficient shock absorber or an adapter to changing terrain. The abnormal supinator usually does not demonstrate a progressive breakdown in tissue (producing a hypermobile foot), such as occurs in the flexible, pronated foot. Rather it is an inflexible foot that causes tissue inflammation and possible joint destruction.

Terminology in the literature describing a high-arched foot is confusing. A pure pes cavus deformity is plantar flexion of the forefoot on the rearfoot.[5,6,16] The pes cavus deformity is usually associated with other deformities of the rearfoot and fore-foot. For example, the calcaneus can be in a varus position, in which case the deformity is referred to as "pes cavovarus." The calcaneus can be in equinus or in plantar flexion, thus described as "pes equinocavus." Finally, the calcaneus can be in a dorsi-flexed position, which is referred to as "calcaneocavus." In all pes cavus deformities, the forefoot is either completely or partially in plantar flexion. Pes cavovarus is plantar flexion of the medial column or first ray. In the standing position, the rearfoot moves into varus to compensate for the forefoot.

Therefore, pes cavus describes deformities of the forefoot and rearfoot in the sagittal or frontal plane. Some of the terms used to describe pes cavus include bolt foot, clubfoot, talipes plantaris, hollow foot, contracted foot, and nondeforming clubfoot.[16]

Classification of Pes Cavus

Earlier studies labeled this high-arched foot "hollow claw foot."[78,79] Steindler[79] clinically described three important aspects of the pes cavus foot: increased height of the longitudinal arch, dropping of the anterior arch with plantar flexion of the forefoot, and some amount of dorsal retraction of the toes, or claw toes (hyperextension of the metatarsophalangeal and flexion of the interphalangeal joints). He reported an interdependency of the toe deformity and the increased height of the medial arch.

Samilson and Dillin[80] classified the pes cavus foot according to the apex of the longitudinal arch. Anterior or forefoot cavus has its apex at the metatarsocuneiform joints. Midfoot cavus has its apex between the metatarsocuneiform joints and the anterior tuberosity of the calcaneus. Hindfoot cavus is characterized by increased vertical height of the calcaneus of 30° or more.[80] The vertical height is measured by the calcaneal pitch (or inclination angle of the calcaneus) on weight-bearing roentgenograms of the foot. The angle is formed by the horizontal line and a line along the plantar aspect of the calcaneus from posterior to anterior calcaneal tuberosity (Fig. 2–26).[5,6,80]

McGlamry and Kitting[81] report plantar flexion of the forefoot on the rearfoot or the apex of the cavus at the tarsometatarsal and the midtarsal joints; however, they call these deformities metatarsal equinus and forefoot equinus, respectively.

McCrea[6] classifies cavus deformities into several categories. Anterior cavus manifests plantar flexion of the forefoot on the rearfoot, occurring at the tarsometatarsal or the midtarsal joint. The second major classification is posterior cavus, which causes changes at the subtalar joint. Posterior cavus also causes an increase in the inclination angle of the calcaneus. The third and most frequent type is a combination of the posterior and anterior cavus, referred to as the global type.[6]

In simple pes cavus, the plantar flexion deformity of the forefoot is equal on the medial and lateral columns. Therefore, weight bearing is evenly distributed over the first and fifth rays. The heel is usually in neutral position, allowing for equal distribution of weight in the rearfoot. The pes cavus foot is often associated with other deformities, such as equinus and varus.

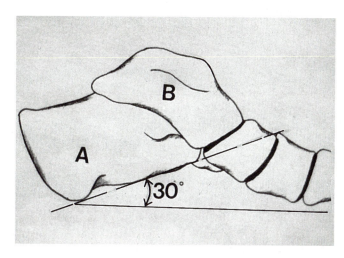

FIGURE 2–26. Inclination angle of the calcaneus is 30°. (A = talus; B = calcaneus.)

Combined Pes Cavus Deformities

Tachdjian[5] delineates three combined deformities: pes cavovarus, calcaneocavus, and pes equinocavus. The combined deformities describe forefoot and rearfoot changes in the pes cavus foot.

PES CAVOVARUS (FOREFOOT VALGUS, RIGID PLANTAR FLEXED FIRST RAY)

Pes cavovarus is plantar flexion of the medial column or first ray (first metatarsal, first cuneiform). The position of the first ray is equinus or fixed plantar flexion. Passive testing of the first ray with the patient in the non–weight-bearing prone position demonstrates limited movement of the first metatarsocuneiform joint into dorsiflexion.[5,82] Because of the interconnection of the first and second metatarsal bones by the transverse metatarsal ligament, plantar flexion of the second ray is also present.[15,83] Mobility of the plantar flexed second ray is restricted to dorsiflexion to a lesser degree. Observation of the fifth ray demonstrates normal mobility and a neutral position.[5] This "stair-stepped" position of the metatarsals, from plantar flexion of the first ray to neutral position of the fifth, is clinically the same as the description of forefoot valgus given by Root et al.[34] Forefoot valgus is defined as eversion of the forefoot on the rearfoot with the subtalar joint in neutral position (Fig. 2–27). As previously noted, DiGiovanni and Smith[57] do not acknowledge forefoot deformities in the frontal plane, such as forefoot varus or valgus. Rather, they attribute these clinical findings to a sagittal plane deformity of the first ray moving into dorsiflexion and plantar flexion, respectively.

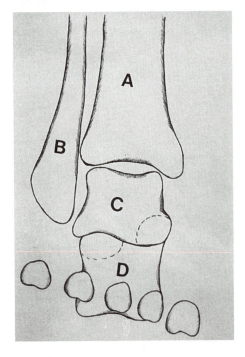

FIGURE 2–27. Uncompensated forefoot valgus. Eversion of the forefoot on the rearfoot with the subtalar joint held in neutral. (A = tibia; B = fibula; C = talus; D = calcaneus.)

In either case, forefoot valgus or a fixed plantar flexed first ray must be compensated for during the stance phase of gait. In a normal foot, the forefoot strikes the ground directly after heel strike. With a fixed plantar flexed first ray, however, the first metatarsal strikes the ground first. Rapid supination of the subtalar joint occurs, immediately shifting the weight laterally (and onto) the fifth metatarsal head (Fig. 2–28).[5,34] As a result of this compensated supination, the foot does not return to pronation during the stance phase of gait. The lack of pronation reduces the ability of the foot to absorb shock and adapt to changing terrain, causing ankle instability. As the rearfoot inverts or supinates, the cuboid pulley becomes a strong lever for the peroneus longus muscle (Fig. 2–15). The muscle now has a mechanical advantage exerting a strong plantar flexion force on the first ray.[34] The deformity may become progressively worse, and soft tissue changes may cause an increased rigidity. Therefore, the rearfoot varus may perpetuate and, in some cases, precipitate forefoot valgus.

Another type of pes cavovarus deformity is flexible forefoot valgus. In this condition, the foot is unstable and develops significant forefoot symptoms.[84] Rearfoot compensation is unnecessary. Flexible forefoot valgus does not promote the locking of the forefoot against the rearfoot and thus produces an instability in push-off.[85] The valgus position of the forefoot (plantar flexed first ray) can be observed in the non–weight-bearing position.

CALCANEOCAVUS

Calcaneocavus deformity describes a dorsiflexion (calcaneus) position of the rearfoot with the forefoot fixed in equinus (plantar flexion).[5] In the weight-bearing position, the subtalar joint does not need to compensate for intrinsic deformities. The rear-

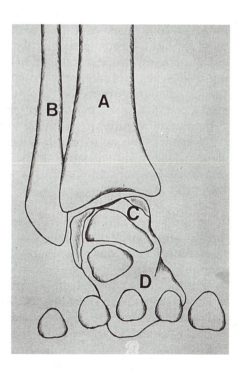

FIGURE 2–28. Compensated forefoot valgus. Inversion of the rearfoot. (A = tibia; B = fibula; C = talus; D = calcaneus.)

foot is usually in neutral or in a position perpendicular to the ground. Calcaneocavus deformity is almost always the result of a neurologic disorder and subsequent weakness or paralysis of the gastrocnemius and soleus muscle groups.[86]

PES EQUINOCAVUS

Pes equinocavus, the third type of pes cavus deformity described by Tachdjian, is an equinus position of the forefoot, hindfoot, and ankle joint. Tachdjian[5] reports that pes equinocavus is secondary to talipes equinovarus or clubfoot.

Causes of Pes Cavus Deformities

The etiology of pes cavus can be divided into three causes: neurologic, contracture of soft tissue structures, and idiopathic.[87–96] The most clinical and scientifically documented article describing the cause of pes cavus was presented in 1963 by Brewerton et al.[87] They reported evidence of central nervous system disorders in 66% of 77 patients followed in a pes cavus clinic over a 5-year period. The neurologic disorders included Friedreich's ataxia, peroneal muscular atrophy, poliomyelitis, spina bifida, cerebral palsy, spinal cord tumors, myelodysplasia, spastic paraplegia, and spastic monoplegia.[87]

Tyan et al[97] investigated the cross-sectional areas of the peroneal and anterior muscle compartments in 41 cases of pes cavus deformities. The causes of the pes cavus deformities included Charcot-Marie-Tooth disease, Friedreich's ataxia, cerebral palsy, status postpoliomyelitis, nerve trauma, and spinal cord tethering. The results demonstrated that the peroneal compartment was enlarged relative to the anterior compartment when compared with normal controls. Overactivity of the peroneus longus in comparison to its antagonist, the tibialis anterior, is proposed as an important factor in the pathogenesis of the majority of symptomatic cases of pes cavus.[97]

Patterns of muscle degeneration in patients with peripheral neuropathies exhibiting pes cavus deformity were studied by computed tomography. Muscle degeneration clearly demonstrated earlier and more severe involvement of the intrinsic muscles of the foot as compared with the extrinsic muscles.[98] The most consistent early degeneration occurred in the pedal lumbricales and interossei.

Causes of pes cavus that may be appropriate for physical therapy include muscle imbalances and weakness of the intrinsic or extrinsic muscle groups of the foot and ankle. Several common muscle groups implicated in the mechanism producing pes cavus are:

1. Weakness of the dorsiflexors of the foot and ankle (anterior tibialis and extensor digitorum muscles), resulting in dropping of the forefoot, which causes contracture of the plantar fascia and shortening of the gastrocnemius and soleus muscle groups.[87,90,92]
2. Unopposed activity of the supinators of the foot, producing a plantar flexed, adducted, and inverted foot position that allows rapid contracture of the plantar fasciae.[87,90] Weakness of the peroneal muscles produces overactivity of the posterior tibialis and anterior tibialis, the antagonist muscle groups.

3. Overactivity of the peroneus longus muscle, producing plantar flexion of the first ray and forefoot pronation. The fixed plantar flexion of the first ray must be compensated by subtalar joint supination or inversion of the calcaneus.[6,34,90,97]

4. Overactivity of the abductor hallucis, flexor digitorum brevis, flexor hallucis brevis, and quadratus plantae has been described as a deforming factor in pes cavus. Garceau and Brahms[91] denervated these muscle groups in 47 cases of pes cavus. Their goal was to stop the progressive increase of pes cavus. The results demonstrated improvement in foot balance, performance, and stability, reducing the pes cavus deformity.

5. Weakness of the gastrocnemius-soleus muscle group, producing a dorsiflexed calcaneus. This weakness may produce a calcaneocavus deformity.[86,87,90] Brockway[95] reports an elongation of the Achilles tendon, with no evidence of weakness in the calcaneocavus deformities.

Contractures of the skin, subtarsal ligaments, and plantar fascia are common in the pes cavus foot.[90,93] The plantar fascia is a strong support to the longitudinal arch and is designed to prevent excessive calcaneal eversion (valgus).[44,90] The deforming force of the plantar fascia (inversion of the calcaneus) is resisted by the Achilles tendon. Once the calcaneus moves into inversion secondary to supination of the subtalar joint, the Achilles tendon becomes an active supinator of the subtalar joint and perpetuates the deformity.[90]

Congenital Talipes Equinovarus (Clubfoot)

Congenital talipes equinovarus is usually a rigid deformity.[5] The clubfoot deformity does not resemble a typical pes cavus foot, although it has several similar characteristics. Three distinctive clinical observations in clubfoot are inversion (varus) of the hindfoot (heel), inversion and adduction of the forefoot, and equinus of the ankle and subtalar joint.[6] The varus heel position and the equinus (plantar flexed) ankle are also found with the pes cavus foot type. As previously noted, Tachdjian[5] reports pes equinocavus secondary to talipes equinovarus.

The exact cause of the clubfoot deformity is unknown. Genetic factors have been implicated by several studies.[5,99–102] Palmar[100] examined four possible inheritance factors: sex-linked, autosomal recessive, multiple gene inheritance, and autosomal dominant. Palmar[100] determined that if there was a family history of the talipes equinovarus deformity, a 10% chance of a recurrence existed.

In addition to the genetic factors, environmental factors may be operational.[5,103] The mechanical theory, or environmental factor, was first advanced by Hippocrates, who proposed that the fetal foot was malpositioned in the uterus and that the equinovarus posture was produced by external forces. As a result of rapid growth in malposition, the ligaments and muscles developed adaptive shortening, and the tarsal bones, especially the talus, responded by changing contour, producing articular malalignment.[5] More recently, a popular explanation for clubfoot involves pressure of the uterine wall increased by the fetus' kicking against it.[103]

The third causal factor in talipes equinovarus is neuromuscular dysfunction—peroneal nerve lesions, peroneal dysplasia, arthrogryposis, or myelomeningocele.[5,103,104]

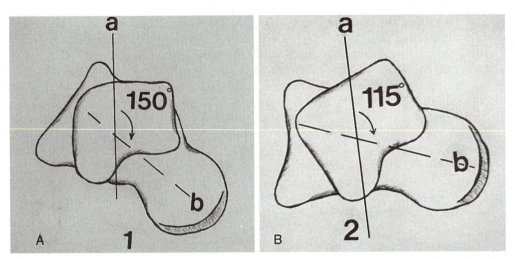

FIGURE 2–29. (1) Long axis of the body of talus, with normal declination angle of the talus from 150° to 160°. (2) Long axis of the head and neck of the talus, with abnormal declination angle of the talus from 115° to 135°. Reduction of the declination angle of the talus is present in the clubfoot deformity.

BONY DEFORMITIES

The talus is the principal bone affected in talipes equinovarus. The anterior end of the talus is medial, and there is plantar deviation.[5,103–108] The long axis of the head and neck of the talus forms an angle with the long axis of the body, called the "declination angle" of the talus.[5] The normal angle in the adult is 150° to 160°. In talipes equinovarus, the angle is decreased from 135° to 115°, representing medial and plantar deviation of the head and neck of the talus.[5] Figure 2–29 demonstrates a normal adult declination angle and an abnormal angle characteristic of a clubfoot deformity. The navicular is displaced mediad and plantad, articulating with the medial aspect of the head and neck of the talus. In severe cases, the navicular bone articulates with the medial malleolus of the tibia.[5]

The contour of the calcaneus is normal. To maintain its articulation with the talus, it must rotate on its long axis inward and downward beneath the talus.[5] The calcaneocuboid articulation is anterior, medial, and plantar deviated, further accentuating the varus deformity.

Soft tissue changes occur as a result of the bone malalignment. The ligaments, capsules, muscles, tendons, tendon sheaths, vessels, and skin are shortened on the medial and posterior aspects of the foot.[5]

SOFT TISSUE DEFORMITIES

Fukuhara et al[109] reported in a study of 16 clubfoot deformities that the talar deformity was not the primary lesion. Histologic and immunohistochemical findings indicated that the cells and collagen fibers of the medial ankle ligaments of clubfeet appeared to be contracted and spatially disoriented. Before the third trimester of gestation, myofibroblastlike cells seemed to create a disorder of the ligaments resembling fibromatosis. Therefore, the ligamentous contracture resulted in a typical clubfoot deformity.[109]

Several studies have demonstrated gross morphologic changes in muscle tissue in congenital idiopathic clubfoot.[110-113] The muscles studied included the triceps surae, the peroneal muscles, and the abductor hallucis muscle. Type I muscle fibers showed an increase in all the muscle groups of the clubfoot deformity. Furthermore, fatty degeneration with fibrosis was observed and postulated to be a consequence of immobilization. Kranicz et al[110] believe that neuromuscular atrophy is a primary cause of congenital clubfoot.

CONSERVATIVE TREATMENT OF CLUBFOOT DEFORMITIES

Physical therapy was used to treat 338 cases of clubfoot deformity. The techniques were based on progressive sequential manipulations at birth. Reduction of the varus and later the equinus component of the clubfoot deformity was performed. Gentle stretching was complemented by active stimulation of the muscles, followed by a simple splint to fix the realignment. Surgery was used in resistant cases. When used alone, the physical therapy techniques achieved 77% good and fair results.[114]

Yamamoto and Furuya[115] treated 91 congenital clubfeet in 59 children using a modified Denis Browne splint over a 6-year period. The children's ages ranged from 4 weeks to 9 months. Operation was later required in 31 feet in 20 children. The other 60 feet in 39 children had excellent or good function. Radiographic assessment indicated that the equinus, adduction, varus, and cavus deformities had all been corrected.[115]

SUMMARY

Pes cavus is a rigid deformity. It may include several combinations of deformities, such as equinus, varus, adductus, and calcaneus (Table 2–2). Pes cavus can be the result of neurologic disease, muscle imbalance, or contracture of soft tissues.

The biomechanics of the foot in pes cavus are the reverse of those in pes planus. The abnormally supinated foot does not act as an effective shock absorber. The rearfoot is prone to instabilities, secondary to compensatory supination of the subtalar

---

TABLE 2–2 Abnormal Supination

I. Pes cavus

    A. Anterior cavus
    B. Posterior cavus
    C. Global

II. Combined pes cavus deformities

    A. Pes cavovarus-forefoot valgus-rigid plantar flexed first ray
    B. Calcaneocavus
    C. Pes equinocavus

III. Congenital talipes equinovarus (clubfoot)

---

joint, as noted in pes cavovarus or forefoot valgus deformities. A varus heel can be a primary deformity, as described in talipes equinovarus. The primary calcaneal varus deformity can produce ankle instability and precipitate plantar flexion of the first ray or forefoot valgus.

CONCLUSION

The foot is an important link in the lower kinetic chain. Abnormal pronation (flat-foot) and abnormal supination (high-arched foot, pes cavus) may produce alterations in the arthrokinematics of the foot and ankle.

Congenital abnormal pronation includes deformities present at birth that produce severe alteration between the talus, calcaneus, navicular, and cuboid articulations. Convex pes valgus, tarsal coalitions, and talipes calcaneovalgus are the most common. Abnormal pronation, however, is usually an acquired deformity resulting from an attempt to compensate for deformities intrinsic or extrinsic to the foot and ankle. Foot deformities are described in relationship to the body planes. The most common frontal plane deformities resulting in compensatory abnormal pronation are forefoot varus, rearfoot varus, and metatarsus varus. The most common sagittal plane deformity causing abnormal pronation is ankle equinus. The transverse plane deformities resulting in compensatory pronation include rotational deformities of the lower extremity and metatarsus adductus.

Abnormal supination is usually a rigid deformity in which the foot lacks shock absorption capabilities. Pes cavus, plantar flexion of the forefoot on the rearfoot, may be combined with other deformities, such as varus and adductus. Pes cavovarus, hypomobile plantar flexion of the first ray, and forefoot valgus are terms that describe a combined deformity of pes cavus that involves plantar flexion and hypomobility of the first ray (sagittal plane deformity) and compensatory rearfoot varus (frontal plane deformity). Although a hypermobile plantar flexed first ray is described as forefoot valgus, it is usually an attempt to compensate for forefoot varus. Calcaneocavus and pes equinocavus are also combined pes cavus deformities. Calcaneocavus is pes cavus with a dorsiflexed calcaneus. Pes equinocavus describes a plantar flexed calcaneus and ankle joint. Both deformities are combined with plantar flexion of the forefoot.

The causes of pes cavus that lend themselves to physical therapy are muscle imbalance and soft tissue contractures. The muscle hyperactivity usually results from neurologic disorders, which may be present at birth or may develop as the child matures.

Abnormal foot and ankle mechanics resulting from abnormal pronation or supination deformities may cause increased weight-bearing forces throughout the lower kinetic chain. The inability to attenuate the increased stress may result in soft tissue breakdown and damage.

GLOSSARY

Positions of the Foot
Abductus: Abducted position or a fixed deformity in the transverse plane.
Adductus: Adducted position or a fixed deformity in the transverse plane.
Calcaneus: Dorsiflexed position or a fixed deformity in the sagittal plane.

Equinus: Plantar flexed position or a fixed deformity in the sagittal plane.
Valgus: Everted position or a fixed deformity in the frontal plane.
Varus: Inverted position or a fixed deformity in the frontal plane.

Deformities of the Foot

Ankle joint equinus: Limited dorsiflexion of the ankle joint with subtalar joint in neutral position.
Calcaneocavus: Dorsiflexed position of the os calcis.
Convex pes valgus: Congenital vertical talus, or rocker bottom foot.
Forefoot valgus: Eversion of the forefoot on the rearfoot with subtalar joint in neutral position.
Forefoot varus: Inversion of the forefoot on the rearfoot with subtalar joint in neutral position.
Hallux abductovalgus: Subluxation in the transverse plane of the first metatarsophalangeal joint.
Hallux limitus: Subluxation of the first metatarsophalangeal joint in the sagittal plane.
Hallux rigidus: The latter stage of hallux limitus, leading to ankylosis of the first metatarsophalangeal joint.
Metatarsus adductovarus: Adduction and inversion of the forefoot.
Metatarsus adductus: Adduction of the forefoot.
Metatarsus varus: Inversion of the forefoot.
Pes cavovarus: Plantar flexion of the first ray, or medial column.
Pes cavus: Plantar flexion of the forefoot on the rearfoot.
Pes equinocavus: Plantar flexion of the forefoot, rearfoot, and ankle joint.
Tailor's bunion: Subluxation in the transverse plane of the fifth metatarsophalangeal joint with the toe in varus position.
Talipes calcaneovalgus: Congenital flatfoot—dorsiflexion and eversion of hindfoot.
Talipes equinovarus: Clubfoot—inversion and plantar flexion of hindfoot and adduction of forefoot.
Tarsal coalition: Congenital union between two or more tarsal bones.

REFERENCES

1. Rose, GK: Correction of the pronated foot. J Bone Joint Surg 44B:642, 1982.
2. Lelievre, J: Current concepts and correction in the valgus foot. Clin Orthop 70:43, 1970.
3. Evans, D, et al: Calcaneo-valgus deformity. J Bone Joint Surg 57B:270, 1975.
4. Purnell, ML, et al: Congenital dislocation of the peroneal tendous in calcaneovalgus foot. J Bone Joint Surg 65B:316, 1983.
5. Tachdjian, MO: The Child's Foot. WB Saunders, Philadelphia, 1985.
6. McCrea, JD: Pediatric Orthopaedics of the Lower Extremity. Futura Publishing, New York, 1985.
7. Thomas, CL (ed): Taber's Cyclopedic Medical Dictionary, ed 16. FA Davis, Philadelphia, 1989.
8. Drennan, JC, et al: The pathological anatomy of convex pes valgus. J Bone Joint Surg 53B:445, 1971.
9. Herdon, CH and Heyman, CH: Problems in the recognition and treatment of congenital convex pes valgus. J Bone Joint Surg 45A:413, 1963.
10. Coleman, SS, et al: Pathomechanics and treatment of congenital vertical talus. Clin Orthop 70:62, 1970.
11. Broughton, NS, Graham, G, and Memelaus, MB: The high incidence of foot deformity in patients with high-level spina bifida. J Bone Joint Surg 76B:548, 1994.
12. DeRosa, PG: Congenital vertical talus: The Riley experience. Foot Ankle 5:118, 1984.
13. Jayakumar, S and Cowell, HR: Rigid flatfoot. Clin Orthop 122:77, 1977.
14. Stormont, DM and Peterson, HA: The relative incidence of tarsal coalition. Clin Orthop 181:24, 1983.
15. Cowell, HR and Elener, V: Rigid painful flatfoot secondary to tarsal coalition. Clin Orthop 177:54, 1983.

16. Jahss, MH: Disorders of the Foot, Vol 1. WB Saunders, Philadelphia, 1982.
17. Turek, SL: Orthopaedics: Principles and Their Application. JB Lippincott, Philadelphia, 1977.
18. Herzenberg, JE, et al: Computerized tomography of talocalcaneal tarsal coalition: A clinical and anatomic study. Foot Ankle 6:273, 1986.
19. Spero, CR, Simon, GS, and Tornetta, P: Clubfeet and tarsal coalition. J Pediatr Orthop 14:372, 1994.
20. Boyd, HB: Congenital talonavicular synostosis. J Bone Joint Surg 26A:682, 1944.
21. Challis, J: Hereditary transmission of talonavicular coalition in association with anomaly of the little finger. J Bone Joint Surg 56A:1273, 1974.
22. Kite, JH: Congenital metatarsus varus. J Bone Joint Surg 332A:500, 1950.
23. Kite, JH: Congenital metatarsus varus. J Bone Joint Surg 49A:388, 1967.
24. Heyman, CH, et al: Mobilization of the tarsometatarsal and intermetatarsal joints for the correction of resistance adduction of the forepart of the foot in congenital clubfoot or congenital metatarsus varus. J Bone Joint Surg 40A:299, 1958.
25. Giannestras, NJ: Recognition and treatment of flatfeet in infancy. Clin Orthop 70:10, 1970.
26. Ferciot, CF: Calcaneovalgus foot in the newborn and its relation to developmental flatfoot. Clin Orthop 1:22, 1953.
27. Kolker, LD: A biomechanical analysis of flatfoot surgery. J Am Podiatr Med Assoc 63:217, 1973.
28. Bleck, EE and Berzins, UJ: Conservative management of pes valgus with plantar flexed talus flexible. Clin Orthop 122:85, 1977.
29. Barry, RJ and Scranton, PC: Flat feet in children. Clin Orthop 181:68, 1983.
30. Rosegger, H and Steinwendner, G: Transverse fetal position syndrome—a combination of congenital skeletal deformities in the newborn infant. Pediatr Pathol 27:125, 1992.
31. McCarthy, DJ: The developmental anatomy of pes valgo planus. Clin Podiatr Med Surg 6:491, 1989.
32. Davids, JR, Hagerman, RJ, and Eilert, RE: Orthopaedic aspects of fragile-X syndrome. J Bone Joint Surg 72A:889, 1990.
33. Rao, UB and Joseph, B: The influence of footwear on the prevalence of flatfeet. A survey of 2300 children. J Bone Joint Surg 75B:525, 1992.
34. Root, ML, Orien, WP, and Weed, JN: Clinical Biomechanics, Vol 2, Normal and Abnormal Function of the Foot. Clinical Biomechanics, Los Angeles, 1977.
35. Mereday, C, Dolan, C, and Lusskin, R: Evaluation of the University of California Biomechanics Laboratory shoe insert in "flexible" pes planus. Clin Orthop 82:45, 1972.
36. Gould, N: Evaluation of hyperpronation and pes planus in adults. Clin Orthop 181:37, 1983.
37. Johnson, KA: Tibial posterior tendon rupture. Clin Orthop 177:140, 1983.
38. Funk, DA, Cass, JC, and Johnson, JA: Acquired adult flatfoot secondary to posterior tibial-tendon pathology. J Bone Joint Surg 68A:95, 1986.
39. Coakley, FV, Samanta, DB, and Finlay, DB: Ultrasonography of the tibialis posterior tendon in rheumatoid arthritis. Br J Rheumatol 33:273, 1994.
40. Karasick, D and Schweitzer, ME: Tear of the posterior tibial tendon causing asymmetric flatfoot: Radiologic findings. AJR Am J Roentgenol 163:1237, 1993.
41. Woods, L and Leach, RE: Posterior tibial tendon rupture in athletic people. Am J Sports Med 19:495, 1991.
42. Mueller, TJ: Acquired flatfoot secondary to tibialis posterior dysfunction: Biomechanical aspects. J Foot Surg 30:2, 1991.
43. Basmajian, JV and Stecko, O: The role of muscles in arch support of the foot: An electromyographic study. J Bone Joint Surg 45A:1184, 1963.
44. Hicks, JH: The mechanics of the foot. II. The plantar aponeurosis. J Anat 88:25, 1954.
45. Hicks, JH: The mechanics of the foot. IV. The action of muscles on the foot in standing. Acta Anat 27:180, 1955.
46. Jones, BS: Flatfoot: A preliminary report of an operation for severe cases. J Bone Joint Surg 57B:279, 1975.
47. Harris, RL and Beath, T: Hypermobile flatfoot with short tendo Achilles. J Bone Joint Surg 30A:116, 1948.
48. Inman, VT, Rolston, HJ, and Todd, F: Human Walking. Williams & Wilkins, Baltimore, 1981.
49. Green, RD: Planal dominance. J Am Podiatr Med Assoc 74:98, 1984.
50. Bordelon, RL: Hypermobile flatfoot in children: Comprehension, evaluation, and treatment. Clin Orthop 181:7, 1983.
51. Duckworth, T: The hindfoot and its relation to rotational deformities of the forefoot. Clin Orthop 177:39, 1983.
52. Taunton, JE, et al: A triplanar electrogoniometer investigation of running mechanics in runners with compensatory overpronation. Can J Appl Sports Sci 10:104, 1985.
53. Perkins, G: Pes planus or instability of the longitudinal arch. Proc Roy Soc Med 41:31, 1847.
54. Hughes, LY: Biomechanical analysis of the foot and ankle for predisposition to developing stress fractures. J Orthop Sports Phys Ther 7:96, 1985.
55. Vetter, LW, et al: Aerobic dance injuries. Phys Sports Med 13:114, 1985.
56. Michael, R and Holder, L: The soleus syndrome: A cause of medial tibial stress (shin splints). Am J Sports Med 13:87, 1985.

57. DiGiovanni, JE and Smith, SD: Normal biomechanics of the adult rearfoot. J Am Podiatr Med Assoc 66:812, 1976.
58. Phillips, RD and Phillips, RL: Quantitative analysis of the locking position of the midtarsal joint. J Am Podiatr Med Assoc 73:518, 1983.
59. Subotnick, S: Biomechanics of the subtalar and midtarsal joints. J Am Podiatr Med Assoc 49:756, 1975.
60. Subotnick, SI: Equinus deformity as it affects the forefoot. J Am Podiatr Med Assoc 61:423, 1971.
61. Melilla, TV: Gastrocnemius equinus: Its diagnosis and treatment. Arch Podiatr Med Foot Surg 2:159, 1975.
62. Anopol, G: Mechanics in weak and flat feet. Am J Surg 7:256, 1929.
63. Bordelon, LR: Hypermobile flatfoot in children. Clin Orthop 181:7, 1981.
64. Sgarlato, TE: Compendium of Podiatric Biomechanics. California College of Podiatric Medicine, San Francisco, 1971.
65. Sarrafian, SK: Anatomy of the Foot and Ankle: Descriptive, Topographic, Functional. JB Lippincott, Philadelphia, 1983.
66. Staehli, LT: Rotational problems of the lower extremities. Orthop Clin North Am 18:503, 1987.
67. Knight, RA: Developmental deformities of the lower extremities. J Bone Joint Surg 36A:521, 1954.
68. Bleck, EE: Developmental orthopaedics III: Toddlers. Dev Med Child Neurol 24:533, 1982.
69. Mittleman, G: Transverse plane abnormalities of the lower extremities: Intoe and outtoe gait. J Am Podiatr Med Assoc 61:1, 1971.
70. James, SL: Chondromalacia of the patella in the adolescent. In Kennedy (ed): The Injured Adolescent Knee. Williams & Wilkins, Baltimore, 1979.
71. Hutter, CG and Scott, W: Tibial torsion. J Bone Joint Surg 31A:511, 1949.
72. Botte, RR: An interpretation of the pronation syndrome and foot types of patients with low back pain. J Am Podiatr Med Assoc 72:595, 1982.
73. Okun, SJ, Morgan, JW, and Burns, MJ: Limb length discrepancy: A new method of measurement and its clinical significance. J Am Podiatr Med Assoc 72:595, 1982.
74. Blustein, SM and D'Amico, JC: Leg length discrepancy: Identification, clinical signs, and management. J Am Podiatr Assoc 75:200, 1985.
75. Beal, MC: The short leg problem. J Am Osteopath Assoc 76:745, 1977.
76. Subotnick, S: Case history of unilateral short leg with athletic overuse injury. J Am Podiatr Med Assoc 70:255, 1980.
77. Anderson, AFA and Fowler, SB: Anterior calcaneal osteotomy for symptomatic juvenile pes planus. Foot Ankle 4:274, 1984.
78. Jones, RA: Discussion of the treatment of pes cavus, section orthopaedics. Proc Roy Soc Med 20:1126, 1927.
79. Steindler, A: The treatment of pes cavus (hollow claw foot). Arch Surg 11:325, 1921.
80. Samilson, RL and Dillin, W: Cavus, cavovarus, calcaneocavus: An update. Clin Orthop 177:133, 1983.
81. McGlamry, DE and Kitting, RW: Equinus foot, an analysis of the etiology, pathology, and treatment techniques. J Am Podiatr Med Assoc 63:165, 1973.
82. Root, ML, Orien, WP, and Weed, JH: Biomechanical Examination of the Foot, Vol 1. Clinical Biomechanics, Los Angeles, 1971.
83. Bossely, CL and Cairney, PC: The intermetatarsophalangeal bursa: Its significance in Morton's metatarsalgia. J Bone Joint Surg 62A:184, 1980.
84. Schoenhaus, HD and Jay, RM: Cavus deformities: Conservative management. J Am Podiatr Med Assoc 70:235, 1980.
85. Green, DR, Sgarlato, TE, and Wittenburg, M: Clinical biomechanical evaluation of the foot. J Am Podiatr Med Assoc 65:732, 1975.
86. Bradley, GW and Coleman, SS: Treatment of the calcaneocavus foot deformity. J Bone Joint Surg 63A:1159, 1981.
87. Brewerton, DA, Sandifer, PH, and Sweetnam, DR: "Idiopathic" pes cavus. Br Med J 2:659, 1963.
88. Todd, AH: Treatment of pes cavus. Proc Roy Soc Med 28:117, 1934.
89. Cole, WH: The treatment of claw-foot. J Bone Joint Surg 22:895, 1940.
90. Dwyer, FC: The present status of the problem of pes cavus. Clin Orthop 106:254, 1975.
91. Garceau, GJ and Brahms, MA: A preliminary study of selective plantarmuscle denervation for pes cavus. J Bone Joint Surg 38A:553, 1956.
92. Hughes, KW: Talipes cavus. Br Med J 2:902, 1940.
93. Rugh, TJ: The plantar fascia: Study of its anatomy and of its pathology in talipes cavus: New operation for its correction. Am J Surg 2:307, 1927.
94. Barenfield, PA, Wedely, MS, and Shea, JM: The congenital cavus foot. Clin Orthop 79:119, 1971.
95. Brockway, A: Surgical correction of talipes cavus deformities. J Bone Joint Surg 22:81, 1940.
96. Jahss, MH: Evaluation of the cavus foot for orthopedic treatment. Clin Orthop 181:52, 1983.
97. Tyan, MC, et al: Investigation of muscle imbalance in the leg in symptomatic forefoot pes cavus: A multidisciplinary study. Foot Ankle 13:489, 1992.
98. Price, AC, et al: Computed tomographic analysis of pes cavus. J Pediatr Orthop 13:646, 1993.
99. Preston, ET and Fell, WT: Congenital idiopathic clubfoot. Clin Orthop 122:102, 1977.

100. Palmar, RM: The genetics of talipes equinovarus. J Bone Joint Surg 46A:542, 1964.
101. Finley, WH, et al: Birth defects surveillance: Jefferson County, Alabama, and Uppsala County, Sweden. South Med J 87:440, 1994.
102. Rebbeck, TR, et al: A single-gene explanation for the probability of having idiopathic talipes equinovarus. Am J Hum Genet 53:1051, 1993.
103. Irani, RN and Sherman, MS: The pathological anatomy of clubfoot. J Bone Joint Surg 45A:45, 1963.
104. Kaplan, EB: Comparative anatomy of the talus in relation to idiopathic clubfoot. Clin Orthop 85:32, 1972.
105. Ponseti, IV and Smoley, EN: Congenital club foot: The results of treatment. J Bone Joint Surg 45A:261, 1963.
106. Ghali, NN, et al: The results of plantar reduction in the management of congenital talipes equinovarus. J Bone Joint Surg 65A:1, 1983.
107. Lovell, WW and Hancock, CI: Treatment of congenital talipes equinovarus. Clin Orthop 70:79, 1970.
108. Kite, JH: Conservative treatment of the resistant recurrent clubfoot. Clin Orthop 70:93, 1970.
109. Fukuhara, K, Schollmeier, G, and Uhthoff, HK: The pathogenesis of club foot. A histomorphometric and immunohistochemical study of fetuses. J Bone Joint Surg 76B:450, 1994.
110. Kranicz, J, Trombitas, K, and Szabo, G: Results of ultrastructural analysis of the calf muscles in clubfoot. Orthopedics 14:73, 1991.
111. Sirca, A, Erzen, I, and Pecak, F: Histochemistry of abductor hallucis muscle in children with idiopathic clubfoot and in controls. J Pediatr Orthop 10:477, 1990.
112. Maffulli, N, et al: Histochemistry of the triceps surae muscle in idiopathic congenital clubfoot. Foot Ankle 13:80, 1992.
113. Gosztonyi, G, et al: Morphometric study of muscle in congenital idiopathic clubfoot. Pathol Res Pract 185:790, 1989.
114. Bensahel, H, et al: Results of physical therapy for idiopathic clubfoot: A long-term follow-up study. J Pediatr Orthop 10:189, 1990.
115. Yamamoto, H and Furuya, K: Treatment of congenital club foot with a modified Denis Browne splint. J Bone Joint Surg 72B:460, 1990.

CHAPTER 3

Normal Development of Gait

Deborah Corradi-Scalise, MA, PT
Wen Ling, PhD, PT

Independent ambulation is the highest form of human locomotion. Clinicians are constantly evaluating both the potential for and the quality of ambulation. To evaluate and treat pathologic gait patterns, it is first necessary to understand the normal development of gait and its components.

Walking (or normal gait) is not an independent occurrence. Rather, it is the ultimate product of a series of developmental changes that begin at birth. Because a typical adult walking pattern does not become evident until age 7,[1–3] one cannot expect the usual components of adult walking to be clinically present before that age. Therefore, descriptions of the gait characteristics of normal children at various ages are presented here as a basis for the effective treatment of children in similar age groups with pathologic gait patterns (Figs. 3–1 to 3–3).

Typically, independent standing occurs at 9.5 months, and at about 13 months,[4] the child is able to use independent walking as a primary means of locomotion. The gait pattern used is an immature (or toddler) form of walking. Initially the toddler maintains a wide base of support, excessive hip and knee flexion as seen during wide-range stepping movements, ankle joint pronation, toe curling, and upper extremity abduction with elbow flexion.[2,5] Progression is in a waddling manner, shifting the weight from side to side, rather than stepping forward. Within several months, maturational changes have already begun to take place. The child now ambulates with a more narrow base of support, better balance, and forward progression using a rhythmic heel-toe pattern with reciprocal arm swing. A mature form of walking eventually develops. The attainment of independent ambulation by the child is the culmination of many complex musculoskeletal and neurophysiologic maturational changes that have been occurring since the neonatal period.

Internal factors that affect maturation of the central nervous system include the completion of central nervous system myelinization and the rapid rate of body and

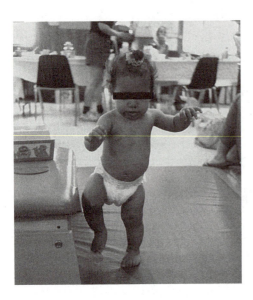

FIGURE 3–1. Toddler gait of a typical 11-month-old child. Child began independent ambulation 2 weeks prior to photograph.

brain growth during the first 3 years. The musculoskeletal system undergoes dramatic changes during the first year of life. The reflexive neonate transforms into a purposeful, independent walker within a 13- to 15-month period.[4] Muscular control develops in a cephalocaudal, proximodistal direction. Many other factors influence the development of a mature gait, including sensation, perception, motivation, and proprioception. As the neuromuscular and musculoskeletal systems develop, motor changes occur in response to environmental needs. The change and variability within the environment require adaptation (and, therefore, maturation) of the human sys-

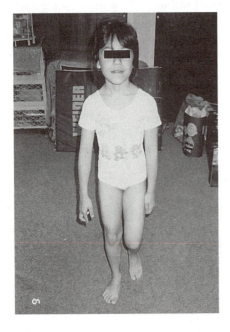

FIGURE 3–2. Mature gait of a typical 8-year-old child.

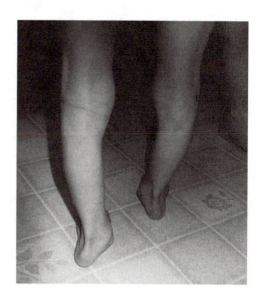

FIGURE 3–3. Pathologic gait pattern of a 4-year-old child with cerebral palsy.

tem. The series of events that change the immature form of walking to the rhythmic heel-toe progression of the adult depend primarily on three developmental processes within the child: the changes that reflect central nervous system maturation, the progression of motor learning, and the increase in physical growth and control of the musculoskeletal apparatus.

COMPONENTS OF GAIT DEVELOPMENT

Neurophysiologic Component

During the first 15 months of life, many changes take place in the nervous and musculoskeletal systems that allow for purposeful, independent walking. These systems develop concurrently and are responsible for the development of a mature gait pattern by the age of 7 years.[1–3]

As postulated by Bobath,[6] the maturation of the central nervous system is a reflection of the integration of primitive reflexes by higher cortical structures. At birth, the neonate displays a host of reflexive movements in response to sensory stimuli. The reflexes directly related to standing and walking are the neonatal placing response of the lower extremity, the positive supporting reflex, and the spontaneous stepping reflex. Movement is therefore said to be a sensorimotor experience. These three reflexes serve as the motor pattern for standing and walking but are modified by the hierarchical control of the central nervous system. The modification of primitive reflexes occurs via the development of the righting and equilibrium reactions.

It is postulated that supraspinal centers inhibit the spinal circuitry of reflexive activities allowing for the adult plantigrade features of heel strike, knee flexion during stance, asynchronous joint movements, and specific precise patterns of muscle activation not identified in either initial independent ambulation or infant stepping.[7]

The righting reactions allow humans to stand erect. They are responsible for maintaining the head and trunk in proper spatial alignment in relation to the ground, with the eyes horizontal. Their major function is to overcome the effects of gravity by moving and stabilizing body parts toward the upright position. Righting reactions are what drive the infant to move and eventually to maintain an upright posture.[8] The delayed achievement of independent standing and walking in the blind child is a direct result of absence of the optical righting reaction. As reported by Adelson and Fraiberg,[9] the achievement of gross motor milestones by blind infants was delayed beyond the normal range. They state that blindness has less of an impact on postural achievements than it does on mobility achievements. The average age for standing alone is 11 months for a blind child as compared with 9.5 months for a sighted child.[4] The average age for independent ambulation is 19.25 months for a blind child compared with 13 months for a sighted child.[4]

The equilibrium reactions, in addition, serve to keep the body's center of gravity balanced within the base of support. In children, during initial independent standing and walking, the base of support is wide. Biomechanically, this allows for stability where muscular and neuromuscular control is lacking. As the body compensates for inefficient muscle activity, the body also increases its energy consumption. As the equilibrium system of the child matures, the walking base narrows, and upright balance is preserved. Functional ambulation can be viewed as the body's ability to maintain an upright position and to respond to a series of rises and drops in the center of gravity by utilization of the righting and equilibrium reactions.[10] The precise use of the righting and equilibrium reaction to catch and balance the center of gravity during forward progression allows a minimum expenditure of energy and therefore an efficient, mature walking pattern.

Children with cerebral palsy display a less than mature gait pattern, owing to disturbances in righting and equilibrium, and inadequate influence by higher brain centers. Leonard et al[7] studied the gait patterns of normal infants and infants with cerebral palsy during treadmill ambulation. Electromyographic and kinematic data were collected. Their results stated that the locomotor characteristics of the infants with cerebral palsy were similar to normal infants during reflexive supported stepping. With maturation, the infants with cerebral palsy retained the synchronous muscle activity, excessive muscle cocontraction and persistence of reflexive foot activity. The lack of inhibitory modulation by supraspinal segments may account for the persistence of primitive reflexive behaviors seen in cerebral palsy.

Without central nervous system dysfunction, the ankle-foot complex naturally responds to a posterior displacement of the center of gravity with ankle dorsiflexion and toe extension. A lateral displacement of the center of gravity elicits ankle inversion. Typically the foot of a child with cerebral palsy serves as a stable, fixed support but is inefficient for balancing.[11] Gunsolus et al[11] evaluated the dynamic foot responses of 50 children, 20 normal subjects and 30 subjects with cerebral palsy. In the normal group, they found that some beginning walkers used toe clawing in response to posterior displacement, but that more than half used medial arch reactions. Advanced walkers demonstrated mature dynamic foot responses. The children with cerebral palsy were more similar to the normal, beginning walkers, as none of the subjects used dorsiflexion during posterior displacement. Additionally, however, none of the dysfunctional subjects used medial arch reactions in response to a lateral displacement. These findings demonstrate the need for efficient equilibrium reactions for the development of mature standing and walking to occur.

Motor Learning Component

Righting reactions allow humans to stand upright, and equilibrium reactions maintain balance and control in the upright posture of bipeds. The initiation of gait can be attributed to the central nervous system's generation of a motor program. Motor programs are "stored sets of motor commands both innate and learned that are synthesized into a desired movement."[12] Of the many theories on motor control, two help to explain the initiation of movement: the closed-loop theory and the open-loop theory of motor control.

The closed-loop theory of motor control is based on the system's ability to learn and perform skilled movements via peripheral feedback. The sensorimotor feedback loop is responsible for modifications or adaptations of the motor program. Stelmach[13] states that this theory is supported by the research of Mott and Sherrington. The researchers completely eliminated afferent pathways to the limbs of monkeys in an attempt to examine the role of sensation in movement. The destruction of the afferent pathways produced a limb that was essentially paralyzed. Functional grasp was lost, which thus emphasizes the importance of an intact sensory system for movement.

The open-loop theory emphasizes a central control mechanism that continuously monitors the peripheral feedback and determines both the spatial and the temporal components of a movement. When a desired performance is achieved, an internal model is established, probably in the neocerebellum, and the feedforward mechanism becomes the dominating force in performing the movement; however, when new stimuli are encountered (e.g., performing the movement in a novel environment, such as walking on uneven terrain), both feedback and feedforward mechanisms are important components in performing the movement.[13] Initially a change in motor control occurs via a response to peripheral feedback; however, "once the peripheral mechanisms are adjusted for, and stored, the system may allow for adjustments in advance of the movement by incorporating the peripheral effects into the motor plan. The central nervous system can then act to correct errors even before they become expressed through the motor act."[14] This allows for the automation seen in a mature walking pattern. Feedback control is the body's response to make postural adjustment to perturbations of the center of gravity, whereas feedforward control involves anticipatory behavior of consequence of postural instability and avoids or accommodates for the instability by voluntary movement.[15]

In physical therapy, after central nervous system insult with subsequent disruption of the ability to walk, the goal of treatment is functional ambulation. Various physical therapy activities and exercises are used to regain motor control, including gait training in health care facilities. These indoor activities are insufficient to allow the individual to regain functional ambulation. Practice for walking should include real-world environments, such as a crowded city street, supermarket, or train station. Owing to the variability between environments, problem solving must occur to develop the appropriate motor programs necessary for successful and efficient walking within different settings. Motor learning occurs in response to a specific need or desire for a skill. Peripheral feedback is necessary, and ongoing problem solving and adjustment must be made to adapt to the variability of each task within different environments. Only with repetition can the variability in the environment be anticipated and feedforward control be developed. It is only by repetition in a variable and functional environment (streets, escalators, train stations) that we can hope to enable patients to problem solve (and thus modify) the motor program to adapt to variable situations and to function independently. In normal development, feedback control develops before the system's ability to use feedforward control.[15]

Brooks[16] has described the neurobehavioral analysis of motor skill learning by stating that intended motor acts are based on perceptions of what is to be done at a particular time, based on sensory information both past and present. The environmental demands placed on the individual motivate the motor act, but it is the combination of cognitive abilities that guides and executes the musculoskeletal system's response. This theory may explain, in part, why children and adults with mental retardation but without primary physical disabilities tend to be awkward or clumsy and tend to display a less than normal pattern of ambulation. Although motor acts (such as walking) are attempted, the cognitive portion of the brain that drives the musculoskeletal system may not be able to acknowledge the most efficient movement pattern for the task. Less than optimal balance in walking is seen owing to the inability to activate an efficient motor program.

Biomechanical Component

Initially the acquisition of independent standing and walking is characterized by inefficient, exaggerated postures and positions that provide stability within the system. "The neural structures that act to control movement must be adapted to the constraints imposed by the structure of the musculoskeletal system (flexibility of muscles) and the physical laws governing movement (gravity, friction)."[17] Therefore, owing to the biomechanical alignment of the infant's lower extremities (anterior pelvic tilt, hip flexion, abduction, and external rotation) and to the structure of the infant's body (short legs, high center of gravity), initial ambulation occurs in a "staccato" manner. The motor program is working within the constraints of the physical structure of the toddler (Fig. 3–4). To ambulate at all, the motor program must adapt to the physical structure of the child.

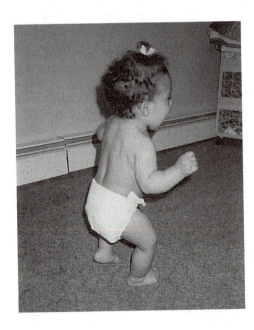

FIGURE 3–4. Sagittal alignment characteristics of a toddler. Note arm posturing, anterior pelvic tilt, wide base of support, and ankle plantarflexion at toe strike.

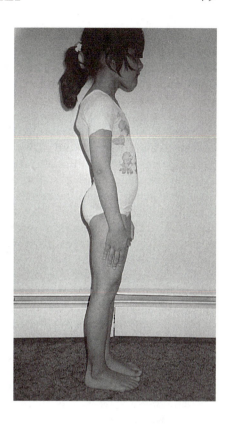

FIGURE 3–5. Typical standing alignment of an 8-year-old child, sagittal view.

As the child's physical structure matures, mechanical and kinesiologic changes occur within the muscles and joints, with a subsequent lowering of the body's center of gravity (Fig. 3–5). Thus, in the more physically mature child, the functional purpose of the motor task remains the same, but the means of attaining the goal changes to a more precise execution, in relation to the body structure. For the infant to progress to independent standing and walking, the musculoskeletal system must possess enough strength and dynamic control to move against the external forces, especially gravity.

Maturation of the musculoskeletal system is an important determinant of the development of a typical adult gait pattern. The soft tissue limitations imposed by the anterior pelvic tilt and hip flexion (seen in the toddler) must resolve, on maturation, to allow for the appropriate proximal and distal joint alignment and muscular function.

Physiologically the neonate displays increased flexion of all joints with a relatively high center of gravity located "at the base of the lower level of the thoracic spine."[18] The wide base of structural support maintained by lower extremity flexion, abduction, and external rotation in the infant allows for the stability on which movement can be initiated. The development of control and movement occurs in a cephalocaudal direction. Head control develops first, followed by trunk control, hip control, and finally leg and foot control. The stabilization pattern of the lower extremities (into hip flexion, abduction, and external rotation) appears initially in all developmental patterns. In the neonate, the posture is primarily due to the intrauterine position and to a physiologic increase in flexor tonus. The lower extremity characteristics of the neonate are a 2 to 1 ratio of external to internal rotation of the hip range of motion, coxa valga of approximately 150°, and the femoral condylar axis facing outward to about 30° to 40°.[19] Once the infant begins to gain control of the musculoskeletal apparatus, the base of support gradually narrows and is replaced by dynamic muscular control.

Initially during independent standing and walking, the child displays limited ability to combine different muscle actions at various joints. Basically, movements are in the "all or none" range, with wide range steps and little availability of various degrees of freedom of combined joint movements. Rather than smooth reciprocal muscle action, much cocontraction is seen around the joints, for stability.[20] The wide base of support for positional stability is exemplified in initial walking. Characteristically, to compensate for a high center of gravity in standing, the toddler widens the base of support so that the center of gravity remains within the base of support, as wide range stepping occurs in conjunction with inefficient pelvic control and coordination. This allows the infant to remain erect and mobile. As the child grows and the physical structure changes, there is a decrease in the anterior pelvic tilt and subsequent hip flexion. The trunk becomes straighter and the lower extremities grow longer. Therefore, a lowering of the center of gravity is seen (Figs. 3–6 and 3–7). The wide range lower extremity propulsive movements become smoother and are now counterbalanced by eccentric muscle contractions, which act to decelerate the body against gravity. Specifically the footdrop of the 1-year-old child disappears as the ankle dorsiflexors develop eccentric muscle control to lower the foot to the ground before midstance. Graded knee control develops during midstance as the hip moves over the supporting foot with the gastrocnemius-soleus muscle group impeding (decelerating) the forward movement of the tibia over the supporting foot.

The importance of musculoskeletal maturation in the development of mature gait was reported by Sutherland et al in 1980[21] and 1988.[22] Sutherland observed that, as the child matures, cadence decreases, while walking velocity and step length increase.

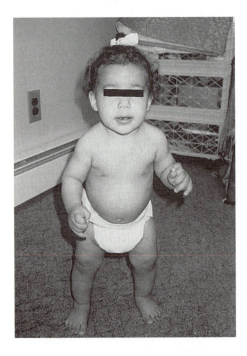

FIGURE 3–6. Typical standing posture of a toddler, frontal view.

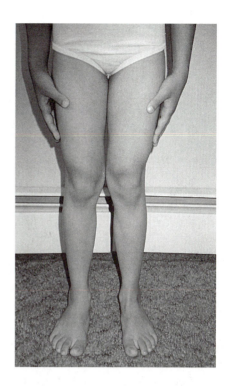

FIGURE 3–7. Typical standing alignment of an 8-year-old child, frontal view.

Important factors in the development of a mature pattern of these determinants are increasing limb length and greater limb stability, manifested by the longer duration of single-limb stance.[21] The work of Sutherland et al in 1988[22] documents the muscular activity about the ankle in early walking. In normal gait, ankle plantarflexion depends upon heel strike. This plantar flexion is absent in 1-year-olds who strike foot flat. At age 1.5 years, there is no consistent integration of the ankle plantar flexors. Dynamic ankle joint range of motion varies from 23° at 1 year old and 31° at 4 years old.

Fewer than half of the 1-year-olds demonstrated heel strike. By 1.5 years old, heel strike was present in nearly all the subjects. In mature walking, the tibialis anterior acts concentrically to lift the foot during swing, followed by an eccentric contraction to decelerate the foot from heel strike to foot flat. In children age 1 to 1.5, the electromyographic activity of the tibialis anterior was prolonged during stance, and there was a delay in the onset of swing phase activity. From 2 to 7 years old, a mature pattern of tibialis anterior phasic muscle activity was present.

The gastrocnemius-soleus functions in mature walking eccentrically to contract to decelerate the tibia during single limb stance, to arrest dorsiflexion, and then to accelerate the ankle joint before opposite foot strike. In children, the gastrocnemius-soleus musculature exhibited swing phase activity (not usually present in adult walking). This activity was described by Sutherland et al[22] as a "wrap around" pattern, beginning near the middle of swing and ending with opposite foot strike. At 2 years old, 25% of the subjects continued to display swing phase muscle activity of the gastrocnemius-soleus musculature. The typical adult firing pattern of the gastrocnemius-soleus musculature, which is present during the single-stance phase of gait, was present in one third of the 1.5-year-olds and three quarters of the 2- to 7-year-old children.

The increase in muscle strength and dynamic muscle control allows the infant to move in and out of a variety of postures. Muscles experience full elongation, concentric contractions, and eccentric contractions in supported positions (such as prone and supine) before the child attempts them while sitting or standing.

"Walking is initiated by inclining the body forward and placing it ahead of its center of gravity. To regain balance, one leg must be brought forward ahead of the shifting center of gravity. Man attempts to minimize the forces that tend to impede effortless motion by attempting to keep his center of gravity on a straight horizontal line during walking."[23] Inman et al[24] discussed the six determinants of gait that are used by the adult to minimize the vertical displacement of the center of gravity during walking. Pelvic rotation forward and backward minimizes the drop in the center of gravity during heel strike. Pelvic tilt laterally minimizes the excessive rise of the center of gravity by dropping the pelvis about 5° during midstance. Knee flexion and the concurrent foot and ankle movement each aid in minimizing the excessive rise and fall of the center of gravity by lengthening and shortening the leg during the stance phase of gait. Lateral motion of the pelvis, which causes the relative adduction of the femur, also aids in minimizing the excessive rise of the center of gravity.

Children gradually learn through muscle functioning to control the center of gravity efficiently. Biomechanical alignment in standing and walking varies with age.

GAIT CHARACTERISTICS BY AGE

Sutherland et al[21] details the following gait characteristics of children: The 1-year-old independent walker is unable to control the displacement of the center of gravity efficiently because of immature musculoskeletal alignment and functioning. Characteristically the pelvis is tilted anteriorly with a subsequent increase in lumbar lordosis; the base of support is wide; and the upper and lower extremities are flexed, abducted, and externally rotated. During walking, the 1-year-old child displays increased knee and ankle flexion in stance, footflat, mild footdrop, decreased duration of single limb stance with the stance leg supporting the body, and the swing leg accelerating the body by rotating the hips. Knee flexion is present during stance, and ankle plantar flexion occurs at foot strike. During the swing phase, there is increased hip flexion, abduction, and external rotation. Hip external rotation is present throughout the entire gait cycle. The typical cadence is rapid (180 steps/min), step length is short (20 cm), and walking velocity is slow (60 cm/sec). The duration of single limb stance is 32% of the gait cycle. The adult mean value is 38%.[22]

The 2-year-old child characteristically displays a decrease in hip abduction, external rotation, and pelvic tilt. The knee moves into flexion after foot strike and then begins to extend before toe-off. Heel strike is present on initial contact, and during swing ankle dorsiflexion is evident. Reciprocal arm swing is present as well as a heel-toe gait pattern. At age 2, the child's cadence has decreased, and step length and walking velocity have both increased. There exists a direct correlation between duration of single-limb support and the ability to balance on one leg. In normal motor development, this ability does not develop until 2.5 years.[22]

By the age of 3, the child displays an adult pattern of joint rotation and has achieved an adult pattern of walking, with the exception of a decreased step length and abnormally high cadence. In comparison to a 3-year-old child, a 7-year-old child has decreased cadence and increased walking velocity, and the duration of single limb stance has increased to 38% of the gait cycle.

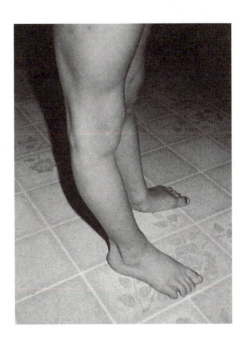

FIGURE 3–8. Pathologic gait, 4-year-old child, sagittal view. Note knee hyperextension, ankle pronation, plantarflexion, and eversion.

The gait characteristics of new walkers are immature, as evidenced by the wide base of support in response to a high center of gravity. As the child develops, the walking velocity and step length increase, as the cadence and double support time decreases. It has been postulated by Sutherland et al[21] that "step length increases in a linear manner with leg length." As the child's leg length increases, so does the child's height. As height is increased, the center of gravity lowers, eventually eliminating the need for a wide base of support seen in the younger child. In combination with more controlled muscle function, this results in the maturation of the gait cycle.

When the physical structure is less than optimal, as in cerebral palsy, mature gait is sacrificed. The child with cerebral palsy who has spastic hamstring muscles (and subsequent limitation of active knee extension) displays a shortened step length. Tightness and shortening of the Achilles tendon elicit toe-walking, footflat gait with calcaneal eversion, or toe-heel gait (Fig. 3–8). Strotzky[25] in 1983 documented the gait patterns of 39 normal children and 6 children with cerebral palsy, using high-speed cinematography. She found that all of the children with cerebral palsy walked more slowly than the normal children. She concluded that the slower gait was due to restricted stride length rather than to decreased cadence. The child with cerebral palsy cannot activate the proper motor program for ambulation owing to musculoskeletal problems and poor righting and equilibrium reactions.

RESEARCH

Much controversy exists in current literature regarding the age at which children display a mature gait pattern similar to normal adults (Table 3–1). This is primarily due to the investigation by researchers of different characteristics of the gait cycle using many methods of gait analysis. Sutherland et al[21] suggest that a mature gait

TABLE 3–1 Age of Acquisition of Mature Gait

Author	Date of Publication	Gait Parameter(s) Studied	Age of Gait Maturation
Okamoto & Kumamoto[1]	1972	Phasic muscle activity	7 years
Berger et al[3]	1984	Phasic muscle activity Knee and ankle joint angles	6–7 years
Sutherland et al[21]	1980	Walking velocity Cadence Step length Duration of single limb stance Ratio of pelvic to ankle spread	3 years
Burnett & Johnson[26]	1971	Heel strike Flexion at midstance Mature foot and knee mechanism	40–50 weeks after the initiation of independent ambulation
Norlin et al[28]	1981	Velocity Stride length Cadence	8–10 years
Corradi-Scalise & Ling[27]	1987	Phasic muscle activity	At least by 8–10 years
Takegami[29]	1992	Ground reaction forces	~8 years
Katoh et al[30]	1993	Ground reaction forces Ankle joint kinematics	Most intense up to 5 years

pattern is well established by age 3 with only minor changes occurring between ages 3 and 7. They identified five important determinants of a mature gait pattern: duration of single-limb stance, walking velocity, cadence, step length, and the ratio of pelvic to ankle spread. These characteristics were analyzed throughout the walking cycle using high-speed cinematography, a Graf-Pen sonic digitizer, a computer, and a plotter as well as electromyograms. Burnett and Johnson[26] state that mature gait (described by heel strike and synchronous arm movements) is constant 22 weeks after the beginning of independent walking, as observed through film analysis. Hip flexion at midstance and a mature foot and knee mechanism appear within 40 to 55 weeks following the initiation of independent gait.

Okamoto and Kumamoto[1] studied the learning process of walking and the process of ambulation as it developed with age, using electromyography, foot switches, and observational records. They conclude that by the end of the second year, the arm swing, push-off motion of the foot, and decrease of forward body sway (which are found in the adult) could be recognized. From this point, the ambulation began to lose the characteristics of infant walking and began to acquire adult walking patterns. The adult walking form was nearly accomplished by 7 years of age. Corradi-Scalise and Ling[27] described the gait characteristics of 8- to 10-year-old children by analyzing phasic muscle activity via electromyographic telemetry and ground reaction forces on the sole of the foot. They concluded that children ages 8 to 10 years clearly display a typical gait pattern similar to that of adults. In addition, Norlin et al[28] studied the gait patterns of 230 children with the use of foot switches. The parameters studied were velocity, stride length, cadence, and temporal phases of the stride as well as leg length of the subjects. Their results stated that the gait characteristics change with age and that the changes are most pronounced up to 8 to 10 years. Thereafter, only minor changes take place through age 16 years, and leg length becomes the dominant factor. Takegami[29] studied the gait pattern of 241 normal 4- to 10-year-old children by analyzing wave patterns of the ground reaction force. The results stated that significant changes in the gait parameters occur up to 8 years of age. In addition, Katoh et al[30] studied the ankle joint kinematics and ground reaction forces of 109 4- to 10-year-old normal children. They reported that maturation of the gait cycle occurred at about 5 years of age. This was related to the maturation of the ankle plantar flexors, which gain the ability to restrain dorsiflexion and improve balance leading to a decreased duration of stance and acceleration phases. Dorsiflexion control and maturation during early stance phase occurred at 8 years of age.

Such discrepancies in the literature lead to difficulty in assessing and comparing gait in childhood. To make relevant comparisons between pathologic gait and normal gait, it is necessary to know more about the development of gait in childhood. The literature reports that many changes occur within the gait pattern between the inception of walking and age 3. After that, only minor changes occur in refinement of movement and in the characteristics of step length, cadence, and walking velocity, which seem to be somewhat dependent on leg length. The consensus in the literature seems to be that by age 7,[1-3] a mature gait pattern has developed that is similar to the adult pattern.

A definitive statement regarding the maturation of gait in childhood is imperative if relevant comparisons between pathologic gait and normal gait are to be made. If children in the age range of 8 to 10 years display a mature gait pattern, their gait studies can be compared with adult studies of normal gait. If the gait patterns of children younger than 8 years old vary with age, children ages 1 through 7 should be compared with children their own age. This is an important concept when children with pathologic gait or developmental delays, or both, are to be compared with the gait of healthy children.

NORMAL VERSUS TYPICAL

Throughout the literature on gait analysis, "normal" joint angles and biomechanical alignments are given. It is important to remember, however, that normal alignment may not, in fact, be typical of the alignment seen in the population. Although there are accepted alignment characteristics of adult walking, because of the innate variability of humans, typical alignment characteristics should be documented as well as optimal alignment or normal patterns. The quality of walking that achieves the goal of bipedal locomotion can vary widely. Terms such as "normal," "optimal," and "typical" must be clearly defined and applied consistently to identify and qualify pathology accurately (Figs. 3–9 to 3–11).

We examined 20 normal 8- to 10-year-old children to determine whether children in that age range display a gait pattern similar to that of adults. A lower extremity examination was performed on each child. Of the 20 children, only 25% displayed no musculoskeletal abnormalities, 50% displayed subtalar joint pronation on weight bearing, 40% displayed genu valgum (either unilateral or bilateral), and 10% displayed genu recurvatum. This clearly adds controversy to the term "normal" as it is applied to the musculoskeletal system of children in this age group. Although 75% of these children did not display "normal" biomechanical alignment, all are considered normal children. Based on comparison with normal walking patterns, 75% never achieved a biomechanically mature gait pattern. Although all these children are func-

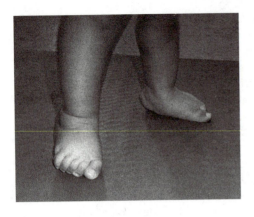

FIGURE 3–9. Ankle joint pronation on weight bearing observed in an 11-month-old child as a reflection of immaturity.

tional walkers, and to the untrained eye possess "normal" ambulation patterns, clinically it is useful to describe these typical gait characteristics and apply them to clients who have so-called pathologic gait.

Typically, in the literature, gait studies have focused on alignment and phasic muscle activities, two important characteristics of gait. Our study attempted to address the maturation of gait in children using these parameters and through theories of motor learning.

Motor control depends on central nervous system maturation and musculoskeletal development. The parameter most suited to address maturation of the human gait pattern is muscle activity. Mature gait can be described through the characteristics of phasic muscle activity corresponding to designated phases of the gait cycle: stance, swing, and double stance. We studied 20 healthy children, 11 boys and 9 girls in the 8- to 10-year age range. A developmental questionnaire was administered to the parents concerning birth history, developmental history, and pertinent medical and surgical history. The short form of the Bruininks-Oseretsky Test of Motor Proficiency (American Guidance Service, Circle Pines, MN 55014) was administered to each child to ensure developmental normalcy. A descriptive study was conducted to analyze phasic muscle activity about the ankle joint and the ground reaction forces on the sole of the foot. An eight-channel electromyography telemetry unit was used to measure phasic muscle activity about the ankle joint. The muscle groups used were the ankle dorsiflexors (including the tibialis anterior, extensor digitorum longus, peroneus ter-

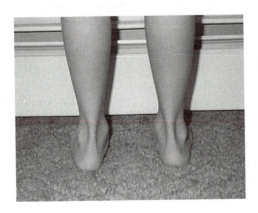

FIGURE 3–10. Ankle joint pronation on weight bearing noted in a typical 8-year-old child. This typifies the variability of biomechanical alignment in normal children.

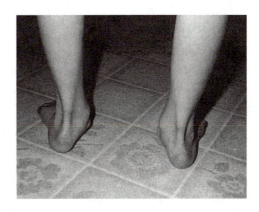

FIGURE 3–11. Severe ankle joint pronation on weight bearing in a typical 4-year-old child with cerebral palsy.

tius, extensor hallucis longus) and the ankle plantar flexors (including the gastrocnemius, soleus, flexor hallucis longus, peroneus longus, tibialis posterior, flexor digitorum longus, and peroneus brevis muscles). An electrodynography system (The Langer Biomechanics Group, 21 East Industry Ct, Deer Park, NY 11729) was interfaced with the electromyography for the data collection on double stance, stance, and swing phases of gait.

The results of the study indicated that children in the 8- to 10-year age range did display a mature gait pattern similar to that of adults. The skilled coordination of muscle groups about the ankle joint, necessary to perform both the mobility phase of gait (swing) and the stability phases of gait (stance and double stance) were evident. During the stance phase of gait, the left lower extremity demonstrated greater firing of the ankle plantar flexors compared with the ankle dorsiflexors. "The inhibition of one set of muscles, while opposing muscles are in excitation, is a condition for effective movement."[31] The right lower extremity in stance demonstrated no variability between firing of the ankle plantar flexors and dorsiflexors, demonstrating cocontraction. Cocontraction is a more primitive pattern than skilled muscle movement. The left lower extremity was, therefore, more skilled than the right for the stance phase of gait.

During the swing phase of gait, the reverse was observed. The right lower extremity demonstrated reciprocal inhibition, and the left lower extremity demonstrated cocontraction of agonist and antagonist. The right lower extremity was, therefore, more skilled during the swing phase of gait than the left.

Analysis of these findings is of great interest. The screening evaluation of the short form of the Bruininks-Oseretsky Test of Motor Proficiency revealed 90% of the subjects to be right-dominant, as determined by preference of throwing and kicking a ball. The conclusion that can be drawn is that the subjects possessed greater coordination and skill of the right versus the left extremities. This statement in itself is misleading. In 95% of the subjects, during the activity of kicking a ball, which is similar to the swing phase of gait, the right lower extremity performed the mobility activity of kicking the ball, while the left lower extremity performed the stabilizing activity of weight bearing to support the body. These results are consistent with the functions of the lower extremities during gait. The left leg displayed greater skill during the stance phase (skill in weight bearing), and the right leg displayed more skill during the swing phase of gait (skilled in kicking). Although the subjects were termed "right-footed," foot dominance can be further classified as that lower extremity best coordinated for the specific activity by describing the mobility and stability characteristics of the task.

During double stance, there was no variability between agonist and antagonist of either leg. Cocontraction occurred bilaterally. The balance of muscle activity around the ankle joint provides the stable base seen in the double stance phase of gait.

The results of this study demonstrate that children in the 8- to 10-year age range display a mature gait pattern similar to that of adults. The skilled coordination of muscle groups about the ankle joint necessary to perform both stance and swing phases of gait efficiently was observed. Right versus left preference of the lower extremities has also been established in this age group. In support of our data, Wheelwright et al[32] also observed asymmetry to exist in normal childhood gait. They studied the spatial and temporal gait parameters of 134 normal children. It was noted that the asymmetry in the double support phase was great with a definite bias between the two sides. The double support time following the left stride was significantly shorter than that following the right. A similar bias existed for both step length and swing time. They related right and left differences to individual laterality and developed dominance.

The results of our study indicate that children in the age range of 8 to 10 years display a mature gait pattern. In analyzing this information, the authors conclude that the motor program specific for ambulation was intact in all 20 subjects. Specifically the differences obtained between skill of right and left lower extremities, regarding efficiency of mobility and stability tasks, were evident. This preprogramming of specificity within the leg movements allows intended movements to be performed efficiently with each leg being preprogrammed for specific functions.

SUMMARY

Many factors influence the development of gait in children. The maturation of the neuromuscular system provides the posture and balance necessary to walk. The development of learning and problem solving provides the motivation for the initiation of gait. The maturation of the physical structure of the bones and muscles allows for the optimal interaction of the body with the outside environment, including the force of gravity.

Initially the gait pattern of the beginning walker is characterized by a wide base of support, anterior pelvic tilt, hip flexion, external rotation and abduction, wide-range stepping movements, ankle joint pronation, toe curling, and upper extremity abduction with elbow flexion. With central nervous system and musculoskeletal maturation, the motor program innate to humans is activated efficiently for functional, mature ambulation. If there is a deficit in biomechanical alignment, postural control, or motor control, the motor program specific for efficient ambulation is not expressed and the pattern of walking is less than normal.

Typical adult gait usually develops by age 7. In a certain percentage of the population, however, mature gait patterns of biomechanical alignment never develop owing to the innate variability of humans. Therefore, although functional ambulation exists in this population, a normal gait pattern is never really achieved as determined by optimal or normal standards. In childhood, typical, normal, and optimal standards must be clearly identified within age ranges to qualify pathology accurately.

REFERENCES

1. Okamoto, T and Kumamoto, M: Electromyographic study of the learning process of walking in infants. Electromyogr Clin Neurophysiol 12:149, 1972.
2. Sutherland, DH: Gait Disorders in Childhood and Adolescence. Williams & Wilkins, Baltimore, 1984, p 10.
3. Berger, W, Altenmueller, E, and Dietz, V: Normal and impaired development of children's gait. Hum Neurobiol 3:163, 1984.
4. Furno, H, et al: Help Checklist. VORT Corporation, Palo Alto, CA, 1984.
5. McGraw, MB: Neuromuscular development of the human infant as exemplified in the achievement of erect locomotion. J Pediatr 17:747, 1940.
6. Bobath, B: Abnormal Postural Reflex Activity Caused by Brain Lesions, ed 3. Aspen, Rockville, MD, 1985, p 1.
7. Leonard, CT, Hirschfel, H, and Forssberg, H: The development of independent walking in children with cerebral palsy. Dev Med Child Neurol 33:567, 1991.
8. Alon, Z: Unpublished material, 1986.
9. Adelson, E and Fraiberg, S: Gross motor development in infants blind from birth. Child Dev 45:114, 1974.
10. Plack, M: Personal communication, 1984.
11. Gunsolus, P, Welsh, C, and Houser, C: Equilibrium reactions in the feet of children with spastic cerebral palsy and normal children. Dev Med Child Neurol 17:580, 1975.
12. Stelmach, GE (ed): Motor Control Issues and Trends. Academic Press, New York, 1976, p 202.
13. Stelmach, GE (ed): Motor Control Issues and Trends. Academic Press, New York, 1976, p 2.
14. Carr, JH, et al: Movement Science Foundations for Physical Therapy in Rehabilitation. Aspen, Rockville, MD, 1987, p 131.
15. Haas, G, et al: Development of feedback and feedforward control of upright stance. Dev Med Child Neurol 31:481, 1989.
16. Brooks, VB: Brain functions in motor skill learning. Conference on the Neurobehavioral Analysis of Motor Skill Learning. Teacher's College Columbia University, New York, 1987.
17. Carr, JH, et al: Movement Science Foundations for Physical Therapy in Rehabilitation. Aspen, Rockville, MD, 1987, p 25.
18. Palmer, CE: Studies of the center of gravity in the human body. Child Dev 15:99, 1944.
19. Resseque, B: Conference Lecture Material, The Dynamic Components of Foot Function. Langer Biomechanics Group, Deer Park, NY, 1984.
20. Carr, JH, et al: Movement Science Foundations for Physical Therapy in Rehabilitation. Aspen, Rockville, MD, 1987, p 93.
21. Sutherland, DH, et al: The development of mature gait. J Bone Joint Surg 62A:336, 1980.
22. Sutherland, DH, et al: The Development of Mature Walking. Clinics in Developmental Medicine. MacKeith Press, London, 1988.
23. Cailliet, R: Foot and Ankle Pain. FA Davis, Philadelphia, 1968, p 45.
24. Inman, VT, Ralston, HJ, and Todd, F: Human walking. In Lieberman, JC (ed): Human Walking. Williams & Wilkins, Baltimore, 1981, p 1.
25. Strotzky, K: Gait analysis in cerebral palsied and nonhandicapped children. Arch Phys Med Rehabil 64:291, 1983.
26. Burnett, CN and Johnson, EW: Development of gait in childhood: Part II. Dev Med Child Neurol 13:207, 1971.
27. Corradi-Scalise, D and Ling, W: Gait patterns of normal school-aged children. Master's Thesis, New York University, 1987.
28. Norlin, R, Odenrick, P, and Sandlund, B: Development of gait in the normal child. J Pediatr Orthop 1:261, 1981.
29. Takegami, Y: Wave pattern of ground reaction force of growing children. J Pediatr Orthop 12:522, 1992.
30. Katoh, P, Mochizuki, T, and Moriyama, A: Changes of sagittal-plane ankle motion and ground reaction force (fore-aft shear) in normal children aged four to ten years. Dev Med Child Neurol 35:417, 1993.
31. Payton, OD, Hirt, S, and Newton, RA: Scientific Basis for Neurophysiologic Approaches to Therapeutic Exercise: An Anthology. FA Davis, Philadelphia, 1978, p 105.
32. Wheelwright, EF, et al: Temporal and spatial parameters of gait in children. I: Normal control data. Dev Med Child Neurol 35:102, 1993.

CHAPTER 4

Closed Kinetic Chain and Gait

Leslie N. Russek, PhD, PT

Locomotion is the ability to move from place to place; *gait* is the more specific act of moving by foot. Human, bipedal gaits include the walk, run, and hop. Walking is characterized by a double limb support phase, in which both feet are in contact with the ground. Running has no double limb support but instead has an airborne phase. Some distinguish jogging from running by initial contact with the forefoot, rather than the heel. Each is a controlled loss of balance, in which a person catches himself or herself from falling forward by redirecting the downward energy into forward progression. Thus, walking and running are states of dynamic equilibrium.

Walking, jogging, and running are all out-of-phase gaits, in which the relative motion of the legs is in different directions. Hopping is an in-phase gait with symmetric leg movement. Because quadrupeds have four legs, they have more possible patterns of movement, generating six gaits: walk, trot, pace, canter, transverse gallop, and rotary gallop. Flying and swimming are forms of nonterrestrial locomotion, and each has various patterns as well.

Closed kinetic chain motions are those in which the terminal body segment is weight bearing. Terrestrial locomotion differs fundamentally from flying and swimming because it requires the alternation between open and closed kinetic chain phases. In humans, the lower kinetic chain is composed of the lumbar spine, pelvis, hip, knee, ankle, subtalar, midtarsal, and metatarsophalangeal joints. The constraints provided by closed kinetic chain motion play a large role in the patterns of gait. This constraint merely reflects the importance of gravity and the biomechanics of the body.

Bipedal gait has played an important role in the intellectual evolution of the human species by freeing the upper limbs for the use of tools. The human musculoskeletal system evolved to permit bipedal gait: The sacrum enlarged to tolerate the increased weight transmission through the rear legs and to take on a role in supporting the viscera. Bipedal gait is not uniquely human, however, and humans are not necessarily the best at it. Ostriches are the fastest bipeds, with a running speed 23 meters per second (52 mph), almost as fast as the renowned cheetah, at 29 meters per second (65 mph).[1] Hopping kangaroos are probably the most energy efficient, using their large Achilles tendons and tails to store elastic energy between bounds.[2]

This chapter reviews the most salient features of human walking, with an emphasis on interactions along the kinetic chain. The chapter begins with the descriptive terminology for gait, with definition of relevant terms. Our limited knowledge about the neurologic control of locomotion is then discussed. An analysis follows of the determinants of gait and energy transfer. The chapter then reviews current understanding of gait kinematics, muscle activity, and kinetics. The concepts of the chapter are brought together with a case study and discussion of clinical implications. The Appendix describes and critiques, in greater detail, methods of gait analysis. The present discussion includes the whole lower kinetic chain but does not duplicate discussion of subtalar and foot mechanics in Chapters 1 and 2.

The goal of animal locomotion is to move the body in an energy-efficient manner, while maintaining appropriate mechanical loads on body structures and tissues and maintaining adequate control for safety. The natural transition from one gait to another as speed increases, such as switching from walking to running, occurs to minimize energy consumption at any given speed.[3] For each gait, the biomechanics of the human body change; the natural, most efficient movement pattern also changes. Although this chapter emphasizes the science of gait, it is well to contemplate the insight of Holzreiter and Köhle:[4] "Gait is not merely a mechanical problem, it is also a personal expression."[4]

CHARACTERISTICS OF GAIT

Figure 4–1 shows the two primary phases of gait, stance and swing, with some of the various terms used to identify events during the cycle. Terms coined by the gait laboratory at Rancho Los Amigos are most generic, whereas the other terminologies are more descriptive of normal gait. The gait cycle is usually considered to begin with the initial contact of one foot. *Initial contact* is normally with the heel and frequently is called *heel strike* or *heel contact;* the general term of initial contact also encompasses pathologic gaits in which contact is not made with the heel. After initial contact, the leg accepts or loads weight as the foot comes down to make full, foot flat contact. *Double limb support* begins with initial contact of one limb and ends with toe-off of the contralateral limb. The body then pivots over the weight-bearing foot; the moment when the center of gravity is directly over the weight-bearing foot is *midstance.* Midstance usually occurs after push-off with the contralateral foot. As the body continues to move forward, the heel raises from the ground (hence *heel-off*) and the body prepares for push-off with this foot. Again, the Rancho Los Amigos terminology, *terminal stance,* is more generic and allows comparable description of pathologic gaits. Initial contact of the contralateral foot usually occurs soon after heel-off. The moment at which the toe loses contact with the ground is called either *toe-off* or *preswing.* The *swing phase* is broken up into three components: *initial swing,* or the acceleration phase; *midswing;* and *terminal swing,* or the deceleration phase. Stance makes up about 60% of the stride and swing 40%. *Double limb support,* which is also the *weight acceptance* or transfer phase, thus constitutes two 10% periods of the stride in adults.

The phases of gait may also be described by the primary type of *energy transfer.* Initial contact is a time of energy absorption, both at the ankle complex and at the

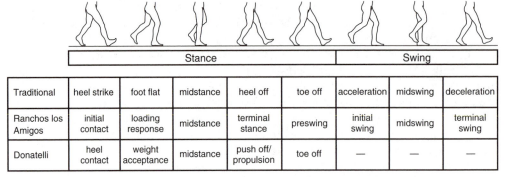

			Stance				Swing	
Traditional	heel strike	foot flat	midstance	heel off	toe off	acceleration	midswing	deceleration
Ranchos los Amigos	initial contact	loading response	midstance	terminal stance	preswing	initial swing	midswing	terminal swing
Donatelli	heel contact	weight acceptance	midstance	push off/ propulsion	toe off	—	—	—

FIGURE 4–1. The named phases of gait, with several of the nomenclature systems: traditional, Rancho Los Amigos, and the nomenclature used in previous chapters.

knee. This *absorption phase* acts both to soften the force of initial contact and to store energy to be released to facilitate forward progression. Push-off, from heel-off to toe-off, is the *propulsion phase*. The force of propulsion is almost entirely from the ankle plantar flexors and is responsible for 80% to 85% of the energy generated during the stride.[5] Mechanisms of energy transfer are discussed in greater detail in a later section.

NEUROLOGIC CONTROL

Although gait, for humans, is normally learned in the first year of life, locomotion appears to be controlled by a central program in the nervous system.[6] In animals, this central program for locomotion is present even before the animal has had an opportunity to learn or practice.[7] Little is known about the higher levels of neurologic control of gait in humans. Consequently the following discussion includes results of animal research.

Locomotion is normally mediated through a combination of central control and peripheral feedback. Interneurons within the spinal cord can produce reciprocal limb movement through a *neural oscillator* or *pattern generator* even without input from higher brain centers. As a result, most of the detailed pattern generation takes place at the level of the spinal cord. In all vertebrates that have been studied, the spinal pattern generator is able to modulate the complex activation among all four limbs. Animals with spinal cord transections can locomote on a treadmill and even make the appropriate transitions from one gait pattern to another (e.g., trot to gallop) as the treadmill speed increases.[8] Such animals, however, lack equilibrium, power, and endurance. The central pattern generator at the spinal level appears also to be paramount in humans, about whom much less detailed information about neurologic control is known.[6,9]

In all animals studied, gait is normally initiated in the brain stem. The basal ganglia (globus pallidus) and subthalamic and pars reticulata of the substantia nigra generate output to the caudal pole of the cuneiform nucleus.[7] From the cuneiform nucleus, signals pass down to the central pattern generators in the spinal cord. Little is known about the higher control of gait in humans, but decorticate cats are not only able to locomote, but also retain many other goal-directed behaviors. Cats with cerebellum transected are able to initiate free walking but have limited ability to respond to obstacles such as walls. Cats with spinal transections are able to locomote if supported and can respond appropriately to basic obstacles to paw movement. Afferent information about movement normally travels, via the ventral and dorsal spinocerebellar tracts, to the cerebellum. The cerebellum, although not necessary for gait, improves the quality and coordination by comparing the efferent central pattern generator plan with afferent input about actual movement. The cerebellum then adjusts the central program to refine movement. Although normal gait uses higher neurologic systems, the spinal pattern generator in animals that have been studied can activate and control the limbs and relevant trunk musculature without higher input. In humans, spinal reflexes are similar to those seen in other animals and are likely to be hardwired in similar ways. The presence of cortical input for humans, as for other animals, provides more flexible responses and allows adaptation to environmental factors.[9]

Proprioceptive and sensory information is normally used to influence the central pattern generator, adjusting movement to avoid obstacles and improve coordination. The basic, monosynaptic stretch reflex is inhibited during gait in humans as well as other animals.[9,10] The simple stretch reflex is supplanted by a more complex spinal reflex involving both the weight-bearing and non–weight-bearing limbs. In humans, the polysynaptic reflexes depend on an intact supraspinal system, as the reflexes are not present in spastic paresis.[9] Joint position information normally contributes to timing of the gait cycles. In spinal animals, if limb movement is obstructed, the muscles remain active in an attempt to complete that gait cycle. The most proximal joint appears to dominate, although distal joints provide input as well.[8] Cutaneous sensory input can also modulate the central pattern. If the front of a cat's paw pad is touched during the swing phase, the cat demonstrates a flexor synergy to raise the paw above the obstacle. As noted previously, afferent input normally goes to the cerebellum as well as to interneurons in the spinal cord.

The importance of sensory input and the ability of animals to locomote, even with spinal cord transections, might suggest that the motor pattern is purely reflex. This notion is not true, however. Although normal locomotion uses afferent input from muscle spindles, tendon organs, and joint afferents when available, locomotion retains the complex timing patterns among all involved muscles even if afferent input is removed. With higher neurologic levels intact, gait can be essentially normal without sensory input. Coordination would be compromised slightly, owing to lack of cerebellar feedback. In animals with spinal transections as well as deafferentation, motor patterns are essentially normal but less stable; perturbation easily disrupts the pattern of muscle activation.

TEMPORAL AND SPATIAL DESCRIPTORS OF GAIT

Time, distance, and speed measures of gait are the simplest to understand and to obtain but remain extremely useful.[11] Figure 4–2 shows spatial measures of a stride. A step goes from one heel strike to the contralateral heel strike and is named by the foot accepting weight. The right step is thus the distance from left heel strike to right heel strike. A stride extends from heel strike to ipsilateral heel strike, such as right to right. A stride is thus comprised of a left and a right step. If average forward velocity is constant, stride length is identical whether measured from right to right or left to left. The stride width is the perpendicular distance between the lines of progres-

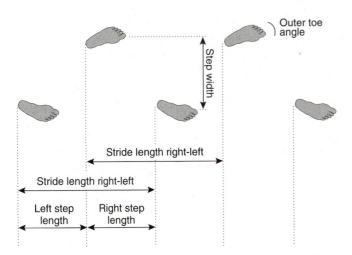

FIGURE 4–2. The spatial parameters of gait. Stride length is the distance from heel strike to ipsilateral heel strike. Step length is the distance from contralateral heel strike to ipsilateral heel strike. Step width is the distance, perpendicular to direction of motion, between heel strikes. The out-toe angle is formed between the line of progression and the longitudinal axis of the foot.

sion; this is also the base of support, unless an assistive device is used. The out-toe angle is the angle between the axis of the foot and the line of progression.

Figure 4–3 shows the various temporal parameters of gait. Stride and step time correspond to the spatial parameters. Stance and swing times are also analogous. Double limb support is the overlap of stance phases, and is not necessarily equal between sides. Winter[12] defines right *double limb support* as left foot contact to right foot toe-off; this definition also applies to left weight acceptance. *Cadence* is the number of steps per minute. *Velocity* is the distance traveled per unit time. Velocity normally oscillates during the stride, as kinetic and potential energy are exchanged; reported velocity is usually the average through the stride, or the net forward velocity.

DETERMINANTS OF GAIT

Saunders and colleagues[13] originally identified essential components of gait, which they defined as determinants. Inman and others[14] later refined these into six determinants, which still provide a helpful framework for interpreting the complex movements of gait. The model is primarily determined by gravity and mechanics; it is frequently called the *inverted pendulum model of gait* because the body moves over the weight-bearing leg like a pendulum. It is also called the *ballistic model of gait* because the swing leg moves freely through space.

Figure 4–4 shows the first determinant: hip flexion and extension. With only this movement, the pelvis moves stiffly over the fixed foot like a hinged compass. This compass motion makes for a bumpy ride, as the pelvis is highest at midstance, then low with an abrupt direction change at double limb support. This abrupt change in direction is both inefficient, as it dissipates energy, and stressful to the musculoskeletal system structures. *Compass gait* does allow for forward progression of the body, however.

Pelvic rotation around a vertical axis (i.e., in the transverse plane) constitutes the second determinant. Figure 4–5 shows how pelvic rotation tends to increase the effective length of the leg, decreasing the rise and fall of the center of gravity. Also, decreasing the height of the vertical arcs decreases the potential energy changes, making the stride more efficient. Because the movement is closed chain, pelvic rotation

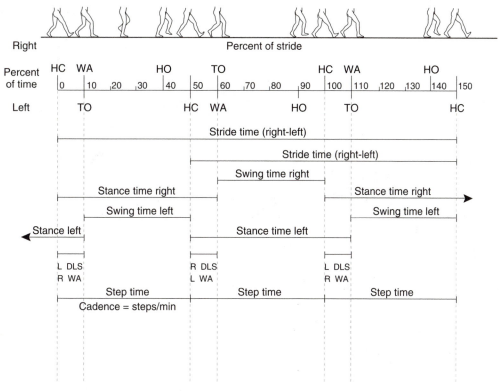

FIGURE 4–3. The temporal parameters of gait for a full right and left stride. Stride time is measured from heel contact to ipsilateral heel contact; for constant velocity, right stride time equals left stride time. Stance time is measured from initial contact to ipsilateral toe-off; swing time is from toe-off to ipsilateral initial contact. Stance and swing time may differ, right to left. Double limb support, or weight acceptance, is the time when both feet are in contact with the ground: initial contact to contralateral push-off. Winter[12] defines the convention that right double limb support is the period between left initial contact and right push off; this is also left weight acceptance. Phases of gait are as defined in Figure 4–1, and also the glossary (DLS = double limb support; WA = weight acceptance).

necessarily entails hip rotation. The total amount of pelvic rotation is about ±4° at normal speeds but increases with speed.[15]

The third determinant is *pelvic obliquity,* a drop in the swing side hip. As depicted in Figure 4–6, pelvic obliquity further smoothes the vertical excursion of the center of gravity, smoothing the stride. The drop of the swing side hip necessitates flexion of the swing leg knee for it to clear the ground. The hip abductors on the weight-bearing side must stabilize the pelvis; if they do not control the amount of hip drop, a Trendelenburg gait results. The normal amount of obliquity is also about ±4°.[15]

The fourth determinant adds *stance leg knee flexion* after initial contact to smooth energy absorption after initial contact and to decrease the vertical rise of the center of gravity at midstance (Fig. 4–7). Decreased vertical oscillation of the center of gravity reduces the stress to musculoskeletal structures up the kinetic chain. In running, the amount of knee flexion at initial contact is greater, to absorb further the compressive forces, which can be four to five times body weight.[16]

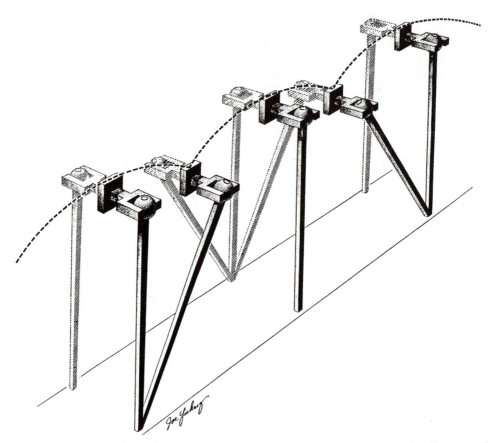

FIGURE 4–4. Compass gait: the first determinant includes only a hinge at the hip, allowing only hip flexion/extension. The pelvis remains perpendicular to the line of progression, and moves up and down in a series of abrupt arcs, traced by the *dashed line*. (From Inman, Ralston, and Todd [1981], with permission. Originally published in a slightly different form in Saunders et al. [1953].)

The foot with ankle dorsiflexion and plantar flexion during stance constitute the fifth determinant and are shown in Figure 4–8. Each of the first four determinants has decreased the vertical distance traveled by the center of gravity. The transition between each arc, at initial contact and push-off, has remained abrupt, however. The presence of a foot, in the fifth determinant, decreases the abrupt direction change at initial contact by allowing the lower leg to rock over the base of support. Plantar flexion during push-off decreases the abrupt direction change at push-off by effectively lengthening the lower leg. The fifth determinant thus softens the vertical arcs into oscillations. With the addition of active force generation by the muscles, plantar flexion also imparts momentum to the leg for swing.

The final determinant is *lateral displacement of the center of gravity over the base of support* (Fig. 4–9). Skaters and cross-country skiers exaggerate this lateral movement, and may glide for a great distance on the supporting leg. By decreasing the torque across the pelvis that the hip abductors must resist, this weight shift increases the stability of gait while decreasing the demand on the muscles.

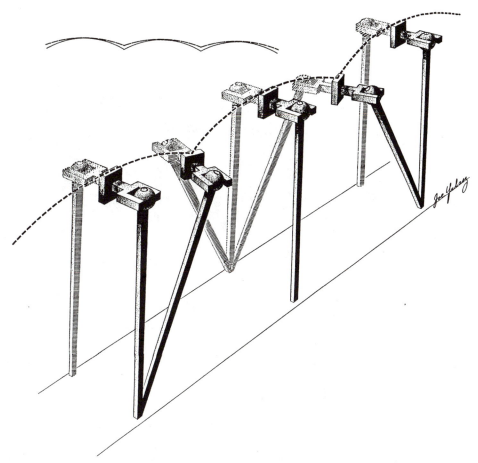

FIGURE 4-5. The second determinant of gait adds pelvic rotation in the horizontal plane. Pelvic rotation acts to lengthen the step by effectively lengthening the legs. By allowing the legs to remain more vertical at contact, pelvic rotation decreases the vertical drop in the center of gravity during double-limb support. The inset on top left shows a tracing of the center of gravity with only the first determinant (*solid line*) and the smoothed path when the second determinant is added (*dashed line*). (From Inman, Ralston, and Todd [1981], with permission. Originally published in a slightly different form in Saunders et al. [1953].)

Movement of the pelvis accounts for three of the determinants, and the position of the pelvis is key to economy and dynamic stability of movement.[15] Although the determinants of Saunders et al[13] do not describe the body above the pelvis, the trunk is also important. Trunk rotation occurs almost exactly out of phase with the pelvic rotation. The arms also swing out of phase with the legs: Forward swing of one arm occurs with forward step of the opposite leg. Anterior and posterior rotation of the pelvis produces extension and flexion of the lumbar spine. A lordotic lumbar spine at push-off aligns the facets in a closed packed position, locking them for stability.[17] This rigid spine extends the rigid lever produced by the foot and ankle as they supinate at push-off. Lateral trunk stabilization is also essential in maintaining balance.[18]

The determinants of gait provide a rationale for some of the complexity: Movement at each of the joints along the kinetic chain is progressively invoked to allow a

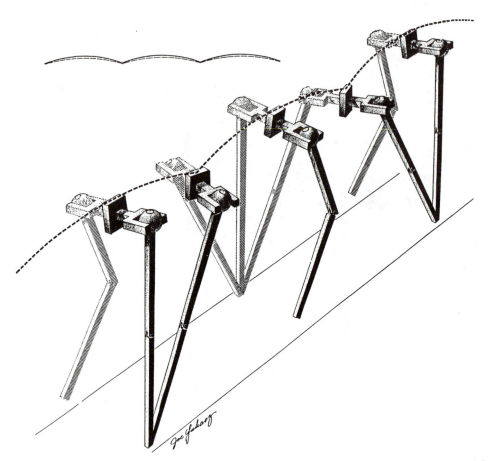

FIGURE 4–6. The third determinant of gait adds pelvic obliquity and swing-knee flexion. The pelvis drops on the swing-leg side, just before toe-off, then gradually returns to neutral by double limb support. Whereas the center of gravity is lower during swing, the vertical rise of the center of gravity is decreased at midstance. The knee of the swing leg must flex to clear the ground. The inset on top left shows the tracing of the center of gravity height with the first two determinants (*solid line*) and with the third determinant added (*dashed line*). (From Inman, Ralston, and Todd [1981], with permission. Originally published in a slightly different form in Saunders et al. [1953].)

smooth translation of the body during the gait cycle. Minimizing vertical displacement of the body during walking improves the economy of gait and reduces the amount of stress and strain on the musculoskeletal system.

ENERGY CONSERVATION AND TRANSFER

The metabolic cost of gait is naturally minimized through optimal use of gravity and mechanical energy exchange. McMahon[19] uses a hinged pendulum model of gait, based on the determinants noted previously, to describe most of the characteristics of human walking at normal speeds. Once set into motion at push-off, the swing leg requires little muscle input and responds to gravity as a pendulum would. Just as an

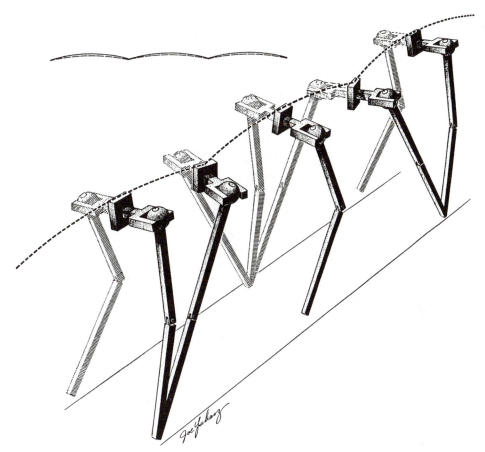

FIGURE 4–7. The fourth determinant of gait adds a small amount of stance-knee flexion. Knee flexion at initial contact absorbs the initial impact, whereas flexion at midstance decreases the center of gravity rise. The inset on top left shows a tracing of the center of gravity height with the first three determinants (*solid line*) compared with the fourth determinant added (*dashed line*). (From Inman, Ralston, and Todd [1981], with permission. Originally published in a slightly different form in Saunders et al. [1953].)

FIGURE 4–8. The fifth determinant of gait adds the foot, with dorsiflexion and plantar flexion at the ankle. The presence of the foot softens the abrupt direction change at initial contact by allowing the shank to rock over the foot. As a result, the vertical direction change up the kinetic chain is less abrupt and less jarring. Ankle plantar flexion during push-off further smoothes the trajectory of the knee. This acts to lengthen the leg at heel contact and toe-off. (From Inman, Ralston, and Todd [1981], with permission. Originally published in a slightly different form in Saunders et al. [1953].)

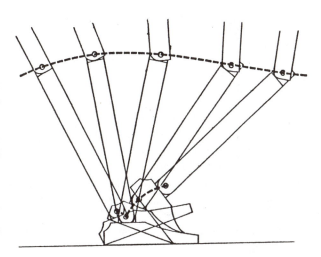

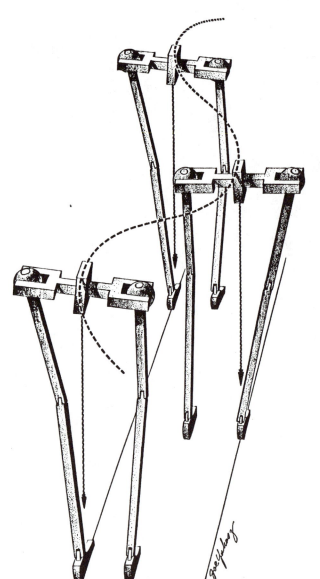

FIGURE 4–9. The sixth determinant of gait adds horizontal oscillations of the pelvis. Shifting weight over the base of support (stance leg) improves stability and narrows the base of support. (From Inman, Ralston, and Todd [1981], with permission. Originally published in a slightly different form in Saunders et al. [1953].)

oscillating pendulum has a resonant frequency, humans have a preferred cadence. Indeed the metabolic cost of walking is the lowest at this resonant frequency.[20] When people walk at speeds and cadences well above or below their preferred ones, the metabolic cost of walking becomes high. The energy-storing mechanisms of walking become inappropriate and inefficient at high velocities, whereas those of running become relatively more efficient. The transition between walking and running thus occurs to minimize the energy demand.[21,22]

In walking, the greatest amount of energy in the body is in the form of potential energy and kinetic energy. Because these energy forms are both related to mass, they are dominated by the bulk of body mass in the head, arms, and trunk. Kinetic and potential energy are exchanged so that the total body energy does not change significantly. The body moves from the potential energy maximum at midstance (maximum vertical height) to the kinetic energy maximum at double limb support (maximum forward velocity). Facilitation of this energy exchange can be used in gait reeducation of stroke patients.[23]

Energy transfer also occurs within and between body segments. Caldwell and Forrester[24] describe four mechanisms of energy transfer: (1) pendulum, (2) joint force transfer, (3) whip, and (4) tendon. The transfer of energy tends to be proximal to distal at pushoff, then distal to proximal at terminal swing. The pendulum mechanism operates both in the swing leg and as an inverted pendulum in the stance leg. The determinants of gait and many of the ballistic models of gait are based on the pendulum characteristics. Whip occurs when the upper leg is used to accelerate the lower leg during early swing, then again when the deceleration of the leg propels the body forward at the end of swing.[25] Joint force transfer uses the rigid body dynamics of the joint surface to transfer energy from one bony segment to an adjacent segment. Joint transfer is important because it frequently changes the direction of movement. Muscle contraction and gravity both apply linear forces on bones, which are constrained to rotate around joint axes: around the proximal joint in open chain or around the distal joint in closed chain. Yet the ultimate goal of rotational motions are the linear translation of the body.[26] Torque can be transmitted not only in the sagittal plane, but also through torque conversion in the transverse plane, as discussed in Chapter 1. Finally, all muscles and tendons can store elastic energy. One-joint muscles can transfer energy from one segment to another, whereas two-joint muscles can also transfer energy from one joint to another. The importance of muscle elasticity is supported by evidence that nonpathologic muscle tightness correlates to decreased oxygen uptake and thus to increased efficiency, in both walking and jogging.[27]

Because the dynamics of running are different than those for walking, the mechanisms of energy storage and transfer are different. In running, in contrast to walking, the peak in potential and kinetic energy occurs together at the peak of the airborne phase. Consequently, there is no exchange between kinetic and potential energy. Running therefore uses elastic energy storage to a greater degree: The human Achilles tendon stores up to 35% of the kinetic and potential energy lost and regained between strides, and ligaments in the arch of the foot store another 17%.[28]

KINEMATICS

Measurement of and treatment to affect joint ranges are fundamental to physical therapy. The most obvious component of locomotion is motion, both of the body as a whole and of the body segments relative to one another. Joint movement is the result of the sum of all forces acting around the joint, including gravity and the ground reaction force as well as muscle action. The functional range of motion present during gait is usually less than the total available range because the individual may not have the strength, time, or coordination to achieve full range.

Before discussing actual joint ranges, it is important to note that a great deal of variability exists in quantitative values reported from different laboratories (see discussion in Appendix). Kadaba and coworkers,[29] comparing ranges reported in the literature, found variation from 19° to 28° in ankle dorsiflexion/plantar flexion, 57° to 68° in knee flexion/knee extension, and 30° to 52° in hip flexion/hip extension.

The following discussion relates kinematics to phase of gait, rather than the percent of stride, because phase of gait is more easily visualized. Heel contact defines the beginning of a stride. Weight acceptance occurs from 0% to 15% of stride.[12] Midstance occurs at about 30%, heel-off at 35%, and toe-off at 60% of stride. Swing goes from 60% to 100% of stride, with midswing at about 85%.

Figure 4–10D shows sample kinematic data for the ankle from Kadaba and coworkers.[29] Between heel contact and weight acceptance, the ankle plantar flexes eccentrically from 0° to 5°. This eccentric deceleration assists knee flexion in dissipating compressive forces at heel contact. From weight acceptance to heel-off, dorsiflexion to 10° takes place as the tibia is carried forward over the fixed foot. From heel-off to toe-off, the ankle plantar flexes concentrically to 15°. From toe-off to midswing, the ankle dorsiflexes to 2° to 3° to allow the foot to clear the ground. Finally, from midswing to heel contact, the ankle plantar flexes just enough to reach neutral, preparing for contact.

At heel contact, the knee flexes eccentrically from 5° to 15° to 20° (Fig. 4–10C). This, the fourth determinant of gait, allows smooth absorption of weight. From

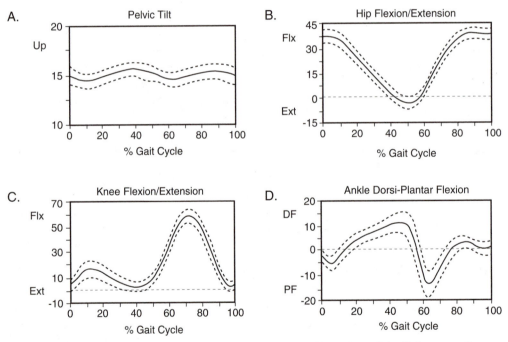

FIGURE 4–10. Sagittal plane kinematic data. (*A*) Anterior/posterior pelvic tilt has a small range of about 3°. (*B*) The hip attains maximal flexion of 35° to 40° at initial contact, steadily extends to about 5° in late stance, and flexes again during swing. (*C*) The knee eccentrically flexes to about 20° in early stance, extends prior to midstance, then flexes to about 60° during swing. (*D*) The ankle plantar flexes to 10° during weight acceptance, and dorsiflexes to 10° to 15° as the leg passes over the foot. The ankle then plantar flexes to 15° during push-off, and returns to neutral during swing. Mean (*solid line*) and standard deviation (*dotted line*) of 40. Heel contact (HC) defines the beginning of a stride. Weight acceptance occurs from 0% to 15% of stride. Midstance occurs at about 30%, heel-off at 35%, and toe off at 60% of stride. Swing goes from 60% to 100% of stride, with midswing at about 85%. (From Kadaba et al.[29], with permission.)

weight acceptance to midstance, the knee extends almost fully, to allow the contralateral swing leg to clear the ground. From midstance to initial swing, the knee flexes rapidly to about 60°, to decrease the inertial moment and to allow this leg to clear the ground during swing. During swing, the knee extends to 0°, then flexes to about 5° immediately before heel contact, to smooth the joining of foot and ground at contact. Measurements of knee motion in the transverse and coronal planes have been inconsistent, probably because of the technical difficulty in observing these subtle changes (see Appendix for description of sources of error). The most definitive study used intracortical pins fixed in the femur and tibia.[30] In this study, Lafortune and coworkers[30] challenged the traditional view of the screw-home mechanism occurring during gait. They found that the tibia was externally rotated about 5° at heel contact, rotated internally to just over 6° at toe-off, then externally rotated again during swing. They found that the knee remained stable at 1.2° of abduction throughout stance, then increased to 6.4° of abduction during swing.

At heel contact, the hip is maximally flexed to 35° to 40° (Fig. 4–10B). From heel contact to heel-off, the hip steadily extends through neutral as the body moves forward over the fixed foot (the first determinant of gait). From heel-off to toe-off, the hip attains maximal extension, of 5° to 10° extension. After toe-off, the hip steadily flexes to approximately 35° to 40°, where it remains until heel contact. The hip also moves in the coronal plane. The hip passes through neutral near heel contact and toe-off and travels to approximately 7° adduction in early stance and 5° abduction at the beginning of swing. Figure 4–11 shows hip motion in the transverse plane: Hip external rotation is maximal at 5°, just before heel contact. The hip passes through neutral just before toe-off and continues to rotate internally until it reaches a peak of 7° at midswing. The hip then rotates rapidly out, to reach 5° at terminal swing.

The pelvis moves about equally in all three planes. Anterior-posterior tilt is only to a total of about ±3° (Fig. 4–10A). Transverse rotation, the second determinant of gait, is ±4°. Pelvic obliquity, the third determinant of gait, also has a total range of ±4°, tilting down from the stance leg (see also Fig. 4–6, third determinant). Trunk rotation occurs in the direction opposite the pelvis, with approximately 5° total range in each of the transverse and coronal planes and 3° in the sagittal plane.[15]

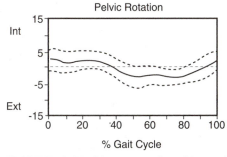
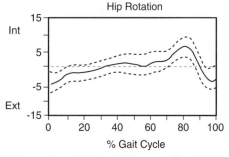

FIGURE 4–11. Transverse plane kinematic data. Pelvic rotation (*left*) and hip rotation (*right*). Mean (*solid line*) and standard deviation (*dotted line*) of 40. Heel contact defines the beginning of a stride. Weight acceptance occurs from 0% to 15% of stride. Midstance occurs at about 30%, heel-off at 35%, and toe-off at 60% of stride. Swing goes from 60% to 100% of stride, with midswing at about 85%. (From Kadaba et al.[29], with permission.)

Although usually emphasizing joint angles, kinematic analysis may also examine movement of body segments. Angular velocities of limb segments, for example, show proximal to distal sequencing during swing phase of gait as well as in kicking and throwing motions.[31] Also, inertial analysis of the lower limb segments helps explain how forward propulsion of the body is achieved.[25]

MUSCLE ACTIVITY AND FUNCTION

Although many of the characteristics of gait can be explained through passive mechanical properties, the driving force ultimately comes from muscles. Muscles act to accelerate, stabilize, and decelerate body segments through concentric, isometric, and eccentric activation.[14] Concentric activity generates energy for propulsion, primarily at pushoff. Isometric energy not only provides stability during stance, but also transmits energy up and down the kinetic chain throughout the stride. Eccentric activity decelerates segments not only to provide cushioning, but also to assist energy transfer along the kinetic chain. Eccentric muscle activity may be dominant during as much as 34% of the support phase.[32] In addition to force production, muscles also provide proprioceptive information through muscle spindles and Golgi tendon organs.[19]

The following overview briefly describes the complex interplay among muscles controlling gait. As with kinematics discussed previously, no single data set can be considered "truth" (see Appendix). The present data have been taken, with permission, from Winter,[12] to whom the reader is referred for more detailed analysis. Dykyj[33] also provides an excellent overview of muscle activity during gait. Again, discussion relates muscle activity to phase of gait, with heel contact defining the beginning of a stride. Weight acceptance occurs from 0% to 15% of stride, midstance at about 30%, heel-off at 35%, and toe-off at 60% of stride. Heel-off and toe-off together make up push-off. Swing goes from 60% to 100% of stride, with midswing at about 85%.[12]

The primary roles of muscle activity at the ankle are for weight acceptance during stance and propulsion at push-off. Between heel contact and weight acceptance, the dorsiflexors (tibialis anterior, extensors digitorum and hallucis longus, and peroneus tertius) control eccentric plantar flexion at the ankle (Fig. 4–12A). The gastrocnemius muscle (Fig. 4–12B) also acts at heel contact to control knee flexion, preventing hyperextension at the knee.[33] From weight acceptance to heeloff, the plantar

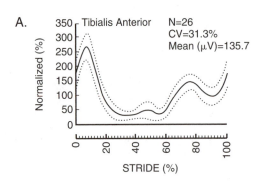

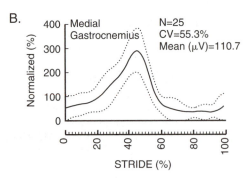

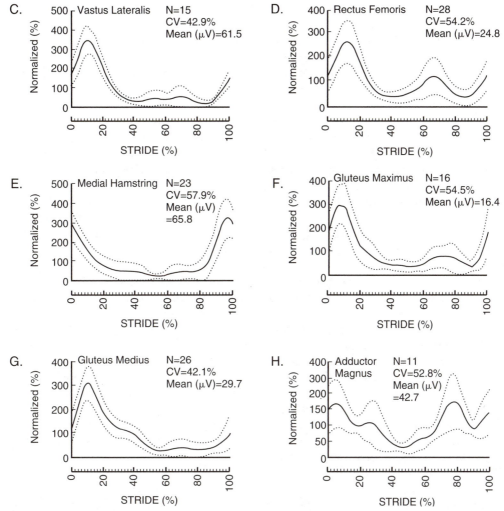

FIGURE 4–12. EMG data for primary lower extremity muscles. (*A*) Tibialis anterior shows a strong burst of activity immediately after heel strike, as it eccentrically resists plantar flexion. Activity then remains low until the ankle is isometrically maintained at neutral during swing. The extensor digitorum longus also acts as a dorsiflexor, and demonstrates similar activity patterns. (*B*) The medial gastrocnemius muscle is typical of the plantar flexor muscles, with a gradual increase in activity as it eccentrically resists dorsiflexion as the leg passes forward over the foot and a strong period of concentric activation during push-off. (*C*) The vastus lateralis, similar to the vastus medialis, shows activity increasing immediately prior to heel strike and peaking during early stance as it eccentrically resists knee flexion and extends the knee during stance. (*D*) The rectus femoris parallels the other quadriceps during late swing and stance, but also shows activity during swing while the rectus acts as a hip flexor. (*E*) The medial hamstrings show activity beginning in late swing to decelerate knee extension in preparation for heel strike, and continuing through early stance to extend the hip. The lateral hamstrings show similar activity. (*F*) The gluteus maximus is active just prior to heel strike and as the hip extends during stance. (*G*) The gluteus medius is active during stance to control pelvic obliquity. (*H*) The adductor longus stabilizes the stance leg through cocontraction with the hip abductors and flexors. During swing, the adductor longus assists in hip flexion. The muscles shown in this figure were selected because they tended to have the greatest amount of activity from their respective groups (e.g., vastus lateralis among quadriceps). The data have been normalized to 100% before ensemble averaging of 25 muscles. (From Winger[12], with permission.)

flexors (gastrocnemius, soleus, posterior tibialis, plantaris, and flexors halucis and digitorum longus) decelerate forward rotation of the tibia. Forceful concentric activity in the plantar flexors produce push-off between heel-off and toe-off. The toe flexors become most active in the later portion of push-off to stabilize the toes. As noted in the section on energy, push-off contributes 80% of the total ankle energy during stride. After push-off, the dorsiflexors again become active to allow the foot to clear the ground.

The knee must absorb weight during the loading phase and carry momentum during swing. The greatest activity in the knee extensors (quadriceps) extends from heel contact to weight acceptance, when the quadriceps act eccentrically to control knee flexion and cushion weight acceptance (Fig. 4–12C, D). The hamstrings are also active at heel contact (Fig. 4–12E), as they act as hip extensors. During midstance, little muscle activity is present around the knee, as the body is carried forward by the momentum of the propulsion phase. Knee muscles become active again toward the end of swing, as the hamstrings decelerate knee extension and the quadriceps stabilize knee extension in preparation for heel contact.

The muscles around the hip not only move the hip, but also stabilize the pelvis on a changing base of support. The pelvis must also provide a stable base from which the trunk muscles can control forward acceleration of the trunk. At heel contact, muscles all around the hip are activated to provide stability to the leg as it accepts weight (Figs. 4–12D through H). Hamstring activity peaks at, or just before, heel contact (Fig. 4–12E), whereas the gluteus maximus activity increases from heel contact to weight acceptance (Fig. 4–12F). Both act to resist the flexion moment at the hip and to extend the hip. Gluteus medius activity (Fig. 4–12G) also peaks at weight acceptance, to control pelvic obliquity as the support of the contralateral leg is lost. The peak in hip adductor activity at weight acceptance produces stance limb stability via cocontraction around the hip (Fig. 4–12H). During midstance and late stance, the hip extensors become relatively silent as the body is carried forward over the fixed leg (into greater hip extension) by momentum. The adductors and rectus are active at toe-off, assisting the hip flexors in accelerating the thigh forward (Figs. 4–12D, H). Finally, the hamstrings and gluteus maximus become active during late swing, decelerating the swing leg, transmitting energy in the swing leg back up into the trunk, and again preparing for heel contact.

The goal of running is speed, rather than efficient use of gravity and momentum, and so the muscle activation patterns are somewhat different. At the hip, the gluteus maximus and hamstrings produce a more forceful extension,[34] rather than allowing momentum to carry the body forward. Also, the adductors are more active in pulling the leg forward during swing and in stabilizing the stance leg.[35] Knee extensors play an even greater role in absorbing energy at heel contact and in extending the knee during the propulsion phase.

KINETICS

The science of kinetics addresses the interaction between motion and the forces causing that motion, including ground reaction forces, joint torques, energy, and power. The primary forces that affect motion during gait include gravity, muscles, and the ground reaction force. These forces may be transmitted through bone, ligament, or muscle. According to Newton's law, the sum of all the forces acting around a joint

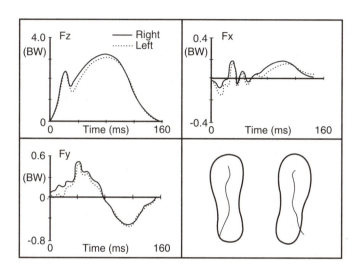

FIGURE 4–13. Ground reaction force and center of pressure data for an elite female runner classified as a rearfoot striker. The running speed was 5.21 meters per second. Fz is the vertical component, and has the greatest amplitude. Fy is the antero-posterior component, showing a decelerating force after heel strike, but an accelerating force during push-off. Fx is the medio-lateral component of force, and remains small. The *line* superimposed on the footprint shows the center of pressure progressing from rearfoot to forefoot during stance phase. (From Williams et al.[36], with permission.)

accelerate or decelerate that joint. Although kinematics told only of the motion itself, kinetics tell about the forces that cause motion. While much of the energy is directed into forward propulsion, some energy is also expended in balancing the forces acting on the body to maintain balance during locomotion.[18] The Glossary reviews some of the mechanical concepts and terms germane to the following discussion.

The basic source of data in studying kinetics is the *ground reaction force*, which has vertical components (holding the body up) and two perpendicular horizontal components (preventing the foot from slipping). Figure 4–13 shows the three dimensions of ground reaction for a running stride, along with the center of pressure patterns.[36] The vertical component (Fz) shows an initial peak, at heel contact, followed by a bell-shaped loading and unloading pattern. The A-P component (Fy) shows a period of braking followed by a period of push-off. The lateral force (Fx) is much smaller than the other two. The pressure pattern shows heel contact at the lateral aspect of the rearfoot, with the pressure peak moving forward and medial. Data for walking are qualitatively similar.[37] Alignment of the ground reaction vector with the hip may minimize the metabolic cost of locomotion by requiring minimal muscle activity.[22] Although the ground reaction vector can itself be analyzed,[38] the ground reaction force data are more often combined with kinematic data to compute the torque, energy, and power at each joint along the kinetic chain.

The ankle provides the greatest propulsive power in walking. Figure 4–14A shows the joint angle, moment, and resulting power at the ankle. The phases of power absorption and generation have been labeled. The initial eccentric plantar flexion phase, occurring as a result of the small dorsiflexion moment, absorbs little power and is not named. As the tibia rotates forward over the foot during stance, the ankle has a dorsiflexion moment, and dorsiflexion occurs. Consequently the plantar flexors absorb energy during what is called the A1 phase. After heel-off, strong plantar flexion during the major propulsive phase, A2, generates 80% of the total energy during the stride.[12] During swing, the ankle has little torque and power associated with it.

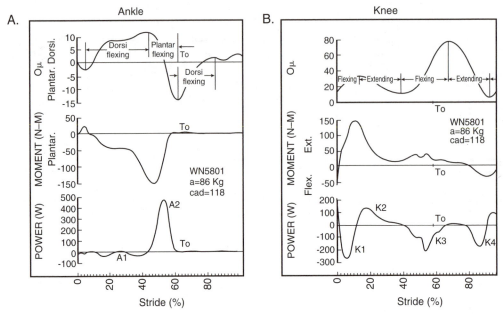

FIGURE 4–14. Kinetic data for (*A*) the ankle and (*B*) the knee. The figure includes joint angular position (*top*), joint moment (*middle*), and power generation or absorption (*bottom*). The primary burst of power production in the ankle occurs during A2, as the ankle forcefully plantar flexes during push-off. The knee absorbs more power than it produces, with the largest power absorption occurring after heel strike as the knee eccentrically flexes to accept body weight. The other power phases are discussed in the text. (From Winter[12], with permission.)

In walking, the knee absorbs more power than it generates. Fig. 4–14*B* shows knee flexion occurring during the flexion moment from heel contact to weight acceptance; this power absorption phase is labeled K1. From weight acceptance through midstance, the knee extends against the flexion moment, so generates the power labeled K2. The K2 phase is the only power generation by the knee. From heel-off to toe-off, the knee extensors control the knee flexion under pressure of the flexor moment, and absorb power in the K3 phase. The knee extensors do not contribute to knee extension during swing, as the energy for knee extension comes primarily from whip and pendulum actions. Toward the end of swing, the knee flexors decelerate the extending knee, absorbing energy during the K4 burst.

Winter[12] found power levels at the hip to be small and quite variable. In general, a small power generation phase, H1, was observed as the hip extended against the flexor moment from heel contact to weight acceptance. The H1 phase also serves to stabilize the trunk, preventing trunk flexion. Between weight acceptance and heel-off, the hip moment is small as the body is carried forward by momentum, absorbing a small amount of power, H2. The largest power burst occurs at pushoff and the acceleration phase of swing. This H3 phase is called *pull-off* for the hip because the hip flexes strongly to pull the leg off the ground and to give the leg momentum needed to complete swing. The low and variable power levels at the hip during stance support the role of the hip as a stabilizer of the pelvis and trunk.

GAIT ABNORMALITIES

This chapter has emphasized normal gait. Table 4–1 lists a number of common gait abnormalities, along with the possible cause and the correlated kinematic, kinetic, and electromyographic (EMG) data. For example, increased step time may occur because of poor energy transfer owing to weakness or because of excessive cocontraction. Kinematic data for both would show decreased joint ranges throughout the lower kinetic chain. Kinetic analysis would show decreased power peaks, in both cases. EMG activity, however, would be different in the two cases: decreased in weakness but increased in cocontraction. In this case, EMG testing would be most helpful in identifying the cause. In other cases, kinematic or kinetic testing might be most informative. Table 4–1 ties together some of the complex information presented in this chapter. It provides a framework for thinking about gait deviations and for analyzing possible causes. Table 4–1 is not intended to be a comprehensive listing nor to be a checklist for evaluation.

CASE STUDY

The case study demonstrates some of the ideas discussed in this chapter. The patient is a 20-year-old woman who sustained a grade 2 right ankle sprain 10 months previously. Although her clinical examination is unremarkable, with normal strength and range in both ankles, she felt that her ankle still "wasn't right." Gait analysis was undertaken to identify abnormalities and to guide further treatment.

Temporal and spatial parameters are within normal limits except for double limb support. Figure 4–15 presents these data, as a percent of normal values for young women. Velocity, step time, stride length, and step length are quite close to normal values. Cadence is slightly fast, which is also suggested by the short step time. Percent of time in stance is slightly higher than normal, with the involved foot hanging on the ground longer than the uninvolved foot. Double limb support, hence weight transfer, takes much longer (30% to 40%) than normal. The asymmetry in stance time is also seen in the double limb support, with the weight transfer off of the involved foot occurring more slowly than off the uninvolved foot.

The patient's overall movement pattern showed excessive weight shift toward the uninvolved side throughout stride, with the center of gravity passing well to the right within the base of support (Fig. 4–16). This weight shift is produced by a right trunk lean, balanced by a drop in the left hip (Trendelenburg) during right stance (Fig. 4–17). Figure 4–17 also shows how the patient uses left arm abduction to counterbalance her right lean.

The total joint ranges during the gait cycle, as a percent of normal, are shown in Figure 4–18. The dominant feature is excessive pelvic rotation, which is more than four times normal. This increase in the second determinant of gait compensates for the decrease in the first determinant: hip range (by 49% and 17% on the left and right). This overreliance on rotation tends to occur in individuals with poor dissociation between the pelvic and shoulder girdles, who thus swing the whole body. Total hip obliquity range is increased, in addition to

TABLE 4–1 Abnormal Adult Gait Patterns

Abnormality	Possible Cause	Kinematic	Kinetic	Electromyogram
Increased step time	Poor energy transfer; weakness Muscle cocontraction	→ Ranges likely → Ranges likely	↓ Power peaks ↓ Power peaks	→ Electromyogram activity ↑ Electromyogram activity
Short step length	→ Pelvic rotation → Swing momentum → Stance leg strength Compensation for balance deficit	→ Pelvic or trunk rotation → Plantar flexion or hip flexion at toe-off ↑ Knee extension during swing → Stance hip extension, ↑ knee flexion All joint ranges ↓	→ A2, ↓ H3 ↑ K4 → Moments → Moments	→ Plantar flexion or hip flexor at toe-off ↑ Hamstring during swing ↑→ Hip extension, ↓ quad, ↓ plantar flexion LE cocontraction
Broad base of support	→ Joint mobility, balance, sensation, proprioception	All sagittal joint ranges ↓ Lack of smooth pattern	↑ Moments in coronal plane	
Increased DLS	Poor energy transfer Compensation for poor balance	↑ Dorsiflexion in midstance; ↓ plantar flexion at push-off Lack of smooth pattern	→ A2 → Moments	→ Amplitude range LE cocontraction
Initial contact Flat foot	Compensation for weak plantar flexion Heel pain → Step length	→ Plantar flexion during loading response Steppage gait → Plantar flexion at push-off	0 plantar flexion moment at heel contact → Ankle moments → A2	→ Plantar flexion at heel contact ↑ Duration of dorsiflexion → Plantar flexion at contralateral push-off
Digigrade	Plantar flexion contracture or spasticity Compensation for leg length discrepancy Pain with knee extension	→ Dorsiflexion → ankle and knee range of motion ↑ Knee flexion	Dorsiflexion moment at heel contact → K1 and A1 ↑ K3	→ Plantar flexion ↑ Plantar flexion and quadriceps → Quadriceps
Lack of knee extension	Edema, pain, instability at knee Quadriceps weakness	Lack terminal extension, ↓ knee range of motion Rapid knee flexion after IC	→ K4 ↑ K1	→ Quadriceps in late swing → Quadriceps at heel contact

Loading response				
Foot slap	Weak eccentric dorsiflexion, toe extension	Rapid plantar flexion after IC	↑ Ankle absorption at heel contact	↓ Dorsiflexion at heel contact
Stiff knee	Weak eccentric quadriceps control	↓ Knee flexion after IC	↓ K1	↑ Hip extension, ↓ quadriceps
Midstance				
Trendelenburg	Weak stance leg abductors; Hyperactive adductors	↑ Pelvic obliquity, trunk lean; Hip adduction	↑ Hip absorption	↓ Hip abduction on stance leg
Lateral trunk lurch	Abdominal weakness; ↓ Mobility of contralateral leg joints	Lateral trunk lean	↑ Moments in coronal plane	↓ Hip abduction on stance leg
Extensor lurch	Hip extensor weakness	Posterior trunk lean	↓ Hip extension moment	↓ Hip extension on stance leg
Pushoff				
Lack of heeloff; poor pushoff	Weak plantar flexion (pushoff)	↓ or slowed plantar flexion	↓ A2	↓ Plantar flexion
	Painful toe extension, ↓ toe range of motion	↓ Toe extension		↑ Toe extension; ↓ toe flexion
	↓ Plantar flexion range of motion	↑ Ankle plantar flexion	↓ A2	Normal plantar flexion activity
	Weak hip flexors (pulloff)	↓ or slowed hip flexion	↓ H3	↓ Hip flexion
Swing				
Circumduction; Vaulting; Hip hiking	Knee flexion painful; Weak stance hip abductors; Swing leg hip flexion or ankle dorsiflexion	↑ Hip abduction, hip height; ↓ hip, knee, ankle range of motion in sagittal plane		↑ Knee extension; ↓ TA, hip or knee flexors
Steppage gait	Footdrop, heel pain	↑ Hip and knee flexion, ankle plantar flexion	↓ ankle moments	↓ Dorsiflexion, ↑ hip flexor
Knee hyperextension	Weak eccentric hamstrings	Rapid knee extension in swing	↑ K4	↑ Hamstring in swing

↑ = Increased; ↓ = decreased.

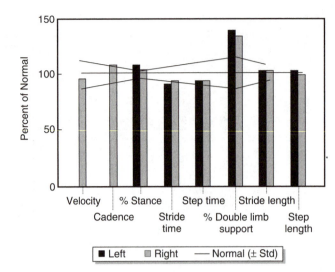

FIGURE 4–15. Temporal and spatial measures for patient 10 months after a left ankle sprain. Dark colored bars indicate values for the left (involved) ankle and the light bars indicate values for the right (uninvolved) ankle. Velocity and cadence are global parameters, independent of side, and so are represented only once. Graphic data are presented as a percent of normal to allow the range of values to be plotted against a single axis and to facilitate identification of abnormal values. The horizontal lines around 100% indicate normal values plus or minus standard deviation. No standard deviation was available for step length. The table below contains the actual data values and normative values from Kadaba, et al.[29]

	Unit	Left	Right	Normal*	std
Velocity	(cm/s)		122	127	16
Cadence	(st/min)		125	115	9.0
% Stance	% of stride	66%	63%	61%	2.6%
Stride time	(sec)	0.96	0.99	1.05	0.08
Step time	(sec)	0.50	0.50	0.53	0.06
Double limb support	% of stride	14%	13%	10%	1.4%
Stride length	(cm)	132	132	130	10
Step length	(cm)	69	66	67	

the Trendelenburg discussed previously. Knee flexion is decreased slightly, on the left. Ankle range is excessive bilateral but more so on the left.

The involved ankle kinematics demonstrate both excessive dorsiflexion range and abnormal pattern (Fig. 4–19). At heel contact, the left ankle plantar flexes more quickly than the right. Weight acceptance during the first 40% of stride shows small oscillations on the left, compared with the smooth, controlled weight acceptance on the right. Dorsiflexion during stance is not well controlled on the left; the left ankle is carried too far into dorsiflexion before heel-off, dorsiflexion occurs more rapidly on the left, and push-off is delayed. Push-off on the left generates slightly less plantar flexion on the left relative to the right. Plantar flexion at push-off is also poorly controlled on the left, demonstrated by the large standard deviation in left ankle position after toe-off. Poor repeatability between strides suggests poor neuromuscular control of the left plantar flexor muscles.

From this analysis, one can conclude the following. The left ankle appears to have poor eccentric control during weight acceptance and as the tibia rotates forward during midstance. The ankle achieves plantar flexion during push-off but late and without adequate control. This poor control results in a slowed weight transfer in both directions but more from the involved to the uninvolved leg. This poor weight transfer causes the left foot to hang on the ground, prolonging double limb support. Other significant abnormalities in gait are also noted: excessive pelvic rotation, a Trendelenburg drop of the left hip, and trunk

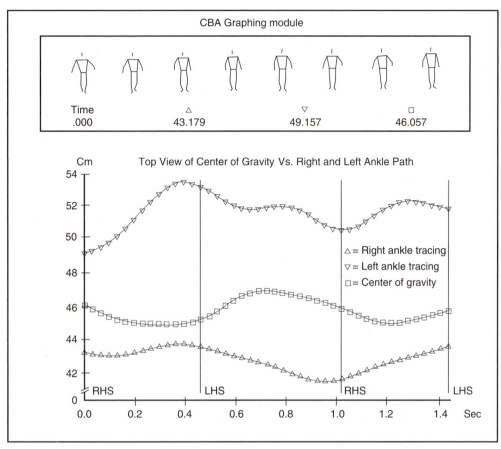

FIGURE 4–16. Top view of the horizontal movement of the center of gravity (*squares*), right ankle (*triangles*) and left, involved, ankle (*inverted triangles*). Time equals 0 and represents right heel strike (RHS); two right heel strikes (RHS) and two left heel strikes (LHS) are marked with vertical lines, and are identified along the time axis. After the initial right heel strike, the center of gravity shifts towards the right foot (the sixth determinant). The left ankle, shown on the top, circumducts before LHS. After LHS, the center of gravity shifts towards the left foot. Note that the center of gravity is biased towards the right (uninvolved) foot, rather than being centered midline to the base of support. Note also the wider lateral motion of the left ankle.

lean to the right. In addition to suggesting balance deficits, this analysis suggests weakness around the pelvic girdle.

The regimen for this patient should emphasize closed-chain exercises, especially single leg balance on the left. Eccentric training at the ankle would improve control at weight acceptance, and concentric training would improve and speed push-off. Gait training should emphasize crisper weight transfer between legs. She should strengthen muscles around the pelvic girdle, particularly the hip abductors, and probably increase trunk flexibility.

Although this analysis considered only temporal, spatial, and kinematic data, predicting the salient features of kinematic or EMG data could be educational. Table 4–1 suggests that increased double limb support time is due to poor energy transfer or poor balance (or both). The excessive dorsiflexion at the left

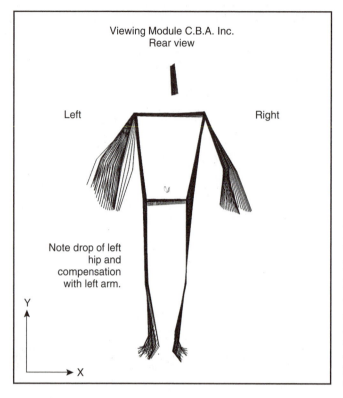

Viewing Module C.B.A. Inc.
Rear view

Left   Right

Note drop of left
hip and
compensation
with left arm.

Y

X

FIGURE 4–17. Rear view of stick figure, from digitized video data, representation of patient going through a full right and left stride. Each joint was digitized at each of 44 video frames; lines connect the digitized joints. The patient's left (involved side) is at the left of the figure. Note the slight drop in the left hip, with a compensating trunk lean right and abduction of the left arm.

ankle during stance may be due to an increased A1 power absorption phase followed by a small A2 propulsion burst. EMG recordings of the gastrocnemius might show decreased activity in early stride, and delayed activation at push-off. The poor control at toe-off might show up as decreased activity in the toe flexors, which normally stabilize the end of push-off.

CLINICAL IMPLICATIONS OF GAIT ANALYSIS

Walking is one of the most fundamental movement patterns in humans. For people who are ambulatory, walking is an essential part of life. Pain with walking is a primary complaint for many with back or lower extremity disorders. Assessment of gait should be part of any trunk or lower extremity evaluation and should be monitored throughout treatment.

Not all differences among individuals indicate abnormality. For example, normal gait patterns change with age. Gait among young children changes with development, until about age 4 years, as discussed in Chapter 3. Older children (aged greater than 5 years) have kinematic and kinetic parameters similar to those for adults, although walking velocity is slower and cadence higher.[39]

Reports of gait parameters among healthy elderly people have been variable. Step length, stride length, velocity, ankle range of motion, center of gravity excur-

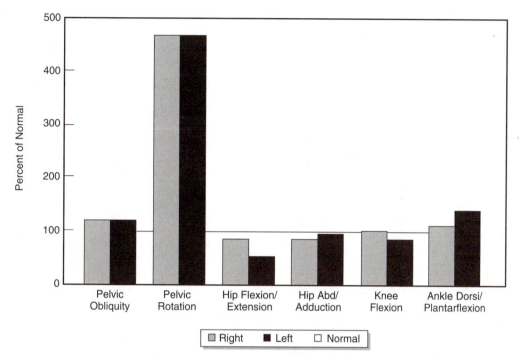

FIGURE 4–18. Total lower extremity joint ranges during the gait cycle, as a percentage of normal. Values are computed as the maximum position for each joint in one direction, in degrees, minus the maximum in the opposite direction. *Dark bars* represent joint range of left (involved) side and *light bars* represent the right (uninvolved) side. As in Figure 7–15, values are presented as percent of normal for young women. Pelvic obliquity and rotation are, by definition, equal on right and left. The dominant feature in this gait is excessive pelvic rotation, which is almost five times normal. Hip range is decreased bilateral, but more on the left than the right. Hip abduction is slightly low, more so on the right. Knee flexion is normal on the right, but decreased slightly on the left. Ankle range is increased on both sides, but more so on the left. (From Kadaba et al.[29], with permission.)

sions, and pelvic obliquity have been found to be the same between paired groups of young and elderly men.[40] Another study found that elderly subjects had decreased step length, decreased double limb support, decreased push-off power, and decreased ankle kinematics.[41] Yet another study found elderly subjects to have decreased lower limb joint ranges and decreased push-off and toe clearance during swing.[42] Any quantitative comparisons of patient gait to normative data must therefore use age-appropriate data.

Although comparing right and left sides of an individual seems a natural way to assess a unilateral involvement, normal gait is not perfectly symmetric. Step time, stance time, step length, joint ranges, and timing are frequently different from one side to the other.[43] In addition, studies have found treadmill and floor walking to have different temporal and spatial characteristics, with a higher cadence and shorter step length on a treadmill than in free walking.[44]

Gait evaluation can (1) provide an objective (whether qualitative or quantitative) measure of function that can be used to monitor progress; (2) identify abnormal function (impairment) and guide identification of underlying cause (the timing of pain

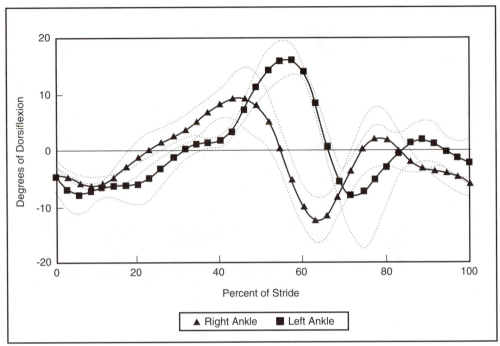

FIGURE 4–19. Ankle kinematics for one stride. Left (*squares*) and right (*triangles*) ankles are both shown beginning at heel strike. Each kinematic is an average of three strides, and one standard deviation above and below are shown. The right (uninvolved) ankle shows a kinematic pattern similar to the normal ankle kinematics shown in Figure 4–10*D*. The left ankle is carried into 10° more dorsiflexion during stance. Toe-off normally occurs at 61% of stride and is normally preceded by a strong push off into plantar flexion. Here, push-off is delayed on the left relative to the right. The amount of plantar flexion is also slightly decreased on the left, suggesting a weak push-off. Also note the greater standard deviation of the left ankle after push-off, indicating less consistency and control of movement. Also note the oscillations in the left ankle after heel strike, during the weight acceptance phase, which also indicate decreased control of movement.

during the gait cycle can implicate dysfunctional structures; abnormal patterns implicate weakness, spasticity, or joint hypomobility or hypermobility, and instability suggests proprioceptive deficits); (3) indicate abnormal stress on joints or soft tissues, either as the primary patient complaint or as a secondary result; (4) indicate inefficient use of energy transfer that may increase the energy cost of gait significantly (this fact is particularly important among elderly, rheumatoid, postpolio, and cerebral palsy patients, for whom energy is limited); (5) warn of safety risks, of reinjury, secondary microtrauma, or macrotrauma from a fall; (6) provide an understanding of gait to allow teaching of compensatory patterns when "normal" cannot be achieved, as after stroke, polio, or multiple sclerosis; and (7) guide surgery, such as for cerebral palsy,[45,46] assess orthotics,[47] prosthetic joints,[11,37] and prosthetic limbs.[48]

Gait evaluation may be undertaken in many ways; the Appendix reviews the most common methods and presents the advantages and disadvantages of each. The method of evaluation must be appropriate to the dysfunction, and the expense in time and money must be proportional to the value of data obtained. Although the new, high-technology analysis methods provide powerful tools, the daily observations of a skilled therapist are likely to remain of paramount importance.

SUMMARY

The goals of locomotion are to move the body forward in an energy-efficient manner while maintaining appropriate mechanical loads on body structures and tissues and maintaining adequate control for safety. These goals are achieved through the smooth alternation between the open and closed kinetic chain phases of gait. The leg functions in closed kinetic chain during stance: from initial contact through weight acceptance, midstance, and terminal stance (heel-off and toe-off). The leg functions open chain during swing.

The neurologic control of gait in humans is still poorly understood. In other animals, locomotion is normally controlled through complex interaction at all levels of the nervous system. In nonhumans, locomotion can be generated and modulated at the spinal level, whereas in humans, the upper levels of the central nervous system appear to play a more important role.

The determinants of gait provide a framework for understanding the essential biomechanical features of gait. The simplest gait pattern is compass gait (first determinant), with only hip flexion/extension. Although compass gait would achieve the goal of forward progression, walking would be inefficient, stressful to body structures, and unstable. The addition of pelvic rotation (second determinant) and pelvic obliquity (third determinant) decreases the vertical excursion of the center of gravity and thus improves efficiency and decreases stress to the body structures. Stance knee flexion (fourth determinant) and ankle dorsiflexion/plantar flexion (fifth determinant) facilitate the smooth transfer of energy up and down the kinetic chain and decrease the biomechanical stress of initial contact. Lateral shift of the center of gravity over the base of support (sixth determinant) further improves the stability and control of walking.

For walking to be efficient, energy must stored or transferred up and down the kinetic chain. Energy transfer occurs through four mechanisms: (1) pendulum, (2) joint force transfer, (3) whip, and (4) tendon (along with muscle). The potential energy lost as the body comes down into initial contact is absorbed through tendon and joint force mechanisms, minimizing stress to the body and redirecting downward energy into forward propulsion. Kinetic energy is then transformed back into potential energy as the body moves like an inverted pendulum over the stance leg during midstance. Energy generation by the muscles occurs primarily during the propulsion phase of push-off and is propagated down the kinetic chain, again through tendons and muscles and joint force transfer.

Even though swing is open chain, energy transfer along the kinetic chain remains important. To move the leg during early swing, energy is transferred proximal to distal through pendulum and whip mechanisms; during late swing, energy is transferred back up the kinetic chain to facilitate the forward progression of the body over the leg.

Joint movement results from all the forces acting on a body segment: muscle torque, gravity, joint reaction, and ground reaction forces. Kinematics is the study of joint and body segment position and motion, and kinetics is the study of the forces that produce movement. Walking is controlled by muscle activation, which harnesses gravity, joint, and ground reaction forces. Muscles may accelerate, stabilize, or decelerate joint motion. Muscles also transmit force or energy from one segment to another.

Physical therapists frequently treat individuals with abnormal gait patterns; injuries caused by poor control during walking; or pain caused by abnormal stress placed on muscles, tendons, and joints. Understanding the biomechanics of gait and interactions along the kinetic chain is essential for proper evaluation and treatment of lower extremity dysfunction in an ambulatory patient.

APPENDIX: METHODS OF GAIT ANALYSIS

Analysis of gait first requires observation or measurement. A variety of methods are available, ranging from simple visual observation to complex computer-assisted analysis of torques and three-dimensional joint motion. Each method offers advantages and disadvantages. Furthermore, each method facilitates collection of certain kinds of information.

VISUAL OBSERVATION

Visual observation, sometimes aided by a stopwatch and tape measure, is the most readily available. The human eye can observe and the human brain can analyze a tremendous amount of information. Even a relatively unskilled observer can qualitatively note the presence or absence of specific events, such as initial heel contact versus forefoot contact, Trendelenburg (hip drop), circumduction, and gross asymmetry. An experienced observer can note a whole wealth of information, including subtle asymmetry and complex interactions along the kinetic chain.[49] Using a stopwatch, one can measure cadence. With a walkway of known length, one can calculate velocity. With a tape measure and pressure-sensitive paper or wet paper towels, one can measure step and stride length.

The most obvious advantage to this low-technology gait analysis is that it requires no special equipment beyond, perhaps, a stopwatch and tape measure. Visual observation can be extremely time efficient because it does not require special setup. Both quantitative and qualitative information can be documented. Because several strides are viewed, the therapist can identify typical patterns and not be misled by the idiosyncrasies of an atypical stride.

The biggest disadvantage is that the amount and quality of information frequently depend on the expertise of the observer. Some of the information, because it is subjective and qualitative, may be difficult to document or to compare at future evaluations. Finally, because the human eye cannot focus on all body segments simultaneously and because different perspectives are necessary to obtain different types of information, thorough observation may require multiple walks. Patients in a great deal of pain or who fatigue easily may be unable to complete multiple walks. Step and stride length information can be cumbersome to measure without fancy equipment but can be obtained more easily with a gait evaluation mat that also measures temporal parameters.[50]

VIDEOTAPING

Videotaping and replay resolves several of the problems of simple observation. A videotape can be replayed, without fatigue, to allow the observer to focus on different segments of the kinetic chain. Video permits observation of subtle phenomena through slow motion and stop action. Videotapes can also be shown to the patient and can allow the patient to perceive and understand better his or her walking pattern. Videotapes can become part of a permanent record and can be viewed at a later date for comparison or for consultation with a gait specialist. Video cameras and videocassette recorders are relatively inexpensive and are readily available. They are portable, convenient, and easy to use. Videotaping is not time-consuming.

The primary disadvantages are lack of quantitative data, the importance of a skilled observer, and the need for at least some special equipment.

SIMPLISTIC DEVICES

Temporal and spatial parameters have been measured using anything from wet paper towels, to foot switches, to specially designed walkways that compute contact time and position.[51] These scalar measures are relatively simple to interpret. The automated systems also have the advantage that they can average multiple strides.

ADVANCED TECHNOLOGIC MEASUREMENT TOOLS

Before going into each of the more technologic gait analysis tools, it is worth considering advantages and disadvantages common to all. The advantages are fairly evident: objective, quantitative data with a high level of detail. Results can be quantitatively compared with normative data or with previous tests of the same individual.

The first common disadvantage is that all tools require elaborate, expensive equipment, which may cost upward of $100,000. Some, such as force plates, require special building construction to minimize artifactual noise. Most are not transportable and thus require the patient to travel to a specialized gait laboratory. Although some fully automated systems complete the analysis within 20 minutes of data collection, many systems require manual intervention for data processing and can require several hours of labor. This, along with the initial capital investment, can bring the expense beyond what is justifiable on a regular clinical basis. With the increased reliance on technology, the interpreter of the final data becomes further removed, and sources of error introduced by the technology itself pose a greater danger. Goniometers or markers, applied to the surface of the limb, may move over the underlying bony structure; external markers may not accurately represent true joint axes.[29,52,53,54] Kinetic data, because it relies on kinematic data input, also face the above-mentioned dangers. Furthermore, kinetic analysis relies on a linked segment model to compute joint torques, and these models continue to be refined.

Any legitimate gait laboratory conducts reliability and validity tests of their data to ensure internal consistency and to remove or compensate for sources of error. A review of the literature suggests, however, that not all clinicians are this thorough. Even for laboratories that are rigorous, the lack of standardized protocols means that each may generate different normative data,[55] and reports from one laboratory may not be directly comparable with those from another. The final data are in the form of complex wave forms, requiring skilled interpretation to extract the meaningful information; neural networks have also been used.[4] Although the final data have a high level of quantitative detail, it is only as valid as the initial data input, as reliable as the data processing, and as meaningful as the quality of interpretation.

Perhaps the oldest of electronic gait measurements is electrogoniometry, using hinged goniometers, some with multiple rotational axes to follow moving joint axes, fixed to the limbs. Wires run from the goniometers to a computer or recording device, where two-dimensional or three-dimensional motion is recorded. Electrogoniometers provide dynamic, quantitative measures of joint movement.[49,56] They can be used to compare quantitatively joint motion right versus left, before and after, and patient versus population norms. They are independent of the viewing axis. Disadvantages of electrogoniometry are primarily related to cumbersome equipment attached to the patient and trailing wires that may interfere with normal gait patterns. Other limitations, of kinematic data itself, are discussed with computerized video analysis.

Computerized video analysis resolved many of the problems of electrogoniometry, by eliminating the need for cumbersome equipment attached to the patient. Instead, small reflective or light emitting markers are fixed at the joint axes. Multiple video cameras record the gait cycle from different perspectives, and the recording is digitized either manually or by computer algorithm. The computer then generates either a two-dimensional or three-dimensional image, similar to a stick figure. This stick figure can then provide information about joint position, joint angle, segment angle, velocity, and acceleration. The computer can also compute energy, power, and center of gravity.

Advantages include a comprehensive supply of information about the body movement, in three dimensions if two or more cameras are used. The information is objective and quantitative and can be compared with later measurements or normative data. It requires only a single stride sample and so does not fatigue a patient.

Several of the disadvantages have been discussed previously. Additionally, kinematic data has been criticized as merely a descriptor of gait patterns, not as a source of information about the causes.[12] Therapists interested in restoring normal gait patterns are frequently interested in the causes of any abnormality, and a given set of kinematic data may have multiple combinations of causative factors.

Force plates can be used to measure the three-dimensional force components of the foot on the ground. When combined with kinematics, as described previously, and a linked segment model, a computer can calculate torques of all lower kinetic chain joints. As with the kinematic analysis, force plates provide objective, quantitative data. Because torques around joints are what cause movement, torque data provide information about the cause of any abnormal movement. Human movement is overdetermined; that is, several combinations of torque patterns can produce the same outcome in joint position and movement.[12] Force plates have been developed, which measure the force distribution across the foot.

Again, many of the disadvantages, shared with other technologic tools, have been discussed previously. The strength of kinetic analysis, in providing information about the cause of movement, also means that there is greater interindividual variability. That is, different individuals use different muscle combinations to achieve the same movement.[12] Consequently, comparing one individual with population norms is more difficult.

EMG analysis uses surface or indwelling electrodes to measure electrical activity of muscle directly. Data may be transferred to the computer either by wire or by telemetry. Data are processed, and several constructs can be analyzed. The most obvious advantage of EMG is that it provides direct information about actual muscle activation. This can identify firing pattern abnormalities and cocontraction. This, therefore, provides more direct information about neural control. EMG data are also objective and quantitative.

In addition to the common disadvantages, indwelling electrodes are invasive and may provide information that is so localized it is no longer representative. Surface electrodes provide information only as good as their placement and stability. Finally, because EMG data must be processed, different smoothing procedures may yield qualitatively different results (compare data of Kadaba, et al[29] to Winter[12]).

For each of the aforementioned measurement techniques, other than force plate kinetics, the patient can walk either freely or on a treadmill. Treadmills offer the advantage that they require less space and are easier to view from a static vantage point. Treadmills constrain the patient to the selected velocity and may obscure temporal asymmetries present in natural walking. Finally, some stride characteristics and even gait patterns may be different in treadmill walking.[44]

This list of methods is not exhaustive: Many other techniques and variations have been used. The method of gait analysis should be chosen not only by what equipment is available, but also by what the goals of evaluation are. Technical advances permit more objective and quantitative data collection. The use of elaborate technology, however, must be justified by the need for a measured parameter that cannot be observed or semiquantified by the therapist.[57] Although repeatability appears to be good for individual laboratories, caution should be taken in comparing an individual patient's data with normative data from another laboratory. Each clinic should determine their own normative data.

GLOSSARY

Phases of Gait

Acceleration: Early stage of swing, when the swing leg is accelerating. Also called initial swing.
Deceleration: End stage of swing, when the leg decelerates before initial contact. Also called terminal swing.
Heel contact: The normal initial contact of the foot at the beginning of a stride. Also called heel strike or initial contact. Initial contact also applies to pathologic gaits in which the heel does not strike first.
Midstance: When the body is directly over the stance foot.
Midswing: Middle of the swing phase.
Push-off: When the heel raises from the ground. Also called heel-off or terminal stance.
Toe-off: When the toe loses contact with the ground. Also called preswing.
Weight acceptance: When the foot makes full contact with the ground. Also, the time at which the contralateral foot reaches toe-off. Also called foot flat and loading response.

Mechanical Terms

Energy: Energy is equivalent to work; energy can be used to do work. Consequently, kinetic energy (1/2 mass × velocity^2), potential energy (mass × height × gravitational constant) and work (force × distance) all can be expressed in units of joule (equivalent to Nm or to Kg × m^2/s^2). Although these units are the same as for torque, work and energy are scalar variables and thus do not have direction.

Force: According to Newton's law, force (measured in Newtons, N), equals mass × acceleration (=kg × m/s²). Force is a vector, with direction as well as magnitude.

Moment: See torque.

Power: Power is work per unit time = energy per unit time = force × velocity. It is measured in watts (=N × m/s = kg × m²/s³) and is also scalar.

Torque: Moment and torque are the same: rotational force produced at a distance around a joint. Because torque is a force × distance, it is measured in Nm (=kg × m²/s²). Torque is the rotational equivalent of force; work, energy, and power also have rotational equivalents.

Vector: A value that has both magnitude and direction, as distinct from a scalar, which has only magnitude.

Work: See energy.

REFERENCES

1. Hill, AV: The dimensions of animals and their muscular dynamics. Science Progress 35:209–230, 1950.
2. Dawson, TJ and Taylor, CR: Energetic cost of locomotion in kangaroos. Nature 246:313–314, 1973.
3. Margaria, R: Sulla fisiologia e specialmente sul consumo energetico della marcia e della corsa a varie velocità ed inclinazioni del terreno. Atti Accad Naz Lincei Memorie, serie VI 7:299–368, 1938.
4. Holzreiter, SH and Köhle, ME: Assessment of gait patterns using neural networks. J Biomech 26:645–651, 1993.
5. Winter, DA: Energy generation and absorption at the ankle and knee during fast, natural and slow cadences. Clin Orthop Rel Res 175:147–154, 1983.
6. Kandel, ER and Schwartz, JH: Principles of Neural Science. Elsevier, New York, 1981, pp 316–321.
7. Grillner, S: Neural control of vertebrate locomotion—central mechanisms and reflex interaction with special reference to the cat. In Barnes, WJP and Gladden, MH, eds: Feedback and Motor Control in Invertebrates and Vertebrates. Croom Helm, Dover, NH, 1984, pp 35–56.
8. Grillner, S: Control of locomotion in bipeds, tetrapods and fish. In Brookhart, JM and Mountcastle, VB, eds: Handbook of Physiology. American Physiological Society, Bethesda, 1981, pp 1179–1236.
9. Dietz, V: Afferent and efferent control of posture and gait. In Bles, W and Brandt, T, eds: Disorders of Posture and Gait. Elsevier, New York, 1986, pp 69–81.
10. Quintern, J, Berger, W, and Dietz, V: Afferent control of posture and gait. In Gantchev, GN, Dimitrov, B, and Gatev, P, eds: Motor Control. Plenum Press, New York, 1987, pp 135–140.
11. Berman, AT, Quinn, RH, and Zarro, VJ: Quantitative gait analysis in unilateral and bilateral total hip replacements. Arch Phys Med Rehabil 72:190–194, 1991.
12. Winter, DA: The Biomechanics and Motor Control of Human Gait: Normal, Elderly and Pathological, 2nd ed, University of Waterloo Press, Waterloo, Ontario, 1991.
13. Saunders, JB, Inman, VT, and Eberhart, HD: The major determinants in normal and pathological gait. J Bone Joint Surg (Am) 35:543–558, 1953.
14. Inman, VT, Ralston, HJ, and Todd, F: Human Walking. Williams & Wilkins, Baltimore, 1981.
15. Stokes, VP, Anderson, C, and Forssberg, H: Rotational and translational movement features of the pelvis during adult human locomotion. J Biomech 22:43–50, 1989.
16. Cavanagh, PR, Rogers, MM, and Ilboshi, A: Pressure distribution under symptom-free feet during bare-foot standing. Foot Ankle 7:262–276, 1987.
17. Slocum, MDB and Bowerman, W: The biomechanics of running. Clin Orthop Rel Res 23:39–45, 1962.
18. MacKinnon, CD and Winter, DA: Control of whole body balance in the frontal plane during human walking. J Biomech 26:633–644, 1993.
19. McMahon, TA: Muscles, Reflexes, and Locomotion. Princeton University Press, Princeton, 1984.
20. Holt, KG, Hamill, J, and Andres, RO: Predicting the minimal energy costs of human walking. Med Sci Sports Exerc 23:491–498, 1991.
21. Margaria, R: Biomechanics and Energetics of Muscular Exercise. Clarendon Press, Oxford, 1976.
22. Alexander, RM: Energy-saving mechanisms in walking and running. J Exp Biol 160:55–69, 1991.
23. Olney, SJ, Jackson, VG, and George, SR: Gait re-education guidelines for stroke patients with hemiplegia using mechanical energy and power analysis. Physiother Can 40:242–248, 1988.
24. Caldwell, GE and Forrester, LW: Estimates of mechanical work and energy transfers: Demonstration of a rigid body power model of the recovery leg in gait. Med Sci Sports Exerc 24:1396–1412, 1992.
25. Dillingham, TR, Lehmann, JF, and Price, R: Effect of lower limb on body propulsion. Arch Phys Med Rehabil 73:647–651, 1992.

26. Jacobs, R and van Ingen Schenau, GJ: Intermuscular coordination in a sprint push-off. J Biomech 25:953–965, 1992.
27. Gleim, GW, Statchenfeld, NS, and Nicholas, JA: The influence of flexibility on the economy of walking and jogging. J Orthop Res 8:814–823, 1990.
28. Ker, RF, Bennett, MB, Bibby, SR, et al: The spring in the arch of the human foot. Nature 325:147–149, 1987.
29. Kadaba, MP, Ramakrishnan, HK, and Wootten, ME: Measurement of lower extremity kinematics during level walking. J Orthop Res 8:383–392, 1990.
30. Lafortune, MA, Cavanagh, PR, Sommer, HJ, and Kalenak, A: Three-dimensional kinematics of the human knee during walking. J Biomech 25:347–357, 1992.
31. Putnam, CA: A segment interaction analysis of proximal-to-distal sequential segmental motion patterns. Med Sci Sports Exerc 23:130–144, 1991.
32. Williams, KR: Biomechanics of running. In Terjung, R, ed: Exercise and Sports Science Reviews. MacMillan, New York, 1985, pp. 389–401.
33. Dykyj, D: Anatomy of motion. Clin Podiat Med Surg 5:477–490, 1988.
34. Mann, RA: Biomechanics of running. In Mack, RP, ed: Symposium on the Foot and Leg in Running Sports. St. Louis, CV Mosby, 1982, pp. 1–29.
35. Dillman, CJ: Kinematic analysis of running. Exerc Sports Sci Rev 3:193–217, 1975.
36. Williams, KR, Cavanagh, PR, and Ziff, JL: Biomechanical studies of elite female distance runners. Int J Sports Med 8:107–118, 1987.
37. Ilde, H and Yamamuro, T: Kinetic analysis of the center of gravity of the human body in normal and pathological gaits. J Biomech 20:987–995, 1987.
38. Begg, RK, Wytch, R, and Major, RE: A microcomputer-based video vector system for clinical gait analysis. J Biomed Eng 12:383–388, 1990.
39. Ounpuu, S, Gage, JR, and Davis, RB: Three-dimensional lower extremity joint kinetics in normal pediatric gait. J Pediatr Orthop 11:341–349, 1991.
40. Blanke, DJ and Hageman, PA: Comparison of gait of young men and elderly men. Phys Ther 69:144–148, 1989.
41. Winter, DA, Patia, AE, Frank, JS, and Walt, SE: Biomechanical walking pattern changes in the fit and healthy elderly. Phys Ther 70:340–347, 1990.
42. Kaneko, M, Morimoto, Y, Kimura, M, et al: A kinematic analysis of walking and physical fitness testing in elderly women. Can J Sport Sci 16:223–228, 1991.
43. Gundersen, LA, Valle, DR, Barr, AE, et al: Bilateral analysis of the knee and ankle during gait: An examination of the relationship between lateral dominance and symmetry. Phys Ther 69:640–650, 1989.
44. Murray, MP, Spurr, GB, Sepic, SB, et al: Treadmill vs. floor walking: Kinematics, electromyogram, and heart rate. J Appl Physiol 59:87–91, 1985.
45. Patrick, J: Gait laboratory investigations to assist decision making. Br J Hosp Med 45:35–37, 1991.
46. Lee, EH, Goh, JCH, and Bose, K: Value of gait analysis in the assessment of surgery in cerebral palsy. Arch Phys Med Rehabil 73:642–646, 1992.
47. McCulloch, MU, Brunt, D, and Vander Linden, D: The effect of foot orthotics and gait velocity on lower limb kinematics and temporal events of stance. J Orthop Sports Phys Ther 17:2–10, 1993.
48. Colborne, GR, Naumann, S, Longmuir, PE, and Berbrayer, D: Analysis of mechanical and metabolic factors in the gait of congenital below knee amputees. Am J Phys Med Rehabil 71:272–278, 1992.
49. Gronley, JK and Perry, J: Gait analysis techniques. Phys Ther 64:1831–1838, 1984.
50. Berman, AT, Zarro, VJ, Bosacco, SJ, and Israelite, C: Quantitative gait analysis after unilateral or bilateral total knee replacement. J Bone Joint Surg (Am) 69:1340–1345, 1987.
51. Friedman, LW: Methods of gait evaluation. Rehabilitation 29:16–18, 1990.
52. White, SC, Yack, HJ, and Winter, DA: A three-dimensional musculoskeletal model for gait analysis: Anatomical variability estimates. J Biomech 22:885–893, 1989.
53. DeLuzzio, KJ, Wyss, UP, Li, J, and Costigan, PA: A procedure to validate three-dimensional motion assessment systems. J Biomech 26:753–759, 1993.
54. Clayton, HM: Advances in motion analysis. Vet Clin North Am Equine Pract 7:365–382, 1991.
55. Shiavi, R: Factors in automated gait evaluation. IEEE Eng Med Biol Mag 29–33, 1988.
56. Chao, EY: Justification of triaxial goniometer for the measurement of joint rotation. J Biomech 13:989–1006, 1980.
57. Davis, RB III: Clinical gait analysis. IEEE Eng Med Biol Mag 35–40, 1988.

CHAPTER **5**

Clinical Assessment
of the Foot

R. Luke Bordelon, MD

This chapter addresses assessment of the foot from a clinical standpoint. It deals with the foot as a functional unit. The importance of the foot as a functional unit is obvious when one realizes that its function is what has allowed humans to walk upright on two feet.[1-5] Laitman and Jaffe[3] observe that the three things that distinguish humans from other primates are the cerebral cortex, the vocal cords, and the lower extremity and foot. Clinicians need to understand that the foot is a special organ.

During the early part of the stance phase, the foot is supple enough to allow adaptation to the contour of the ground and to maintain balance. During the latter part of stance phase, it converts to a rigid lever for push-off (Fig. 5–1). This motion is obligatory during the gait cycle, being initiated by changes in position of the talocalcaneal and the midtarsal joints of the foot, but it is not dependent on muscle action. Rather, changes in the position of the foot occurring during the gait cycle dictate this motion. Support of the foot and conversion of the foot from a supple to a rigid structure for push-off depend on the axes of motion of the joints of the foot and ankle, the shapes of bones, and the tension of the ligaments. When these structures are normal, the foot supports the body and allows bipedal gait with conversion of the foot from the supple to the rigid position at a proper time during the gait cycle.[2,7-9]

NORMAL FOOT

The normal foot is defined as one that is supple during the early stance phase and converts to a rigid lever during push-off, in accordance with the obligatory motions of unrestrained gait.[2,7-9] The foot functions in two modes. The first is

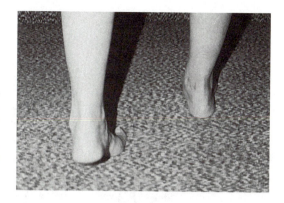

FIGURE 5–1. Demonstration of the changes that occur in the foot during the act of walking. The foot everts to become supple during the early part of stance phase in order to adapt to the ground (as shown by the right foot) and converts to a rigid lever for push-off by the end of stance phase (as shown by the left foot).

non–weight bearing, during which the muscles of the foot move it freely in space. The second is the weight-bearing mode, when the foot is fixed to the floor by the ground reaction and the body moves over the foot.[5,20] To understand the function of the foot, one must understand the normal components of the foot and their motions. This section discusses the clinical evaluation of the foot in both the non–weight-bearing and weight-bearing modes.

Clinical Evaluation: Non–Weight Bearing

The foot examination is performed initially with the foot bearing no weight (Fig. 5–2). The neutral position of the subtalar joint is identified as the position in which the talus and the navicular are congruous, and it is the midpoint of function of the talonavicular joint.[5,10,11] The neutral position is identified by palpating the talonavicular and moving the loaded foot into adduction and inversion and abduction and eversion while applying ample pressure against the fourth and fifth metatarsal bones

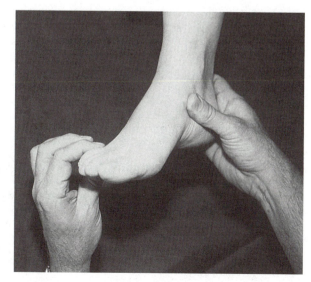

FIGURE 5–2. Examination of placement of the foot in the neutral position by palpating the talonavicular joint with the right thumb and grasping the fourth and fifth metatarsal heads to load and move the foot to ascertain the midpoint of function of the talonavicular joint.

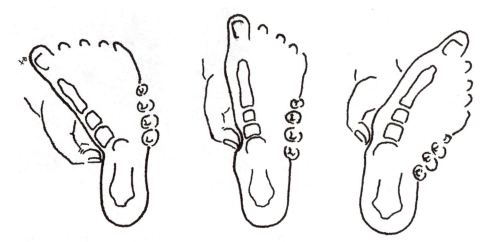

FIGURE 5–3. Demonstration of neutral position of talonavicular joint determined by palpating the relationship of the navicular and the talus. Middle drawing shows a foot with the talonavicular joint congruous, indicating that this is the midposition of function of the subtalar joint complex. (Reprinted with permission from Clinical Orthopedics.)

(Fig. 5–3). The point at which the talus and the navicular bones are congruous is the midpoint of function of the foot, or the neutral position.[2,5,7,8,10,11]

All examinations and measurements of the foot and ankle are performed with the neutral position as the initial reference point (Table 5–1). The foot components are examined first in passive motion, then in active motion.

PASSIVE RANGE OF MOTION

With the foot in the neutral position, passive motion of the foot reveals that, in the transverse plane, the foot can be moved into adduction and abduction. The range of adduction is generally twice that of abduction, approximately 30° and 15°, respectively (Fig. 5–4). The forefoot is moved passively through inversion and eversion into varus and valgus positions. This motion generally ranges from 25° of inversion into varus position of 25° of eversion into valgus position.[2,7]

The heel is then grasped and moved in eversion and inversion. The motion of inversion is generally twice that of eversion, about 20° of inversion and 10° of eversion, and a definite soft tissue end point at the extreme of eversion.[2,5,7]

TABLE 5–1 Elements of Non–Weight-Bearing Assessment

Neutral position subtalar joint: congruous position of talus and navicular, which is determined by palpation of talus

Forefoot transverse plane movement: abduction 30°, adduction 15°

Forefoot frontal plane movement: inversion 25°, eversion 25°

Rearfoot frontal plane movement: inversion 20°, eversion 10°

Position of the first metatarsal in relationship to the lateral four metatarsals

First metatarsal mobility in sagittal plane: dorsiflexion 20°, plantar flexion 20°

Open kinetic chain supination, pronation, adduction, abduction, inversion, eversion, plantar flexion, dorsiflexion

Ankle joint sagittal joint: dorsiflexion 20°, plantar flexion 50° with the knee flexed and extended

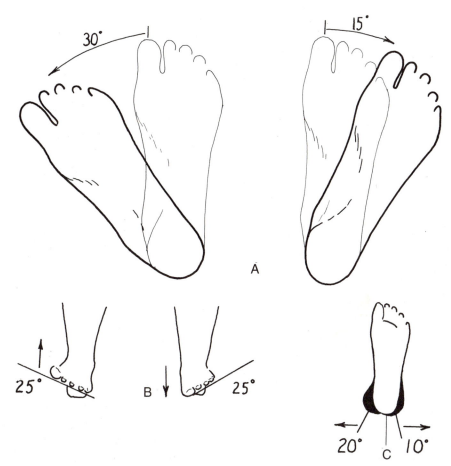

FIGURE 5–4. Passive motion of the normal foot. (*A*) Passive motion in the transverse plane of abduction and adduction usually demonstrates twice as much adduction as abduction with about 30° of adduction and 15° of abduction. (*B*) Passive motion of the forefoot in the frontal plane demonstrates 25° of inversion and 25° of eversion to position of maximum varus and valgus of the forefoot. (*C*) Passive motion of the heel generally demonstrates 20° of inversion and 10° of eversion with a definite end point at the end of eversion.

The position of the first metatarsal bone is then evaluated. This metatarsal should be evaluated first because the motion of the medial segment (the first metatarsal and first cuneiform) has a different range of motion than the lateral four metatarsal bones.[2,7,5,10] The first metatarsal is examined by placing a thumb beneath the metatarsal head and the other thumb beneath the lateral four metatarsal heads (Fig. 5–5). Passive motion of the first metatarsal bone is assessed by pushing the metatarsal bones up and then down. Passive motion should produce equal movement of the first metatarsal bone in dorsiflexion and plantar flexion (Fig. 5–6). Twenty degrees of first metatarsal dorsiflexion and 20° of plantar flexion are considered to be within normal limits.

ACTIVE RANGE OF MOTION

Active motion of the foot and ankle in the non–weight-bearing position is then performed (Fig. 5–7). The motions of the subtalar joint in supination are adduction,

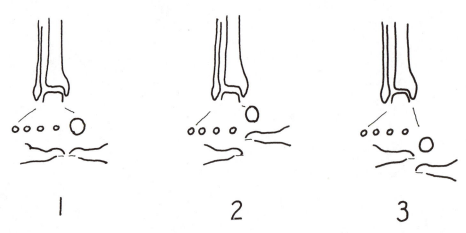

FIGURE 5-5. Position of the first metatarsal is determined by placing thumb under first metatarsal and lateral four metatarsals and observing level: (1) normal position; (2) dorsiflexed position; and (3) plantar flexed position.

inversion, and plantar flexion. The motion of the subtalar joint in pronation are abduction, eversion, and dorsiflexion. The supination and pronation movements are triplanar because of the axes of motion (Fig. 5–7).[2,5,7,10] Active range of motion of the ankle joint is determined next. Normal motion is from 20° of dorsiflexion to 50° of plantar flexion, measured with the knee flexed and extended.[12]

The muscles are then examined with the foot in the non–weight-bearing position. They are tested to determine the muscle strength and the motion produced by the individual contraction of each muscle group.[13] Muscle testing of the extrinsic foot muscles can be divided into anterior, posterior, medial, and lateral compartments. In testing the muscles, it is especially important to determine whether there is normal flexibility of the triceps sural muscle group or whether there is limitation of motion by the gastrocnemius-soleus musculotendinous unit.

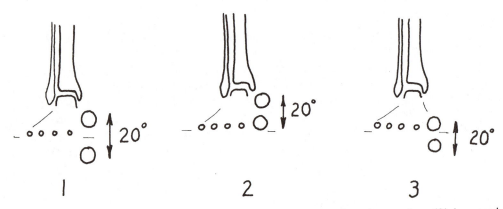

FIGURE 5-6. Passive motion of the first metatarsal: (1) normal passive motion; (2) increased dorsal motion with decreased plantar motion; and (3) increased plantar motion with decreased dorsal motion.

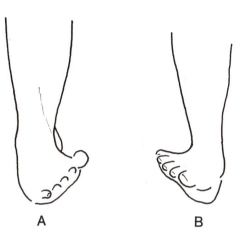

FIGURE 5–7. Active motion of the subtalar joint, non–weight-bearing, is a triplanar motion. (*A*) Supination is active triplanar motion of the subtalar joint complex with the foot moving into adduction, inversion, and plantar flexion. (*B*) Pronation is an active triplanar motion of the subtalar joint with the foot moving into abduction, eversion, and dorsiflexion.

A   B

Clinical Evaluation: Weight Bearing

With the patient standing, the clinician ascertains the relationship of the foot and ankle to the remainder of the lower extremity and the body by assessing the position of the leg, knee, and thigh along with motions of the hip and knee (Table 5–2). Leg lengths should be measured through clinical assessment or by radiographs. When the normal foot is examined while standing in the neutral position, the weight-bearing line passing through the superior iliac spine of the pelvis and the patella also passes through the second metatarsal bone. The forefoot is perpendicular to the tibia in the frontal plane. The heel is in line with the tibia in the frontal plane (Fig. 5–8). The patient's gait is observed next (Table 5–3). With a normal foot and gait, the heel everts during the early part of stance phase and the foot becomes supple. Then the foot converts to a rigid lever for push-off in the later part of stance phase (Fig. 5–1). Evaluation of gait is discussed in detail in Chapter 7.

The position of the components of the foot as well as their motion and structure is the most important consideration in the biomechanical changes of the foot from the supple to the rigid position during gait. One must certainly consider, however, the associated effects of the muscles as in Chapter 1 and should assess the muscle function in both the weight-bearing and non–weight-bearing modes to ascertain whether there is any specific abnormal muscle function that has produced an aberration of gait. For the purpose of this discussion, it is assumed that the muscles are functioning within normal limits, as is generally the clinical situation except for gastrocnemius-soleus muscle tightness, which should have been ascertained during the physical examination and testing of the ankle motion.

TABLE 5–2 Weight-Bearing Assessment

Subtalar joint neutral position
Weight-bearing line through superior iliac spine of the pelvis, patella, and second metatarsal
Forefoot perpendicular to the tibia in the frontal plane
Heel in line with the tibia in the frontal plane, which can be observed from a posterior view

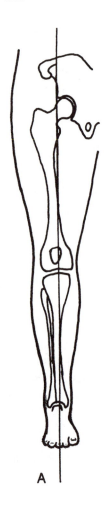

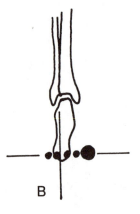

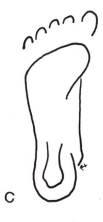

FIGURE 5–8. The position of the components of the normal foot in the neutral position. (*A*) Weight-bearing line through the anterior superior iliac spine and patella passes through the second metatarsal. (*B*) The forefoot is perpendicular to the leg. (*C*) The heel is in line with the tibia.

TABLE 5–3 Gait Assessment During Stance Phase

Heel contact to weight acceptance (early midstance): pronation, shock absorption, torque conversion, balance maintenance, adjust to terrain

Midstance or neutral position of subtalar joint

Late midstance to push-off: supination, rigid lever, propulsion, pulleys established for extrinsic muscles of the foot and ankle

THE ABNORMAL FOOT

The abnormal foot is defined as a foot presenting some aberration that does not have the position, motion, or function of the normal foot described previously. The two types of abnormal foot are pes planus and pes cavus (Fig. 5–9). Flatfoot, or pes planus, is an abnormality that usually tends to make the foot supple (or to collapse) because it lacks supination sufficient to form a rigid lever during push-off in gait.

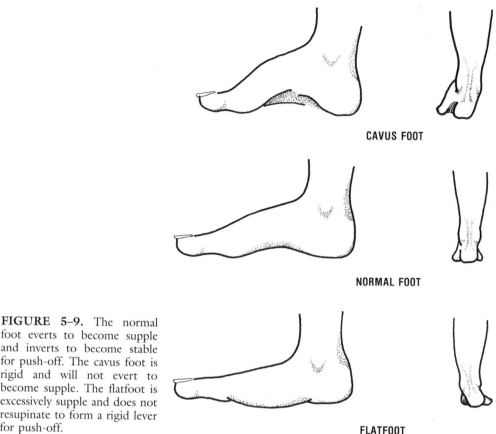

CAVUS FOOT

NORMAL FOOT

FIGURE 5–9. The normal foot everts to become supple and inverts to become stable for push-off. The cavus foot is rigid and will not evert to become supple. The flatfoot is excessively supple and does not resupinate to form a rigid lever for push-off.

FLATFOOT

Conversely, pes cavus is an abnormality in which the foot is rigid and does not become supple on weight bearing.[2,7–9]

Flatfoot Deformity

Examination of a flatfoot with the talonavicular joint in the neutral position generally reveals that the positions of the foot components are (1) abduction of the forefoot in relation to the weight-bearing line in the transverse plane; (2) varus, or inversion, of the forefoot in the frontal plane; and (3) valgus, or eversion, of the heel in the frontal plane (Fig. 5–10).[2,7,9]

Any one of these abnormalities may produce a flatfoot deformity with ambulation, but generally (and especially if the flatfoot deformity is severe) all three are present; that is, forefoot abduction in weight bearing, forefoot varus in non–weight bearing, and heel valgus in standing.

On examination of a flatfoot for motion abduction of the forefoot, forefoot inversion, and heel eversion are generally all increased and the opposite motions are decreased (Fig. 5–11). In a person with flatfoot, the first metatarsal bone is generally dorsiflexed or has an unusually wide range of dorsiflexion motion.

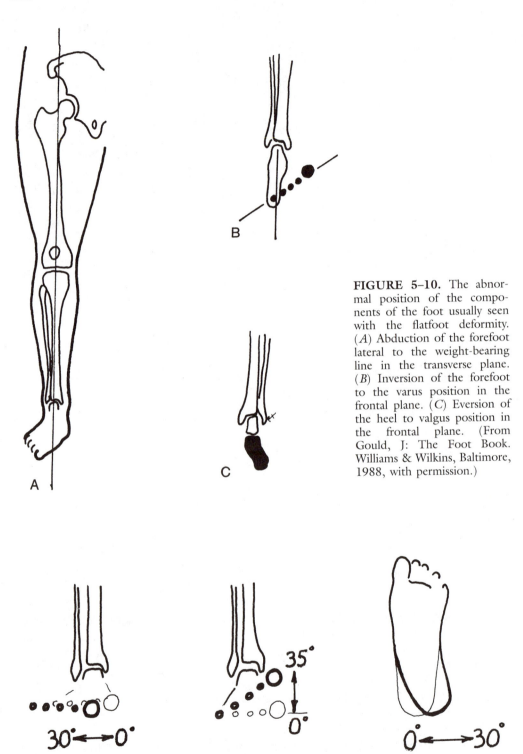

FIGURE 5–10. The abnormal position of the components of the foot usually seen with the flatfoot deformity. (*A*) Abduction of the forefoot lateral to the weight-bearing line in the transverse plane. (*B*) Inversion of the forefoot to the varus position in the frontal plane. (*C*) Eversion of the heel to valgus position in the frontal plane. (From Gould, J: The Foot Book. Williams & Wilkins, Baltimore, 1988, with permission.)

FIGURE 5–11. Depiction of usual motion with flatfoot deformity. Increased abduction motion of the forefoot in the transverse plane (*left*). Increased inversion motion of the forefoot in the frontal plane (*middle*). Increased eversion of the heel in the frontal plane (*right*).

Pes Cavus

Examination of the cavus foot with the talonavicular joint in the neutral position generally reveals three components: (1) adduction of the forefoot relative to the weight-bearing line in the transverse plane; (2) forefoot valgus in the frontal plane; and (3) heel varus in the frontal plane (Fig. 5–12). The first metatarsal bone is generally plantar flexed and has an increased range of plantar flexion.[2,7,9]

Generally, movement in the cavus foot is characterized by increased forefoot adduction in the transverse plane, increased forefoot eversion, and increased heel inversion. Relative to these deformities, the opposite movements are decreased (Fig. 5–13). The more severe the condition, the greater the degree of deformity. It is important to understand that only one of these structural deficits may produce foot cavus when walking, but generally in a severely abnormal foot all of these deformities are present. With ambulation, the cavus foot is rigid because it does not pronate to unlock the midfoot and subtalar joint, so they may become supple. Therefore, the foot cannot adapt to the ground and cushion the impact.

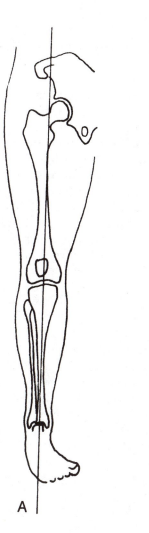
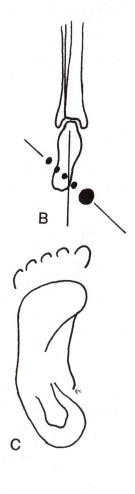

FIGURE 5–12. Position of the components of the foot usually seen with a cavus deformity. (*A*) Forefoot is adducted in the transverse plane relative to the weight-bearing line. (*B*) The forefoot is everted to the valgus position in the frontal plane. (*C*) The heel is inverted to the varus position in the frontal plane.

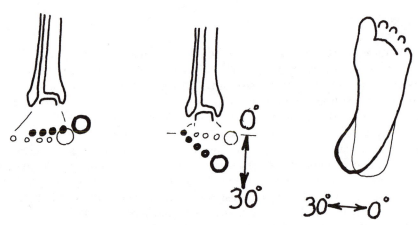

FIGURE 5–13. Depiction of usual motion of cavus foot. Increased adduction of the forefoot in the transverse plane (*left*). The forefoot in the frontal plane (*middle*). Increased inversion motion of the heel (*right*).

ORTHOTICS AND SURGICAL CONSIDERATIONS

If the physical examination reveals normal position and motion of the components of the foot and normal muscle function, the foot should function in a normal manner because there is no structural or gait aberration. If pain is present in a foot of this type, the examiner should search for an intrinsic cause, such as primary tendinitis or interdigital neuroma. Alternatively, something extrinsic may produce an abnormality of the foot: either through the loss of muscle function or through secondary deformities resulting from loss of muscle function. Such a situation occurs with the rupture of the posterior tibial tendon: The foot cannot supinate. Ultimately the foot develops secondary fixed deformities of general forefoot abduction in the transverse plane, varus in the frontal plane, and heel valgus in the frontal plane. In a situation in which the pain is caused by an arthritic joint, such as the first metatarsal cuneiform or talonavicular, pain may limit the joint range of motion. Limitations of joint motion and gait abnormalities depend on how that joint functions during the gait cycle.[2]

Orthotic Devices

An orthotic device is defined as a device that assists the foot to function in a more normal manner.[14,15] Following the clinical classification and considering the types of orthotics used, one can see that the normal foot with normal motion does not need an orthotic device. For flatfoot that is supple and does not invert to become rigid during the late phase of weight bearing, a rigid orthotic is used to support the foot and allow it to resupinate.[6] A cavus foot that is rigid and does not evert to become supple during the early phase of weight bearing requires an orthotic that is soft and absorbs shock while increasing the weight-bearing area.[2] A more detailed biomechanical evaluation of the foot and ankle and biomechanical orthotic prescriptions are discussed in Chapters 7 and 10.

Surgical Treatment of Flatfoot Deformity

In flatfoot that has a single causal component, the treatment may be directed toward correcting that component. For example, flatfoot produced solely by heel valgus can be corrected by performing osteotomy of the os calcis to bring it into the proper position so that the normal subtalar passive motion of the heel is 10° of eversion to 20° of inversion. If the first metatarsal bone is dorsiflexed, a plantar flexion osteotomy may be performed. If the foot is abducted and the forefoot is in varus, the surgeon can bring the forefoot out of abduction or shorten the medial column (or both) to correct these deformities. The surgery involves an opening wedge osteotomy of the cuboid bone with shortening of the navicular bone, closing wedge osteotomy and fusion of the navicular cuneiform joint, or lengthening of the anterior portion of the os calcis between the anterior and middle facets.[6]

All foot components must be assessed before performing surgery for flatfoot if correction of the deformity is to be approached properly. For instance, if the problem is uncompensated forefoot varus with inability of the heel to evert and a varus osteotomy of the heel is performed, the patient may have even greater difficulty because of increased uncompensated forefoot varus.

Surgical Treatment of Pes Cavus

The pes cavus foot is evaluated to see if there is a single specific deformity. If there is, it is corrected. If the first metatarsal is plantar flexed, producing the cavus deformity as well as abnormal gait, a dorsiflexion osteotomy of the first metatarsal bone, soft tissue release, or both are required to correct the problem. If the cavus deformity is the result of heel varus, a closing wedge osteotomy is necessary, which brings the motion of the subtalar joint to as close to normal as possible (20° of inversion and 10° of eversion). If the deformity is associated with or caused by adduction and valgus deformity of the forefoot, the lateral column is generally shortened by a closing wedge osteotomy of the cuboid, the anterior portion of the os calcis, or both. It is more difficult to correct the problem components of the rigid cavus foot than it is to correct the loose hypermobile flatfoot; however, the surgeon attempts to correct either deformity to produce as structurally normal a foot as possible without fusing any major joints. The mobility of the subtalar joint complex, which includes the subtalar and the midtarsal joints, must be maintained.[6]

SUMMARY

This chapter has covered the assessment of the foot from a clinical standpoint, looking at the foot as a functional organ that developed to allow humans to walk with a bipedal gait. The normal foot converts from the supple position during the early part of stance phase to a rigid position during the latter part.

The appearance and motion of the foot with normal parameters for function have been presented. Use of orthotics and surgical considerations based on these parameters are presented, to allow the clinical practitioner to produce a more normally functional foot.

The components of the flatfoot deformity are abduction of the forefoot, varus or inversion of the forefoot, and valgus or eversion of the heel. The first metatarsal bone is dorsiflexed and generally limited in plantar flexion.

The components of the pes cavus deformity are adduction of the forefoot, valgus or eversion of the forefoot, and varus or inversion of the heel. The position of the first metatarsal bone is generally plantar flexed and rigid.

REFERENCES

1. Bordelon, RL: Foot first: Evolution of man. Foot Ankle 8:125–126, 1987.
2. Bordelon, RL: Surgical and Conservative Foot Care. Charles B. Slack, Thorofare, NJ, 1988.
3. Laitman, JT and Jaffe, WL: A review of current concepts on the evolution of the human foot. Foot Ankle 2:284, 1982.
4. Leakey, M: Footprints in the ashes of time. National Geographic 446:446–455, 1979.
5. Root, M, et al: Biomechanical Examination of the Foot, Vol I. Clinical Biomechanics Corporation, 1971.
6. Weaver, K: The search for our ancestors. National Geographic 561, 1985.
7. Gould, J: The Foot Book. Williams & Wilkins, Baltimore, 1988.
8. Bordelon, RL: Hypermobile flatfoot in children: Comprehension, evaluation and treatment. Clin Orthop 181:7, 1983.
9. Bordelon, RL: Management of disorders of the forefoot and toenails associated with running. Clin Sports Med 4:4, 1985.
10. Sgarlato, T: A Compendium of Podiatric Biomechanics. California College of Podiatric Medicine, Los Angeles, 1971.
11. Bordelon, RL: Correction of hypermobile flatfoot in children by molded inserts. Foot Ankle 1:143, 1980.
12. American Academy of Orthopaedic Surgeons: Joint Motion-Method of Measuring and Recording, 1965.
13. Goss, CM: Gray's Anatomy. American ed 29. Lea & Febiger, Philadelphia, 1972.
14. Jahss, MH: Atlas of Orthotics: Biomechanical Principles and Applications. CV Mosby, St. Louis, 1975.
15. Jahss, M: Disorders of the Foot. Vol I. WB Saunders, Philadelphia, 1982, pp 1–36.

CHAPTER 6

Biomechanical Radiographic Evaluation*

George Vito, DPM
Stanley Kalish, DPM

This chapter presents basic radiographic techniques used to evaluate foot deformities and injuries. It does not include all radiographic techniques. Rather it is a short synopsis of basic views, commonly performed angular measurements, and the deformities revealed by the described measurements.

It must be remembered that radiographs are never the sole means of making a diagnosis but are instead just one type of finding that must be integrated with many others to arrive at a pertinent clinical assessment or diagnosis.

The most common clinical views of a foot include the dorsoplantar, lateral, medial, lateral oblique, medial oblique, and the axial sesamoidal.[1-3] Radiographs can be termed either projections or views. Projections refer to the way in which the x-ray generator "sees" the body part to be exposed. The views described are the way in which the film "sees" the part to be exposed.[1] For example, a medial oblique *view* can be the same as a lateral oblique *projection*. To avoid confusion, however, all descriptions in this chapter are presented as projections.

PROJECTIONS

The *dorsoplantar projection* is usually taken with the patient in a weight-bearing or (if the patient is injured) recumbent position. In a weight-bearing position, both feet may be radiographed together, or individually. The generator is positioned 15° from

---

*The authors thank Michael Holvick, DPM for his assistance with this chapter.

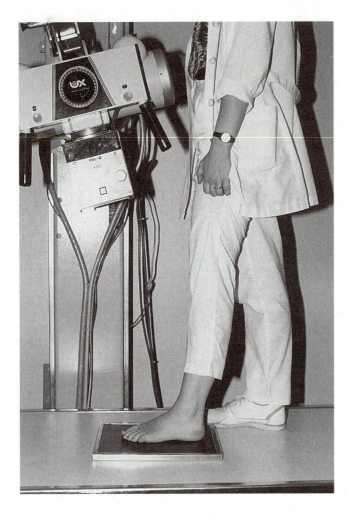

FIGURE 6–1. The generator is positioned 15° from the vertical.

the vertical to ensure proper visualization of the tarsal joints without the generators being in the patient's abdomen (Fig. 6–1). With the patient recumbent, the foot is placed flat on the film, and the knee is flexed 45° with the generator placed perpendicular to the film (Fig. 6–2). With these projections, we are able to examine the transverse plane relationships of the midfoot area, the metatarsals, and the entire forefoot area. The anterior portion of the greater tarsus, Lisfranc's joint, all of the metatarsophalangeal joints, and the interphalangeal joints can be viewed (Fig. 6–3). The articulations and shapes of the navicular, the cuboid, the medial cuneiform bones, and (to a lesser extent) the middle and lateral cuneiform bones can also be evaluated from this projection.

The *lateral projection* is taken with the generator at a 90° angle to the foot.[1] The foot is positioned so that the medial side of the first metatarsal head and the medial side of the calcaneus are against the film. This projection can either be taken weight bearing (Fig. 6–4) or non–weight bearing and gives a proper demonstration of the talus and calcaneus (Fig. 6–5). Most of the cuboid can be seen, and less clearly, visualization of the navicular and the medial cuneiform is also possible. Figure 6–6 clear-

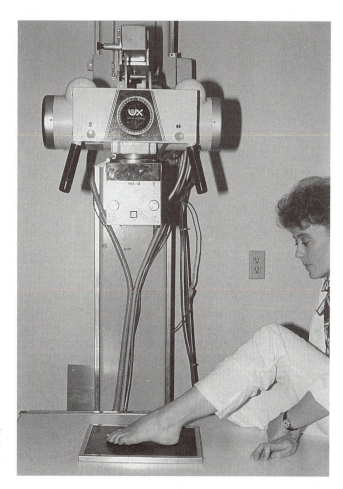

FIGURE 6–2. With the patient in a recumbent position, the knee is flexed at 45°, with the generator perpendicular to the film.

ly identifies the first and fifth metatarsals and the second through fourth metatarsals overlapping each other. The first digit is relatively visible also.

The *lateral oblique projection* is the most popular oblique projection used in podiatry, giving a slightly distorted and slightly magnified representation of most of the bones of the foot.[2] The patient stands on the film, which is angulated 45° from the central beam (Fig. 6–7). The digits, lesser tarsus, cuboid, fourth and fifth metatarsal articulations with the cuboid, and the metatarsals are clearly seen (Fig. 6–8).

The *medial oblique projection* is exactly the opposite of the lateral oblique projection. The patient stands on the film with the central beam angulated 25° from the vertical (Fig. 6–9). The digits, tibial sesamoid, first metatarsal, first cuneiform, navicular tuberosity, and medial calcaneus are seen (Fig. 6–10).

In the *axial sesamoid projection*, the patient stands with the digits against the film. The film holds the digits in extension. The patient first puts weight on the ball of the foot and then, keeping the digits against the film, raises the heel enough so that the central ray clears it (Fig. 6–11). The sesamoids, the cristae of the first metatarsal head, and the inferior aspect of the lesser metatarsals are visualized (Fig. 6–12).

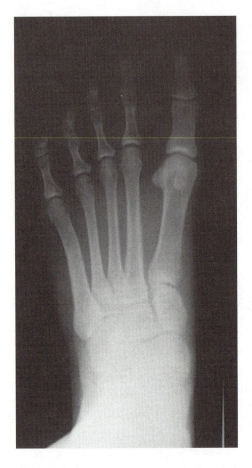

FIGURE 6–3. Dorsoplantar projection.

ANGULAR AND AXIAL RELATIONSHIPS OF THE DORSOPLANTAR PROJECTION

Longitudinal Axis of the Rearfoot

The longitudinal axis of the rearfoot bisects the posterior surface of the calcaneus and the distal anteromedial corner of the calcaneus. If the posterior surface of the calcaneus cannot be visualized, a line parallel to the lateral border of the calcaneus is constructed to represent the longitudinal axis of the rearfoot (Fig. 6–13).[1]

Longitudinal Axis of the Lesser Tarsus

The longitudinal axis of the lesser tarsus (talus, calcaneus, navicular, cuboid) is used to compare the position of the lesser tarsus with that of both the metatarsus and the greater tarsus. First, one must transect the lesser tarsus by locating the medial aspect of the talonavicular joint and the medial aspect of the joint between the first metatarsal and the first cuneiform.[1] The line that connects them is then bisected. Sec-

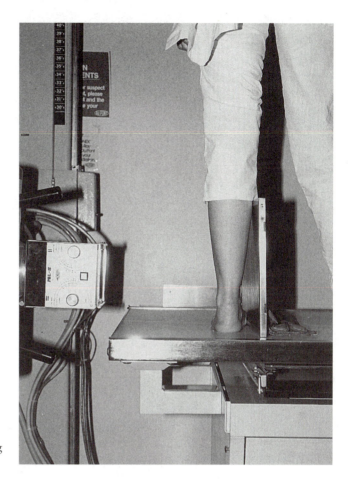

FIGURE 6–4. Weight-bearing lateral projection.

ond, the lateral aspect of the calcaneocuboid articulation and the lateral aspect of the base of the fifth metatarsal are identified. The line connecting them is bisected (Fig. 6–14). The two bisections should then be connected. A line perpendicular to this transection constructs the longitudinal axis of the lesser tarsus.

Longitudinal Axis of the Metatarsal Bones

The longitudinal axis of the metatarsal is constructed by bisecting the neck of the second metatarsal and the base end of the shaft of the second metatarsal. Connecting these two points gives the longitudinal axis of the metatarsals (Fig. 6–15).

Longitudinal Axis of the Digits

The longitudinal axis of the digits is constructed by bisecting the neck of the proximal phalanx of the second toe and the bisection of its base. Connecting these two points produces the longitudinal axis of the digits (Fig. 6–16).

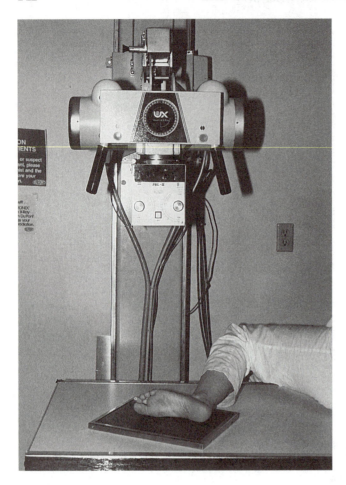

FIGURE 6–5. Non–weight-bearing lateral projection.

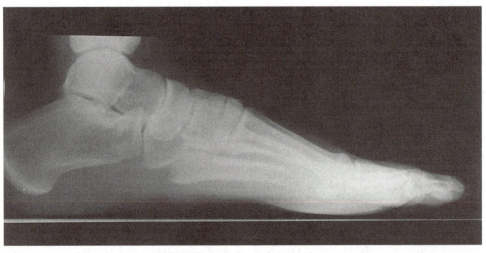

FIGURE 6–6. Lateral projection.

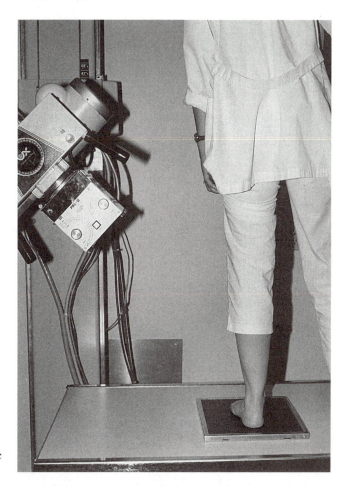

FIGURE 6–7. Lateral oblique projection.

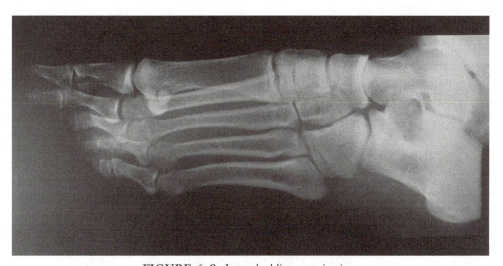

FIGURE 6–8. Lateral oblique projection.

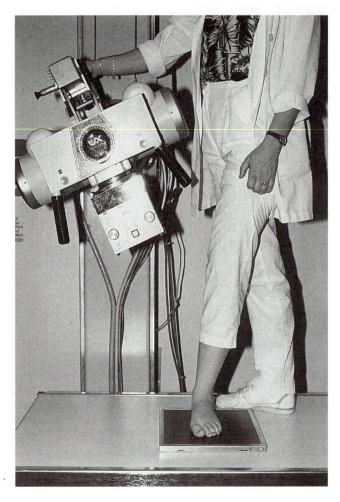

FIGURE 6–9. Medial oblique projection.

Talocalcaneal Angle

The talocalcaneal angle (Kite's angle) has long been used as an index of relative foot pronation and supination. This angle is formed by a line bisecting the head and neck of the talus (collum tali axis) and the longitudinal axis of the rearfoot (Fig. 6–17). The normal range of this angle is approximately 17° to 21°. The articular relationship between the navicular and the talus must also be visualized. Approximately 75% of the head of the talus should articulate with the navicular. Along with this relationship, the axis of the talus should run through the center of the first metatarsal (Fig. 6–18). On pronation, the axis runs medial to the first metatarsal, and on supination, it projects laterally.[1]

The talocalcaneal angle compares the pronation-supination of the rearfoot with that of the forefoot. If the rearfoot is maximally pronated, the forefoot compensates. Therefore, symptoms of overpronation are present in the forefoot; the same is true for supination. In cases of partial pronation of the rearfoot, however, if more pronation is

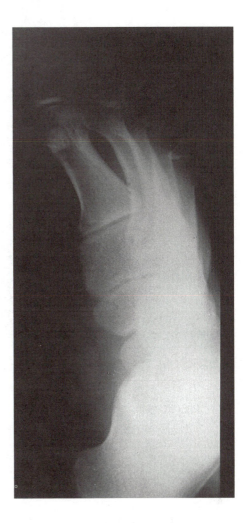

FIGURE 6–10. Medial oblique projection.

needed, the rearfoot accommodates. This deformity in the rearfoot can be corrected, either by posting the rearfoot with an orthotic or by surgery of the rearfoot. Further discussion of biomechanical orthotics appears in Chapter 10.

Cuboid Abduction Angle

The cuboid abduction angle is formed by a line representing the lateral aspect of the cuboid and the longitudinal axis of the rearfoot (Fig. 6–19). The normal range of this angle is 0° to 5°. When the angle is greater than 5°, pronation of the foot has occurred; however, when supination and adduction of the forefoot are seen, this angle may be less than 0°, as a negative value.[6] The angle is a reflection of the rearfoot. When the rearfoot is maximally pronated, the cuboid is abducted because of the forces exerted through the talonavicular and calcaneocuboid joints. When the foot is maximally supinated, the cuboid may be adducted. Therefore, correction of this defor-

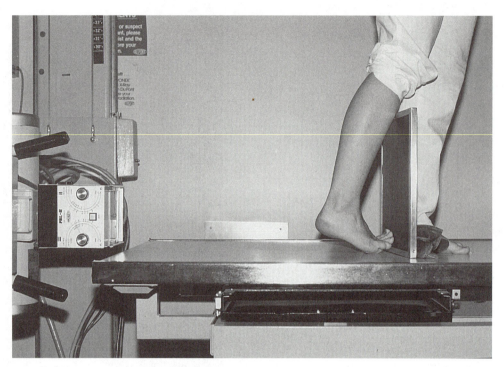

FIGURE 6–11. Axial sesamoid projection.

mity in the rearfoot is accomplished either with orthotic posting or by surgical intervention.

Talonavicular Angle

The talonavicular angle is constructed by using the collum tali axis and the transection of the lesser tarsus. The normal angular relationship should be between 60° and 80° (Fig. 6–20). An angle of less than 60° represents pronation, whereas an angle greater than 60° represents supination.[1] Once again, this relationship reflects rearfoot to midfoot accommodation; however, correction of the deformity occurs with forefoot posting of an orthotic to allow limited motion of the talonavicular articulation. If correction cannot be accomplished with an orthotic, fusion of the talonavicular joint may be considered.

Metatarsus Adductus Angle

The metatarsus adductus angle is formed by the intersection of the longitudinal axis of the metatarsus and the longitudinal axis of the lesser tarsus (Fig. 6–21). The normal range is between 6° and 10°.[1] If the rearfoot is in a maximally supinated position, without midfoot and forefoot compensation, the forefoot is in an adducted posi-

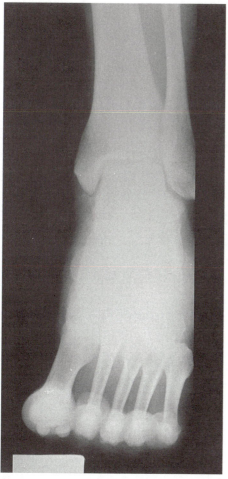

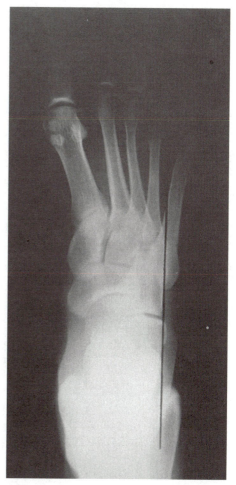

FIGURE 6–12. Axial sesamoid projection.

FIGURE 6–13. The longitudinal axis of the rearfoot.

tion, depending on the age of the patient. If there is mild adductus in a child, an orthotic with a medial flare can be used to allow the foot to rotate laterally at the tarsometatarsal joint, thus permitting the metatarsal to abduct. If the metatarsals are completely ossified and the epiphyseal plates are closed (after age 8 to 10 years), however, surgical correction with osteotomies of the first through the fifth metatarsals may be considered. If the deformity can be recognized early in life, this problem can also be treated, with orthotics and through serial casting to lengthen both the medial capsule and the ligamentous attachments of the tarsometatarsal joints.

Metatarsus Primus Adductus Angle (Intermetatarsal Angle)

The intermetatarsal angle is formed by the transverse plane, angular relationship between the first and second metatarsals (Fig. 6–22). The ideal intermetatarsal angle

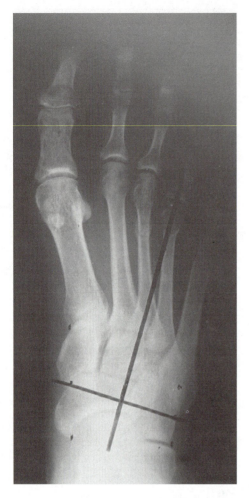

FIGURE 6–14. The longitudinal axis of the lesser tarsus.

is 8°.[1,2] This angular relationship is a principal consideration in determining treatment for bunion deformities. If the forefoot and the metatarsals are adducted, the intermetatarsal angle can be up to 12° and still be considered normal. If there is a high intermetatarsal angle (over 8°) causing a hallux abductus deformity, surgical correction is directed toward the base of the first metatarsal. If the intermetatarsal angle is less than 8°, surgical correction is directed toward the head of the first metatarsal.

Hallux Abductus Angle

The hallus abductus angle is formed by the intersection of the longitudinal axis of the first metatarsal and the longitudinal axis of the proximal phalanx of the hallux. Normal angulation does not exceed 15° (Fig. 6–23).[1,5] If the angle is greater than 15°, a hallux abductus deformity should be considered. If the angle is negative, hallux varus is considered. The angular relationship determines whether a soft tissue release

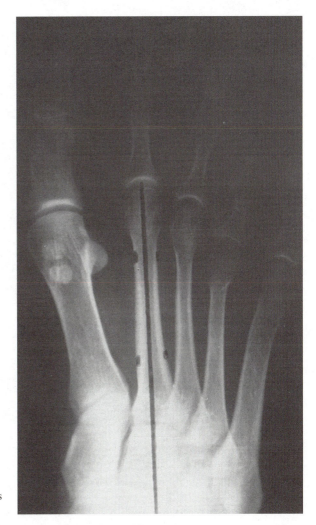

FIGURE 6–15. The longitudinal axis of the metatarsals.

should be performed at the metatarsophalangeal joint of the first metatarsal or if an osteotomy of the distal aspect of the metatarsophalangeal joint should be undertaken. If there is extreme hallux abductus (25° to 30°), osteotomy of either the distal third of the first metatarsal or of the proximal phalanx is considered. If the angle is less than 25°, a soft tissue release of the metatarsophalangeal joint may be all that is needed to reduce the deformity.

Hallux Interphalangeal Angle

The interphalangeal angle of the hallux is formed by the intersection of the longitudinal axis of the proximal and distal phalanges of the hallux (Fig. 6–24). The normal angle is 8° to 10°. When the angle is greater than 10°, the distal portion of the hallux is directed in the lateral position against the second digit. This may cause a ret-

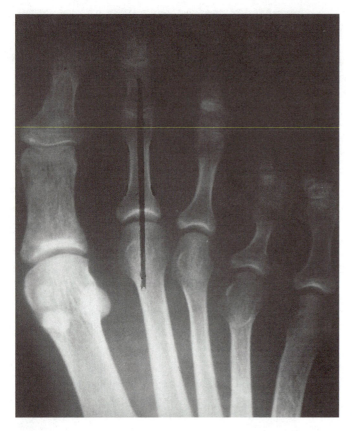

FIGURE 6–16. The longitudinal axis of the digits.

rograde force on the metatarsophalangeal joint, resulting in hallux abductovalgus deformity. Therefore, with a large hallux interphalangeal angle (greater than 10°), surgical correction with osteotomies of the distal aspect of the proximal phalanx or of the proximal aspect of the distal phalanx is needed to reduce this angle.

Proximal Articular Set Angle

The proximal articular set angle is formed by a line perpendicular to the effective articular surface of the first metatarsal head and its intersection with the longitudinal axis of the first metatarsal (Fig. 6–25). This value is then subtracted from 90°. The normal range is 0° to 8°. With a hallux abductovalgus deformity, this angle may be considerably greater. The effective articular surface of the metatarsal head is determined by using the most lateral aspect of the articular surface of the first metatarsal head and the most medial aspect of the functioning articular cartilage on the head of the first metatarsal. If the proximal articular set angle is greater than 8°, the deformity (hallux valgus) is with the head of the first metatarsal; therefore, any correction to be performed is undertaken at this location.

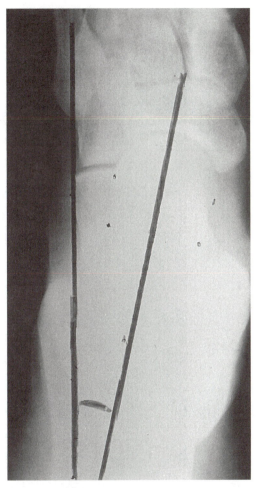

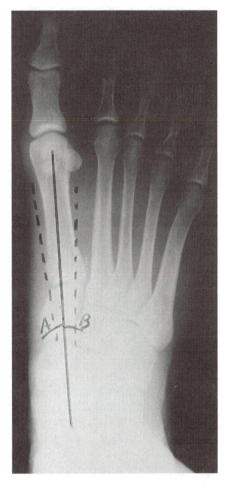

FIGURE 6–17. The talocalcaneal angle.

FIGURE 6–18. The talocalcaneal axis. (*A*) With pronation, the axis will project medially. (*B*) With supination, the axis will project laterally.

Distal Articular Set Angle

The distal articular set angle is formed by a line perpendicular to the effective articular surface of the base of the proximal phalanx of the hallux and its intersection with the longitudinal axis of the proximal phalanx (Fig. 6–26). Again this value is subtracted from 90° and is normally 0° to 8°. If the deformity (hallux valgus) is with the proximal phalanx, surgical correction is performed at this level.

Metatarsal Break Angle

The metatarsal break angle is an obtuse, proximal angle formed by points located at the distal centers of the first, second, and fifth metatarsal heads (Fig. 6–27). The

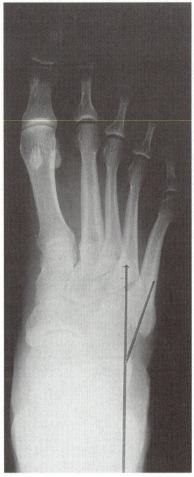

FIGURE 6–19. The cuboid abduction angle.

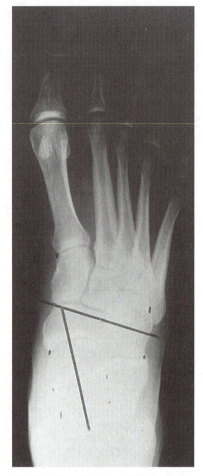

FIGURE   6–20.   Talonavicular angle.

average metatarsal break angle is 142.5°.[1,4,5] This value demonstrates that all the metatarsophalangeal joints are aligned and functioning as a fulcrum over which the body weight is raised.[4,5] When a metatarsal is elongated, excessive stress is exerted through the second metatarsal, causing localized pain. Surgical intervention to the lesser metatarsals should be undertaken with caution. There is a failure rate of 57% when metatarsal osteotomies are performed.[3] Orthotic posting of the forefoot is the procedure of choice at this level to accommodate possible plantar flexion of the second metatarsal or the dorsiflexed attitude of the first and third metatarsals.

Tibial Sesamoid Position

The tibial sesamoid position (TSP) is determined by the relative apposition of the sesamoid to the first metatarsal axis (Fig. 6–28). Seven positions are identified:

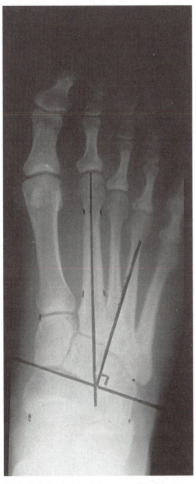

FIGURE 6–21. Metatarsal adductus angle.

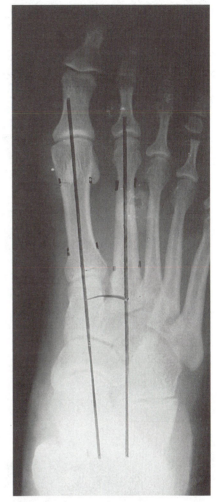

FIGURE 6–22. The intermetatarsal angle.

TSP 1: Tibial sesamoid lies medially, clear of the first metatarsal axis.
TSP 2: Tibial sesamoid laterally abuts the first metatarsal axis.
TSP 3: Tibial sesamoid laterally overlaps the first metatarsal axis.
TSP 4: Tibial sesamoid is bisected by the first metatarsal axis.
TSP 5: Tibial sesamoid medially overlaps the first metatarsal axis.
TSP 6: Tibial sesamoid medially abuts the first metatarsal axis.
TSP 7: Tibial sesamoid lies laterally, clear of the first metatarsal axis.

Patients who have a tibial sesamoid position greater than TSP 3 usually show abnormalities in the crista.[1] The crista makes up the medial wall for the fibular sesamoid articulation and the lateral wall for the tibial sesamoid articulation. With a hallux abductus valgus deformity, the surgeon always considers the position of the tibial sesamoid. In most procedures to correct hallux abductus valgus, the conjoined ten-

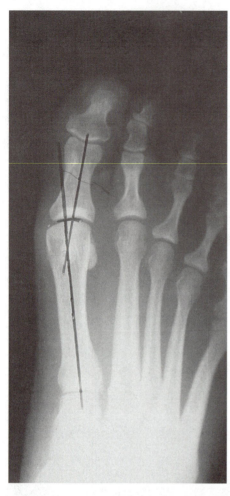

FIGURE 6–23. Hallux abductus angle.

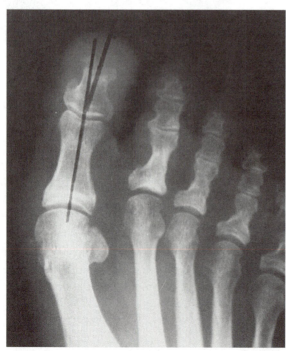

FIGURE 6–24. Hallux interphalangeal angle.

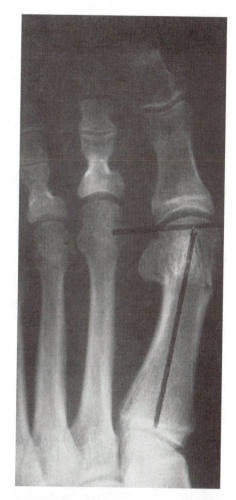

FIGURE 6–25. Proximal articular set angle.

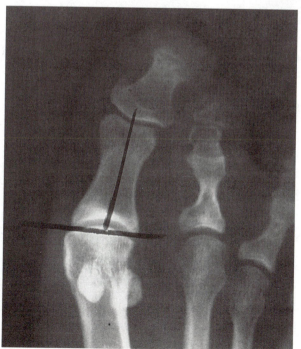

FIGURE 6–26. Distal articular set angle.

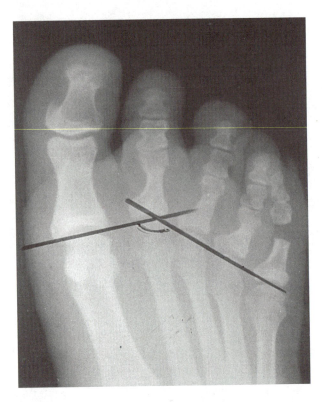

FIGURE 6–27. Metatarsal break angle.

dons of the transverse and oblique hallux adductor are released from their insertions into the fibular sesamoid and the proximal phalanx of the first metatarsophalangeal joint. This procedure relieves the tension forces of the adductor tendon on the joint.

ANGULAR AND AXIAL RELATIONSHIPS OF THE LATERAL PROJECTION

Cyma Line

The Cyma line is the articulation between the talonavicular and the calcaneocuboid, Chopart's joint. In the normal foot, these two articulations form a continuous S-shaped curve (Fig. 6–29A). With pronation, the talus slides anteriorly, creating an anterior break in the Cyma line, with the talonavicular joint being distal to the calcaneocuboid joint (Fig. 6–29B). In supination, the talus moves posteriorly into the ankle mortise, and the Cyma line has a posterior break.[1,5] The talonavicular joint is proximal to that of the calcaneocuboid joint (Fig. 6–29C).

Collum Tali Axis

The collum tali axis is a longitudinal bisector of the neck of the talus. Because of its variable shape, the radiographic plotting of the axis may be difficult (Fig. 6–30).

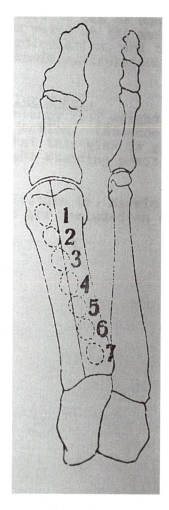

FIGURE 6–28. Tibial sesamoid position.

Plane of Support

The plane of support is determined by the most plantar aspect of the calcaneal tuberosity and the most plantar aspect of the head of the fifth metatarsal (Fig. 6–31).

Calcaneal Axis

The calcaneal axis is determined by connecting a point representing the most plantar aspect of the tuberosity of the calcaneus with the most distal plantar aspect of the calcaneus (Fig. 6–32).

First Metatarsal Declination Axis

The first metatarsal declination axis is determined by bisecting the neck and the base of the first metatarsal and connecting these points. (Fig. 6–33).

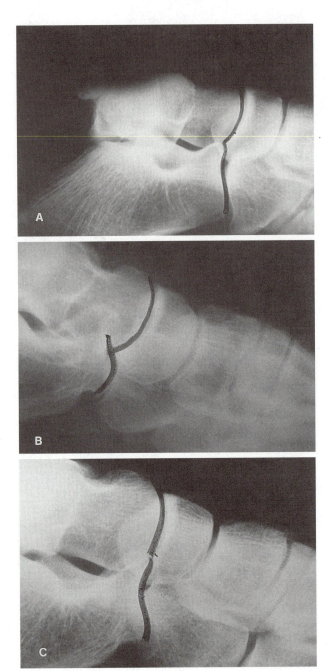

FIGURE 6–29. Cyma line. (*A*) Normal; (*B*) pronated; (*C*) supinated.

Calcaneal Inclination Angle

The calcaneal inclination angle is a determination of relative arch height and is formed by the intersection of the plane of support and the calcaneal inclination axis (Fig. 6–34). This angle is useful in evaluating a pronated or supinated foot. The more pronated the foot type, the smaller the angle, with an increased angle in a supinated foot type. The average value is 15°; however, abnormalities of pronation and supination

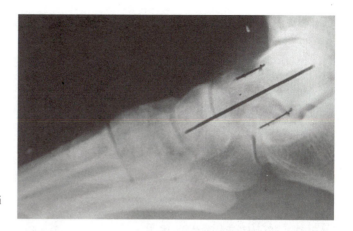

FIGURE 6–30. Collum tali axis.

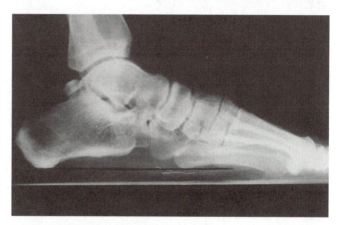

FIGURE 6–31. Plane of support.

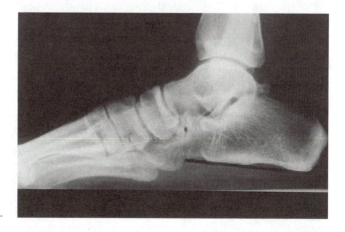

FIGURE 6–32. Calcaneal axis.

are expressed well beyond or well below the average measurement.[1] With a greater angle, the midfoot may compensate, causing midfoot symptoms; therefore, orthotic control may be used. If the deformity is not compensated, however, lateral ankle sprains may occur, potentially necessitating surgical correction. With a small angle, orthotic control may be used if midfoot symptoms occur. With a true uncompensated flatfoot, however, a midfoot arch reconstruction with a calcaneal osteotomy may be performed.

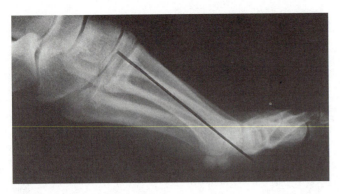

FIGURE 6–33. First metatarsal axis.

Talar Declination Angle

The talar declination angle is constructed by the plane of support and the collum tali axis (Fig. 6–35). This angle averages about 21°.[1,4,5] The collum tali axis should be colinear with the first metatarsal declination axis. Hypermobility in this joint is reflected by symptoms of pain on increased activity. A talar declination angle (greater than 21°) allows for greater pronation, whereas an angle less than 21° allows for supination. With pronation, an orthotic usually controls the pronation if the deformity is flexible. If the deformity is not flexible, a medial arch suspension may be indicated to raise the arch to a functional level. If supination is the problem, calcaneal osteotomies are indicated on the lateral aspect to reduce the amount of supination.

Anterior Projection of the Ankle

The ankle is in a neutral position with the x-ray tube at 90° from vertical, neither internally nor externally rotated (Fig. 6–36). This view is used to evaluate the structural integrity of the tibia and fibula. The articulation of the tibia and fibula is not properly visualized owing to overlap of the tibia on the fibula; therefore, an ankle mortise projection is needed.

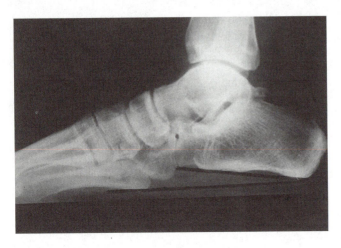

FIGURE 6–34. Calcaneal inclination angle.

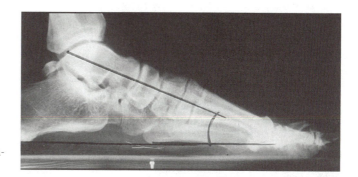

FIGURE 6–35. Talar declination angle.

Ankle Mortise Projection

The ankle is internally rotated 15° with the x-ray tube at 90° from vertical (Fig. 6–36). This view is used to determine the structural integrity of the tibia and fibula. This view is also used to evaluate the articulating surface of the talus in relation to the tibia. It is also used to assess the angular relationships of the ankle (Fig. 6–37).

The axis of the shaft of the tibia is perpendicular to the horizontal plane of the ankle joint and is continuous with the vertical axis of the talus.

The tibial angle is formed by the intersection of a line drawn tangentially to the articular surface of the medial malleolus and a horizontal line drawn along the articular surface of the talus. The normal range of the tibial angle in men is 45° to 61° and in women is 49° to 65°.

The fibular angle is formed by the intersection of a line drawn tangentially to the articular surface of the lateral malleolus and articular surface of the talus. The normal range of the fibular angle in men is 45° to 63°; in women the normal range is 43° to 62°.

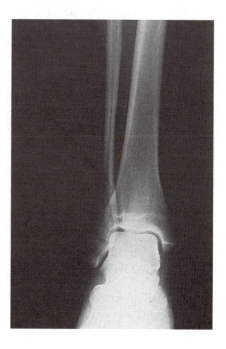

FIGURE 6–36. Anterior-posterior view of normal ankle.

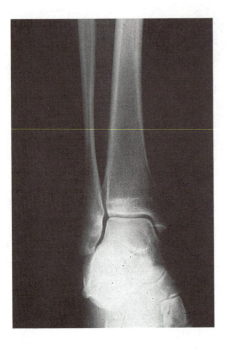

FIGURE 6–37. Ankle mortise projection.

Lateral Projection of the Ankle

This view is used to determine the structural integrity of the tibia, fibula, talus, and calcaneus (Fig. 6–38). The midfoot and forefoot can be visualized in the same view many different ways. The lateral projection of the ankle is taken with the generator at a 90° angle to the ankle. This view is identical to the lateral projection of the foot with the exception that more of the tibia and fibula is visualized.

Stress Inversion Projection of the Ankle

The inversion projection of the ankle is performed when testing the functional integrity of the lateral ligamentous structures of the ankle, specifically the calcaneal fibular ligament (Fig. 6–39). The ankle is placed 12° in internal rotation, and the ankle is inverted either manually or with a mechanical device. A local anesthetic is usually used to block the intermediate dorsal cutaneous and sural nerves. Comparison views should be performed to compare the possibility of bilateral laxity. The angular measurement of laxity is constructed by drawing a line along the articular surface of the talus and the articulating surface of the tibia. These lines should either be parallel or less than 8°. If the angle is greater than 8°, comparison views should be obtained.

Stress Anterior Drawer Projection

The stress anterior drawer projection is performed when testing the functional integrity of the lateral ligamentous structures, specifically the anterior talofibular lig-

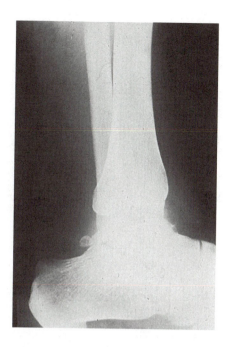

FIGURE 6–38. Lateral projection of the ankle.

ament (Fig. 6–40). The patient is placed in a non–weight-bearing position as in performing a lateral projection of the ankle. Distraction is performed by displacing the calcaneus anteriorly within the ankle mortise, with posterior force placed on the tibia. If excursion of the talus within the ankle mortise is greater than 4 mm as compared with the opposite side, disruption of the anterior talofibular ligament is assumed.

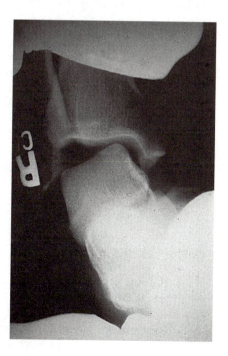

FIGURE 6–39. Stress inversion projection of the ankle.

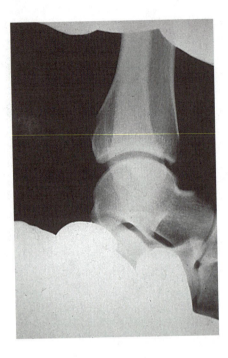

FIGURE 6–40. Stress anterior drawer projection.

SPECIFIC RADIOGRAPHIC STUDIES

Bone Scanning

TECHNETIUM-99M SCANNING

Bone scintigraphy using technetium 99m is excellent for screening because it provides extremely good sensitivity but at the expense of being nonspecific. Increased tracer uptake occurs as a result of hyperemia. A positive bone scan does not necessarily represent an osseous lesion because juxtacapsular joint lesions, periosteal inflammation, or inflammation at tendinous insertions can also produce positive results. The predominant scintigraphic finding is a "hot spot" (increased tracer localization). The exception to this are "cold spots," which are due to no delivery of the tracer as a result of necrosis or fulminant destructive osteomyelitis not accompanied by significant reparative processes.

The four-phase bone scan is used to differentiate osteomyelitis from cellulitis:

Phase 1: at time of injection shows an immediate radionuclide angiogram or dynamic blood flow; osteomyelitis and cellulitis both show increased uptake at this point.

Phase 2: 10 minutes after injection shows focal increases (blood pool image); cellulitis and osteomyelitis are still positive at this point.

Phase 3: 4 hours after injection (delayed static scan or bone image); cellulitis becomes quiescent at this point.

Phase 4: 24 hours later, used for patients with poor vascular flow; focal increases in this phase, are indicative of osteomyelitis.

GALLIUM SCANNING

The isotope, gallium 67 citrate, was originally developed as a marker for certain tumors (i.e., lymphoma) and is considered an inflammatory imaging marker. It is less dependent on blood flow than technetium. There are three mechanisms for gallium 67 localization:

1. Leukocyte localization or incorporation
2. Direct lactoferrin binding at the site of infection
3. Direct bacterial uptake by siderophores

Gallium is valuable in monitoring disease activity and response to treatment in patients with chronic osteomyelitis. Gallium is not as sensitive to bone remodeling as technetium.

INDIUM SCANNING

Indium 111 scan is much more specific for infection (especially acute infections). With this scan, white blood cells are labeled with the tracer and injected intravenously. This technique was developed to detect leukocyte accumulation at sites of inflammation and abscess formation. Scans are performed 24 hours after injection. A positive scan is defined as a focal accumulation of leukocytes that is higher than the surrounding bone activity. This technique is reserved for complicated posttraumatic or postsurgical patients with equivocal conventional bone scans, in cases in which technetium 99m scanning reveals false-positive results because of rapid turnover.

Xeroradiography

Xeroradiography is a process in which an image is produced on a selenium-coated plate. This process tends to emphasize the characteristics of borders between tissues, making detailed information more easily seen. It is sensitive enough to visualize nonmetallic foreign bodies.

Fluoroscopy

An imaging modality in which radiographic images are produced continuously on demand to give a real-time, dynamic image that is displayed on a television screen. The C-arm fluoroscope is the usual unit used intraoperatively.

Arthrography

Following the injection of contrast medium into a joint, radiographs are then taken. Arthrography is used to diagnose capsular or ligamentous tears. Arthrography has essentially been replaced by magnetic resonance imaging (MRI).

Tomography

This procedure requires a complex reciprocal motion of both the radiographic tube and cassette around the patient. It requires a relatively large number of radiation exposures and demands exacting technique but has the advantage of providing excellent bony detail in areas of complex osseous anatomy. The most useful applications of tomography are in the evaluation of osteochondral fractures in the dome of the talus, arthritic changes or loose bony fragments of the subtalar joint and the tarsometatarsal joints, stress fractures of the navicular, union versus nonunion of an arthrodesis site, and the status of metallic implants.

Tenography

Tenography is most often used on the ankle tendons. It can also document calcaneofibular ligament tears because this ligament is contiguous with a part of the peroneal tendon sheath. It has been used to identify irregularities of the peroneal tendons themselves. Tenograms may show irregularity of the involved tendon and the tendon sheaths.

Magnetic Resonance Imaging

MRI gathers information in the form of low-energy radio wave and transduces this energy into images with the use of computers. MRI has been applied with great success to the assessment of a variety of musculoskeletal disorders. The advantages of this technique include an ability to provide sectional images in any plane with excellent spatial and contrast resolution and the capability of revealing considerable physiologic and histologic data. The accurate interpretation of the images provided by magnetic resonance, however, is not accomplished without difficulty, requiring foremost that the examiner have considerable knowledge of the pertinent osseous and soft tissue anatomy. MRI is used specifically for soft tissue deformities (i.e., tendon injuries, soft tissue tumors).

Computed Tomography

Computed tomography (CT) can establish the presence, nature, size, margination, and exact location tumors. Muscle and soft tissue involvement can be determined. If a tumor is located next to blood vessels, a contrast medium is needed to enhance its identification. CT is excellent to evaluate metabolic bone diseases (osteoporosis, aseptic necrosis, osteomalacia). It is excellent in evaluating trauma, especially the calcaneus and the subtalar joint. CT scanning is specifically used for osseous deformities in comparison to MRI. Sectional images in any plane can be performed with excellent visualization of soft tissue structures.

SUMMARY

One must remember that radiographs do not make the diagnosis; the clinician does. Not one but many of the angles of axes described in this chapter contribute to making a diagnosis of pertinent foot pathology. The discussion in this chapter informs clinicians about how radiographs of the foot and ankle are made and interpreted. An understanding of these interpretations permits clarification of the decisions that underlie conservative or surgical intervention for successful podiatric management.

REFERENCES

1. Weissman, S: Radiology of the Foot. Williams & Wilkins, Baltimore, 1984.
2. Whitney, AK: Radiographic Charting Technique. Philadelphia College of Podiatric Medicine, Philadelphia, 1978.
3. Montagne, J, Chevrot, A, and Galmiche, JM: Atlas of Foot Radiology. Year Book Medical Publishers, Chicago, 1981.
4. Gamble and Yale: Clinical Foot Roentgenology. Williams & Wilkins, Baltimore, 1957.
5. Gamble and Felton: Applied Foot Roentgenology. Williams & Wilkins, Baltimore, 1966.
6. Bloom, W and Hollenbach, J: Medical Radiographic Technique. Charles C Thomas, Springfield, MO, 1965.

CHAPTER 7

Biomechanical Evaluation for Functional Orthotics

Michael J. Wooden, MS, PT, OCS

This chapter describes a step-by-step process of biomechanical evaluation of the foot and ankle complex. Using static and gait analysis methods, a system of problem solving for orthotic therapy is provided.

In many clinics, orthotics are made from plaster impressions of feet, sometimes by minimally trained personnel and often without benefit of measurements and gait analysis. The system described in this chapter uses specific observations and measurements that provide many clinical advantages. First, the ideal subtalar joint neutral position is determined, so that deviations from neutral can be observed. Second, limitations and deformities causing these deviations from neutral can be evaluated. Third, measurement reliability can be increased with proper methods and repetition. Fourth, objective data can be obtained. From these data, the clinician can establish a baseline, follow progress, communicate with other clinicians, and determine the appropriate amount of "treatment" to be built in to the orthotic.

Before proceeding with this chapter, the reader is urged to review Chapters 1 and 2, which provide details of normal and abnormal mechanics. Note especially the causes of compensation at the subtalar joint and other joints leading to abnormal pronation or supination. A better understanding of these conditions enhances the ability to evaluate them.

The reader must also realize that this chapter is taken somewhat out of context; that is, only a part of the entire lower quarter screening process is provided. A history must also be obtained, especially if there is evidence of an overuse syndrome related to weight-bearing activities. Evaluation of the spine and lower limb for alignment, range of motion, muscle imbalance, and mobility problems is essential, particularly if the pain complaint is extrinsic to the foot. In some cases, radiographs and evaluation for neurologic and vascular status are needed, as described in other chapters in this book.

This chapter is divided into sections that deal with static and dynamic evaluation procedures. Measurement examples are provided, and a case presentation is offered as a summary. This format is followed in Chapter 10, when biomechanical orthotics are discussed, and more cases are presented, using the measurement techniques and problem-solving process discussed in this chapter.

STATIC EVALUATION

Observation

With the patient standing, relaxed, and with equal weight on each foot, the examiner observes for postural deviations or for signs of lower extremity deviations (Fig. 7–1).[1] These could include:

1. *Transverse plane deviations:* rotation or torsion of the hip, femurs, knees, or tibias, observed from the front or from behind.
2. *Frontal plane deviations:* varus or valgus of femurs or tibias, viewed from behind.
3. *Sagittal plane deviations:* hip flexor tightness or genu recurvatum, viewed laterally.

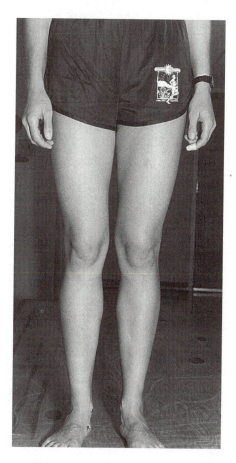

FIGURE 7–1. Observation of the patient in standing, anterior view.

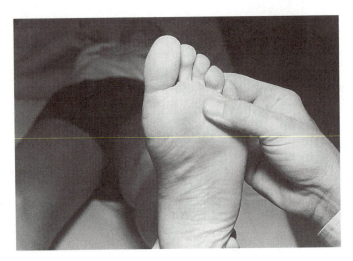

FIGURE 7–2. Check for calluses or other skin lesions.

The examiner also observes for extremes of foot abduction or adduction and for obvious increases in the concavities under the medial and lateral malleoli. Last, the clinician looks for toe abnormalities, such as bunions, clawing, or hammering. Visualization of these abnormalities could be indicative of abnormal mechanics, particularly when there is a history of overuse syndrome or pain secondary to repetitive trauma.

Next, with the patient sitting or supine, inspect the plantar aspect of the feet for calluses, keratoses, and other skin lesions (Fig. 7–2). These indicate abnormal weight-bearing and shearing forces. Calluses under the second, third, or fourth metatarsal heads are associated with abnormal pronation because of the lack of push-off provided by the first ray.[2,3] A callus on the medial aspect of the great toe is a sign that push-off is occurring from that part of the toe rather than the plantar aspect and is usually seen in hallux abductovalgus. Calluses under the first and fifth metatarsal heads as well as along the lateral border of the foot are usually found in abnormally supinated or cavus feet.[2]

Again, these are observations that show tendencies and relationships. The next several measurements help to identify and quantify abnormalities and various compensations.

Lines of Bisection

In this method of static evaluation, many of the measurements employ goniometry. A clear plastic goniometer with a rounded edge and 2° increments is best. Lines of bisection are drawn on the lower third of the leg and on the calcaneus.[3] Drawn correctly, these lines provide the examiner with reference lines for goniometry and later are used to observe movement during gait. Without radiographs, it is impossible to ensure clinically that the lines actually follow the shape of the tibia, talus, and calcaneus. The best that can be achieved are lines visualizing the long axis of the mass of the segments. To reduce but not, unfortunately, totally eliminate the chance of measurement error, the lines must be (1) straight, (2) in the midline of the segments, (3) on the posterior aspect of the segments, and (4) able to be lined up continuously in space. This may require moving the calcaneus a few degrees into inversion or eversion because the foot may not rest with the lines aligned.

PROCEDURE

The patient is prone with the foot to be measured 6 to 8 inches off the table. The leg is rotated so that the foot is perpendicular to the floor, which helps the examiner mark the back of the leg and the heel. The foot and leg can easily be stabilized by flexing and rotating the opposite limb into the "figure four" position (Fig. 7–3).

When visualizing or measuring for the midline, a series of dots is placed on the lower leg and calcaneus (Fig. 7–4A) using a straightedge and, if necessary, moving the calcaneus into a few degrees of inversion or eversion. The dots are checked to see if they provide lines that are continuous in space (Fig. 7–4B). The leg and calcaneus lines are then drawn. To avoid soft tissue distortion, especially in standing, the lines are not connected to each other (Fig. 7–4C). Two reference lines are now available for goniometry.

Subtalar Joint Range of Motion: Neutral Position

In normal gait, the subtalar joint should pronate or supinate only a few degrees from the neutral position, depending on foot position for that subphase of stance.[4] Abnormal pronation and supination are compensations that cause the subtalar joint to function in extreme positions away from neutral.[3] Therefore, when evaluating the feasibility of orthotic intervention, determining the subtalar joint neutral position is critical. Static and dynamic evaluation determines whether the subtalar joint is deviating excessively from the measured neutral position and, ultimately, what orthotic treatment will reduce this deviation. Additionally, some of the static measurements require that the subtalar joint be held in neutral while measuring.

The most common method of finding the neutral position of the subtalar joint is by palpation, which is highly variable.[5–7] Calculations based on subtalar joint range of motion are alternative methods.[8,9] Broussard-Smith and colleagues[9] found both to

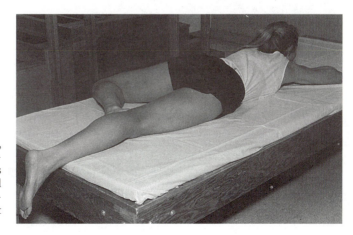

FIGURE 7–3. The prone, "figure four position" for static measurements. The foot is perpendicular to the floor, and the opposite limb helps stabilize against the medial aspect of the knee.

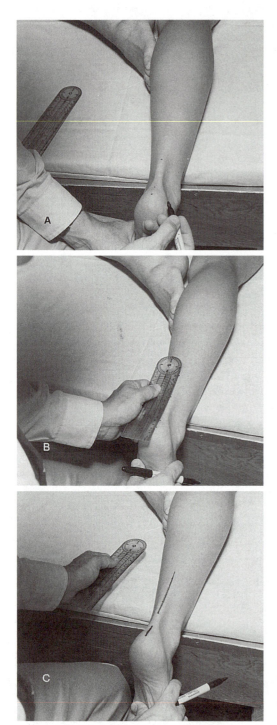

FIGURE 7–4. (*A*) Midline dots are placed on the lower leg and calcaneus, then (*B*) checked to ensure that they are continuous in space, and then (*C*) connected to form two lines of bisection.

be reliable, but the calculation method is more time-consuming.[9] In the author's experience, the palpation method is the most clinically useful.

PROCEDURE FOR PALPATING

To determine the neutral position of the subtalar joint, the anterior aspect of the head of the talus is palpated with the thumb and middle finger of the medial hand while the patient is prone.[5,6] The examiner's lateral hand grasps the foot at the base of the fourth and fifth metatarsals, applying a downward distracting force to remove any resting ankle dorsiflexion. The foot is then passively inverted and everted as talar protrusion is palpated: The talus protrudes laterally with inversion and medially with eversion. The neutral position is that point at which protrusion is felt equally on the lateral and medial sides. Using the bisection lines, this position is measured with a goniometer and recorded in degrees varus or valgus (Fig. 7–5).

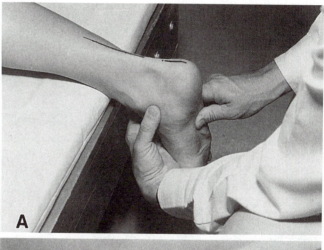

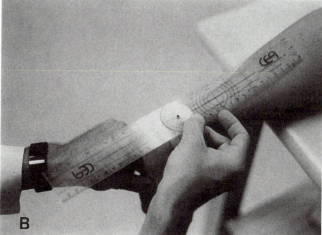

FIGURE 7–5. (*A*) Palpation for the subtalar joint neutral position. (*B*) Measuring the neutral position with a goniometer.

Forefoot/Rearfoot Relationship

As discussed in detail in Chapter 2, abnormal alignment of the forefoot can influence the weight-bearing position of the subtalar joint.[2,3] Forefoot varus is a position of inversion of the forefoot on the rearfoot, with the subtalar joint in neutral.[2,3,10–12] To bring the medial aspect of the foot in contact with the ground during weight-bearing, the subtalar joint pronates (the calcaneus everts). Conversely, forefoot valgus, a position of eversion of the forefoot on the rearfoot with the subtalar joint in neutral, results in subtalar supination (calcaneus inverting).[2,3,10–12]

These forefoot deformities should be visualized and measured in the uncompensated or non–weight-bearing position. Later on, orthotic therapy based on these measurements is designed to keep the subtalar joint from compensating into either abnormal pronation or abnormal supination.

PROCEDURE

To measure forefoot varus (Fig. 7–6), the lateral hand grasps the foot at the base of the fifth metatarsal. The subtalar joint is held in its predetermined neutral position with excessive ankle plantar flexion removed. One arm of the goniometer rests against the metatarsal heads, while the other arm is perpendicular to the heel bisection line. Note that the axis is held laterally. The angle described by the metatarsal

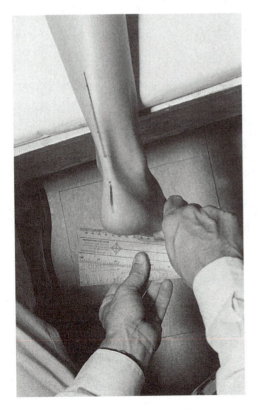

FIGURE 7–6. Measurement of forefoot varus.

heads and the imaginary line perpendicular to the heel line is read and recorded. To measure forefoot valgus, the goniometer axis is held medially, but the rest of the procedure is the same.

With practice, this procedure has shown good reliability.[12,13] Care must be taken, however, to reduce the chance of measurement error. Because the lines describing the forefoot/rearfoot angle are several inches apart (from the heel to the metatarsal heads), the foot must be held carefully and viewed along its long axis. This procedure is aided by gently dorsiflexing the ankle to the point of resistance. Avoid dorsiflexing the foot too forcefully, which may momentarily distort the forefoot/rearfoot relationship being measured.

Ankle Joint Dorsiflexion

Ankle joint equinus is a limitation of dorsiflexion at the ankle joint, which can cause the subtalar joint to compensate in weight bearing by pronating abnormally.[2,3,11] The limitation can be caused by tightness of the gastrocnemius/soleus muscle group, bony abnormality at the ankle, or periarticular connective tissue restrictions brought on by trauma or immobilization. Regardless of its cause, equinus must be determined because it may be a reason for abnormal subtalar joint compensation.

PROCEDURE

With the patient still prone, ankle dorsiflexion is measured by placing the rounded edge of a goniometer at the contour of the heel, while the arms are aligned with the long axes of the fibula and the fifth metatarsal (Fig. 7–7A). The foot is passively dorsiflexed, and the measurement is recorded (plus or minus 90°). The clinician should try to reduce the possibility of measurement error by:

1. Holding the subtalar joint in neutral position and observing the bisection lines; allowing the foot to pronate may give a false-positive recording of dorsiflexion.
2. Pushing dorsally at the midfoot; pushing too far distally on the foot can also give a false-positive recording if the midfoot area is hypermobile, as in talipes equinus.

This measurement can be repeated with the knee in flexion (Fig. 7–7B) to help differentiate between soleus and gastrocnemius tightness.

First Ray Position and Mobility

PROCEDURE

While the patient remains prone, the position of the distal aspect of the first ray is noted. Specifically the clinician looks for either a dorsiflexed or plantar flexed first ray. In the latter, when the subtalar joint is held in neutral, the head of the first metatarsal is in a more plantar flexed position relative to the other four.[1]

Mobility of the first ray is checked by moving it in dorsal and plantar directions while stabilizing metatarsal heads two through five. A plantar flexed first ray is par-

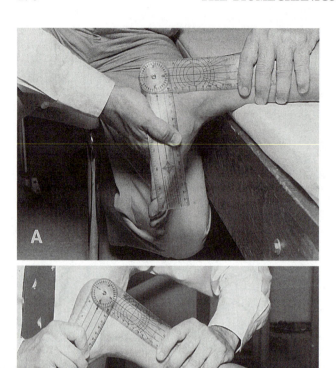

FIGURE 7–7. (*A*) Measurement of ankle dorsiflexion with the knee extended and (*B*) flexed.

ticularly significant if it is fixed or hypomobile because the subtalar joint may have to invert (supinate) to bring the lateral aspect of the foot into contact with the ground.[1] A rigid, plantar flexed first ray can be measured similarly to a forefoot valgus (see forefoot/rearfoot relationship).

First Metatarsophalangeal Joint Range of Motion

A limitation of first metatarsophalangeal joint mobility, especially dorsiflexion, can result in gait deviations that promote excessive pronation.[1] Sixty degrees to 65° of dorsiflexion is sufficient to prevent these deviations at push-off.

PROCEDURE

The foot is stabilized as the arms of the goniometer are placed on the long axis of the first ray and the first proximal phalanx. The hallux is passively dorsiflexed, and the measurement is recorded as shown in Figure 7–8.

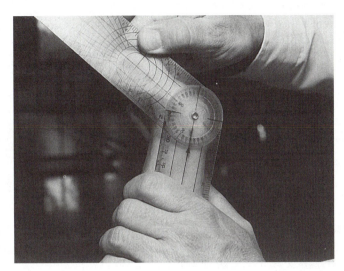

FIGURE 7–8. Measuring dorsiflexion of the first metatarsophalangeal joint.

TABLE 7–1 Summary of Static Measurements

Procedure	Patient Position
Observation	Standing
Check for calluses	Sitting or supine
Subtalar inversion	
Subtalar eversion	
Subtalar neutral	
Forefoot/rearfoot relationship	Prone
Ankle dorsiflexion	
First ray position	
First ray mobility	
Tibia	
Tibia/calcaneus	Standing
Pronation/supination	

Table 7–1 presents a summary of the static evaluation procedures, listed according to patient position.

Standing Tibial Measurement

PROCEDURE

With patient in equal stance on a firm, level surface, the subtalar joint is placed in the neutral position by palpating the talus as described previously; the patient "rolls" the foot into inversion until neutral is palpated. This positioning can be confirmed by measuring with a goniometer. The leg bisection line is now measured in relation to the horizontal—one arm of the goniometer rests on the standing surface, while the other arm is aligned with the leg bisection line (Fig. 7–9). The measurement is recorded as 0° (vertical) or in degrees of varus or valgus.

Standing Tibia/Calcaneal Measurement

Most of the measurements to this point have been taken in the uncompensated, neutral subtalar joint position. The tibial/calcaneal measurement is now taken in the compensated (weight-bearing) position. This measurement is made under the assumption that in equal, relaxed standing, the subtalar joint should be at or near its neutral position and indicates to the clinician what abnormal compensation might be occurring.

PROCEDURE

The tibia/calcaneal angle is formed by the leg and calcaneus bisection lines. With the patient in relaxed standing, the goniometer arms are aligned with the bisection lines (Fig. 7–10). The measurement is recorded as 0° or as degrees of varus or valgus. At this point, the clinician asks two questions:

1. How many degrees from neutral is the calcaneus?
2. In what direction is the calcaneus (and therefore) the subtalar joint oriented?

For example, if the predicted subtalar joint neutral position is 5° varus, and the tibia/calcaneus angle is 8° valgus, the subtalar joint is actually 13° pronated, perhaps because of rearfoot varus, forefoot varus, ankle joint equinus, or other reasons (Fig. 7–11).

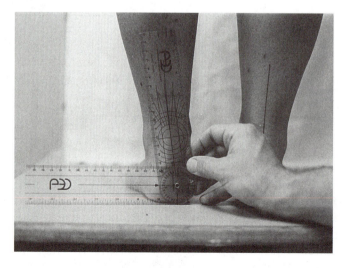

FIGURE 7–9. Standing tibial measurement showing tibial varus.

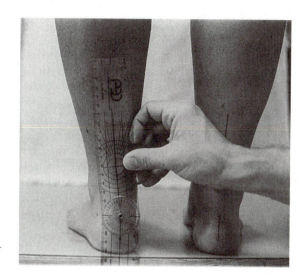

FIGURE 7–10. Standing tibial/calcaneal measurement.

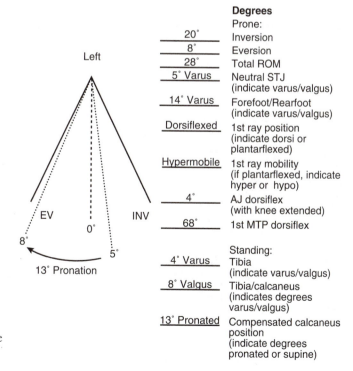

FIGURE 7–11. An example of subtalar joint pronation.

	Degrees
	Prone:
20°	Inversion
8°	Eversion
28°	Total ROM
5° Varus	Neutral STJ (indicate varus/valgus)
14° Varus	Forefoot/Rearfoot (indicate varus/valgus)
Dorsiflexed	1st ray position (indicate dorsi or plantarflexed)
Hypermobile	1st ray mobility (if plantarflexed, indicate hyper or hypo)
4°	AJ dorsiflex (with knee extended)
68°	1st MTP dorsiflex
	Standing:
4° Varus	Tibia (indicate varus/valgus)
8° Valgus	Tibia/calcaneus (indicates degrees varus/valgus)
13° Pronated	Compensated calcaneus position (indicate degrees pronated or supine)

Left

EV   INV

0°

8°   5°

13° Pronation

DYNAMIC EVALUATION: GAIT ANALYSIS

Gait analysis is used to determine deviations from the normal, or at least ideal, gait pattern. The clinician is looking for signs of abnormal mechanics: pronation or supination occurring at the wrong time during the stance phase of gait.

Gait analysis is best accomplished with the patient on a treadmill, so that repeated cycles can be watched easily. The patient should be observed walking on the floor, however, because gait patterns used on a treadmill are often different. Gait should be analyzed when the patient is barefoot, in shoes, and eventually, in shoes with orthotics. To assist in specific observations, additional marks are placed on the medial aspect of the foot at the medial malleolus, the navicular tuberosity, and the first metatarsophalangeal joint. All are easily palpable. The X on the navicular tubercle is observed from the side in relation to the other marks. This observation demonstrates how the medial longitudinal arch rises and falls during various aspects of gait and how the navicular tubercle protrudes to and from the midline. The calcaneal bisection line is used to observe from behind for calcaneal movement, which is primarily in the frontal plane.

Normal Gait

The following discussion briefly summarizes the major characteristics of normal gait.[2,4,11,14]

HEEL STRIKE

The calcaneus is in a neutral to inverted (supinated) position; the navicular is in an upward position along with the medial longitudinal arch; the tibia is externally rotated.

HEEL STRIKE TO FOOTFLAT (NORMAL PRONATION)

The calcaneus everts as the midtarsal joint "unlocks," causing the talus to move medially; the tibia rotates internally. As noted in Chapter 1, these provide shock absorption, accommodation to the walking surface, and attenuation of lower extremity internal rotation. The foot reaches maximum pronation at footflat.

MIDSTANCE

The foot has reached maximal pronation. The navicular and medial longitudinal arch are down and protrude medially; the tibia is rotated internally. In early midstance, a reversal of pronation begins as the tibia is moving anterior to the talus and the subtalar joint passes through neutral. In late midstance, the subtalar joint is supinating.

HEEL-OFF TO TOE-OFF (NORMAL SUPINATION)

The calcaneus inverts from the fully everted position; the midtarsal joint "locks," moving the talus in a lateral direction; the tibia rotates externally; the foot is abducted no more than 10° to 15°. The foot and lower limb are now rigid levers for propulsion.

SWING

The ankle is dorsiflexed to clear the floor; the foot is inverted to prepare for the next heel strike. With a knowledge of what should occur during stance in a normal gait, various types of abnormal pronation and supination can be analyzed.

Abnormal Pronation

Three types of abnormal pronation are seen clinically:

1. *Failure to resupinate.* Normal pronation occurs from heel strike to footflat. During push-off, from heel-off to toe-off, the subtalar and midtarsal joints stay in their pronated positions; therefore, there is a loss of a rigid lever.
2. *Late pronation during push-off.* From heel strike to midstance there is little or no pronatory movement of the subtalar or midtarsal joints. From heel-off to toe-off, the calcaneus suddenly everts, the navicular falls, and the foot whips into excessive abduction; therefore, there is little shock absorption and, again, loss of a rigid lever.
3. *Early excessive pronation.* The subtalar and midtarsal joints are pronated throughout the entire stance phase. Because they are fully pronated at heel strike, there is no range of motion left for normal pronation. The foot does not supinate in push-off or in swing; therefore, both shock absorption and the rigid lever are lost.

Abnormal Supination

The supinated or high-arched foot can be classified as pes cavus, pes equinocavus, or pes cavovarus.[15] In any case, gait analysis reveals a somewhat invert-

TABLE 7–2 Observations During the Stance Phase of Gait

Gait Pattern	Heel Strike		Heel Strike–Foot Flat		Heel-Off–Toe-Off	
	Calcaneus	Navicular	Calcaneus	Navicular	Calcaneus	Navicular
Normal	Neutral to inverted	Up	Everts	Drops	Inverts	Rises up
Abnormal pronation						
Fails to resupinate	Neutral to inverted	Up	Everts	Drops	Stays everted	Stays down
Late pronation at push-off	Neutral to inverted	Up	Stays inverted	Stays up	Everts	Drops
Early, excessive	At or near full eversion	Down	Everted	Down	Stays everted	Stays down
Abnormal supination	Neutral to inverted	Up	Stays inverted	Stays up	Stays inverted	Stays up

ed calcaneus and an elevated navicular and medial longitudinal arch throughout stance. A rigid lever is maintained at push-off, but with no normal pronation after heel strike, there is reduced shock absorption. Table 7–2 is a summary of typical observations noted during gait analysis for normal, pronated, and supinated feet.

CASE STUDY

A 37-year-old factory assembly line inspector presented with a 1-year history of pain on the plantar aspect of the second metatarsophalangeal joint aggravated by walking. This was especially true at work where he walks 8 to 10 hours a day on a concrete surface. Radiographs and an examination by an orthopedist were negative. The diagnosis was capsulitis of the second metatarsophalangeal joint.

Static biomechanical evaluation findings are shown in Figure 7–12. Gait analysis revealed pronation throughout the stance phase of gait, especially on

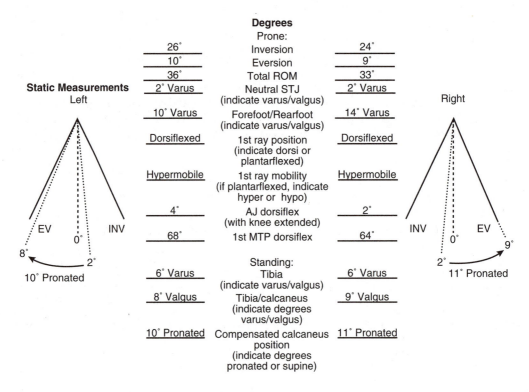

FIGURE 7–12. Case study: summary of evaluation findings.

the right. Specifically the calcaneus was everted, and a collapse of the medial arch was noted at heel strike. The pronated position of the foot was maintained throughout the stance phase of gait. The instability of the foot during push-off caused excessive abduction of the forefoot. These findings indicated early, excessive pronation. Specifically, there was abnormal pronation from heel strike to footflat, which caused a decrease in shock absorption. Additionally, there was no supination during the push-off phase of stance. Therefore, the patient was pushing off from a less than rigid lever. In this case, the first ray was hypermobile because of the pronation and was unable to resist adequately ground reaction force during push-off. Therefore, the second metatarsal joint progressively became more weight bearing. Additionally the second metatarsal head was rotating and shearing against the ground because of the sudden abduction at push-off. At this point, temporary orthotics would be constructed that would enhance shock absorption and help to provide a rigid lever for push-off by reducing the amount of subtalar joint compensation for the various limitations.

REFERENCES

1. James, SL: Chondromalacia patellae. In Kennedy J, ed: The Injured Adolescent Knee. Williams & Wilkins, Baltimore, 1976.
2. Root, ML, Orien, WP, and Weed, JH: Clinical Biomechanics. Vol II: Normal and Abnormal Function of the Foot. Clinical Biomechanics Corp, Los Angeles, 1977.
3. Donatelli, RA: Abnormal biomechanics of the foot and ankle. J Orthop Sports Phys Ther 9:11, 1987.
4. Donatelli, RA: Normal biomechanics of the foot and ankle. J Orthop Sports Phys Ther 7:91, 1985.
5. Johanson, MA, Donatelli, RA, Wooden, MJ, et al: Effects of three different posting methods on controlling abnormal subtalar pronation. Phys Ther 74:149–159, 1994.
6. Elveru, RA, Rothstein, JM, and Lamb, RL: Goniometric reliability in a clinical setting: Subtalar and ankle joint measurements. Phys Ther 68:672, 1988.
7. Wooden, MJ, Catlin, PA, Attebery, D, et al: An examination of subtalar joint motion during the stance phase of gait. Poster presentation, Combined Sections Meeting, American Physical Therapy Association, New Orleans, 1994.
8. Root, ML: Biomechanical Examination of the Foot. Clinical Biomechanics Corp, Los Angeles, 1971.
9. Broussard-Smith, P, Catlin, PA, and Wooden, MJ: Reliability and comparability of the calculation and palpation methods for measurement of the subtalar joint neutral position. Unpublished data. Emory University Division of Physical Therapy, Atlanta, GA, 1992.
10. Digiovanni, J, and Smith, S: Normal biomechanics of the adult rearfoot. J Am Podiatr Med Assoc 66:812, 1976.
11. Subotnik, S: Podiatric Sports Medicine. Futura Publishing, Los Angeles, 1975.
12. Garbalosa, JC, McClure, MH, Catlin, PA, and Wooden, MJ: The frontal plane relationship of the forefoot to the rearfoot in the asymptomatic population. J Orthop Sports Phys Ther 20:200–207, 1994.
13. Cantu, R, Catlin, PA, and Wooden, MJ: A comparison of two measurement tools and two techniques for measuring the forefoot/rearfoot relationship. Unpublished data. Emory University Division of Physical Therapy, Atlanta, GA, 1987.
14. McPoil, TG and Knecht HG: Biomechanics of the foot in walking: A functional approach. J Orthop Sports Phys Ther 7:69, 1985.
15. Tachdjian, MO: The Child's Foot. WB Saunders, Philadelphia, 1985.

APPENDIX: DYNAMIC ASSESSMENT OF FOOT MECHANICS AS AN ADJUNCT TO ORTHOTIC PRESCRIPTION

I. J. Alexander, MD
K. R. Campbell, PhD

Detailed analysis of frontal plane mechanics of the foot through its examination at rest contributes significantly to the effective treatment of patients with foot and ankle complaints. A number of stress phenomena related to frontal plane deformities can be alleviated by the appropriate correction of the foot mechanics through the utilization of orthotics and, in some cases, shoe modification. Currently the assumption is made that static frontal plane deformities produce predictable alterations in the dynamic stance phase mechanics of the foot. Based on the static evaluation, orthotics, which are thought to correct faulty stance phase mechanics, are fabricated and modified. The effectiveness of these orthotics in relieving a variety of stress phenomena in the foot and ankle, or more proximally in the lower limb, supports the belief that the desired alterations in dynamic stance phase mechanics do occur.

Evolving advances in technology will soon provide a means to document foot mechanics objectively with a high degree of accuracy. With the two techniques described here, the usefulness of the static examination as a predictor of stance phase kinematics can be assessed, and the effectiveness of orthotic correction in altering dynamic foot mechanics can be evaluated.

The first of the two techniques measures dynamic foot pressure distribution using force platforms and has evolved over the past 30 years. The second, newer technique of three-dimensional kinematic analysis of limb motion applies to the moving foot. These two techniques make it possible to document accurately the motion characteristics of the normal, the deformed, and the neurologically impaired foot and to assess the effects of both orthotic and surgical intervention.

TECHNIQUE 1: DYNAMIC PLANTAR PRESSURE DISTRIBUTION

The assessment of dynamic plantar pressure distribution has been approached from two perspectives. The devices available record data either from a single step or to a floor-mounted device or from multiple steps sensing pressure from transducers taped to the foot or incorporated in the shoe sole.

Two types of floor-mounted devices exist. One is based on optical recording of pressure-dependent light intensity or wavelength patterns, which, by scaling, can be converted into pressure values. The other technique is dependent on recording from an array of individual electronic transducers that are mounted on the floor. An example of this approach can be seen in Figure 7–13, which illustrates foot pressure distribution from a patient with right rigid forefoot varus and flexible compensatory hindfoot valgus and a normal left foot pressure pattern.

Shoe-mounted transducers present numerous technical problems, and the exten-

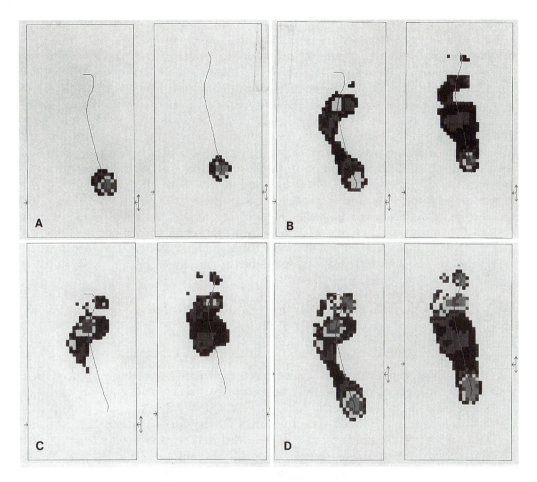

FIGURE 7–13. Sequence of foot pressure distribution in a patient with a rigid forefoot varus and compensatory hindfoot valgus (*right*) matched with stance phase pressure distribution of a healthy subject (*left*). (*A*) Heel strike; (*B*) footflat; (*C*) heel-off; (*D*) summated pressures from entire stance phase.

sive modification necessary to the shoes makes the approach a relatively impractical method of assessing plantar pressure distribution. In-shoe transducers, which are usually taped to the sole of the foot, have been used extensively. The quantitative accuracy of most commercially available transducers has been poor, necessitating frequent calibration. In addition, replacing transducers in the same locations on the sole of the foot can present reliability problems in serial studies.

Assessing dynamic plantar load distribution in barefoot subjects with floor-mounted devices is likely to be most helpful in studying the mechanics of normal and abnormal feet. Normal variations in foot structure and motion are reflected in different patterns of dynamic load distribution under the foot. Correlating these patterns with static structural variations noted on mechanical assessment of the foot will improve our understanding of the importance of these structural differences. In abnormal feet, the differences are magnified and the effects of therapeutic interventions to change load-bearing patterns are more easily recognized. The in-shoe transducers or transducer mats are most useful in evaluating the effectiveness of orthotics and shoe modification in altering weight-bearing patterns under the foot.

The capabilities of currently available commercial devices are impressive. Resolution of the fixed-floor units is as good as 2×3 mm, and sampling rates of the transducer matrices are as high as 70 Hz. Sophisticated software available with some of these units offers automated center of pressure determination, whole-foot and area-specific automated determination of contact time, contact area, peak pressure, load in Newtons per cm^2, and impulse (an integration of total load and contact time). One system is even capable of storing information on preselected areas of interest, to allow comparison of identical areas under the foot before and after therapeutic intervention. Tests of the transducer type matrix have shown that reproducibility of the obtained data is high and that accuracy is within 5%. Two commercially available foot pressure measuring devices with quantitative capabilities are described here.

DEVICES FOR MEASURING FOOT PRESSURE

EMED System

The EMED system (Movelle, Germany) is a capacitance-transducer matrix–based system with a variety of available sensor densities, two sensors per cm^2 and 4 sensors per cm^2 being used most frequently for foot pressure assessment. A calibration device is available to ensure continued sensor accuracy. The system has a number of collection area sizes available and is capable of collecting data at rates greater than 100 Hz. For dynamic foot pressure assessment, the usual sampling rate is 70 Hz. The EMED system can be adapted to connect to an in-shoe transducer mat, which gives in-shoe pressure distribution. Early prototypes of this system do not offer the resolution of the floor-mounted device.

On an experimental basis, the floor-mounted matrices have been mounted on force platforms to allow measurement of simultaneous shear forces under the foot.

F-Scan System

The F-Scan System manufactured by Tekscan, Inc. (South Boston, MA) is an integrated cost-effective in-shoe and floor mat pressure measurement system. The F-Scan consists of data acquisition electronics, software, trimmable in-shoe sensors (sizes range from children's to men's size, 14) and a floor-based system (470 mm $\times$ 320 mm). The ultra-thin (0.007″) reuseable in-shoe sensors consisting of 960 individual sensors are ideal for clinical evaluation of surgical and nonsurgical interventions, which effect gait biomechanics and plantar pressure distribution. Dynamic two-dimensional pressure contours and rotating three-dimensional images enable the clinician to quickly assess changes in segmental contact timing and pressure distribution. Standard software features include 165 Hz sampling rates, real-time and playback capabilities, and quantitative data presentations of force and pressure. Additional add-on capabilities include clinical seating and prosthetic sensor modules.

Pedabarograph

The Pedabarograph is an optics-based system that uses the critical light reflection technique to assess pressure distribution under the foot. The transducer-mounted glass plate of the system is illuminated from the sides and covered with a deformable plastic mat. When pressure is applied to the overlying mat, it is apposed to the glass surface and the normally internally reflected light is allowed to scatter. Greater pressure applied to the mat increases the contact area between the mat and the glass plate, producing more intense emission of light. The image is recorded through stance by a video camera. Using gray scale conversion, which assigns pressure values to different intensities of light, pressure maps are generated at a sampling rate of 30 Hz. This system has the potential for measurement of simultaneous shear forces.

Both systems provide software that allows determination of area-specific peak pressure and impulse, the pressure-time integral. This allows prospective assessment of plantar pressure effects of therapeutic intervention.

TECHNIQUE 2: THREE-DIMENSIONAL KINEMATIC ANALYSIS

Kinematic analysis of stance phase of the foot using gait analysis techniques promises to provide information of even greater value than plantar pressure studies. Although a number of methods of tracking limb motion have been devised, our experience has been with computerized tracking of video camera images of retroreflective markers. The subcutaneous location of many bony landmarks in the foot helps eliminate errors due to soft tissue shear so often experienced in motion studies of the more proximal limb.

For evaluation of each foot, 14 retroreflective markers are used (Fig. 7–14). Two are placed on the anterior tibia, one over each of the malleoli, three on the calcaneus, and one over the base and the head of the first and fifth metatarsals, providing four forefoot markers. To analyze great toe motion, three markers are on wands attached to a plate wrapped over the top of the proximal phalanx of the hallux. Four cameras record the paths of each marker, and computer integration of the multiple two-dimensional pathways formulates a three-dimensional trajectory for each marker. Computerized comparison of marker positions within selected coordinate systems allows determination of the relative motion of selected marked parts. Calcaneal, midfoot, and forefoot inversion-eversion, plantar flexion, dorsiflexion, and transverse plane rotation (calcaneal internal-external rotation), forefoot adduction-abduction can be assessed. Great toe flexion and extension, varus and valgus deviation, and frontal plane rotation can also be analyzed. Although the accuracy of these determinations appears to be great, confirmation awaits studies made with pins placed directly into bone.

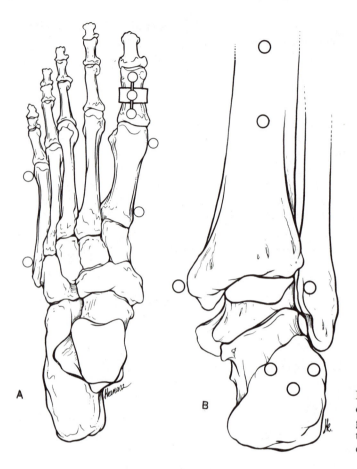

A

B

FIGURE 7–14. (*A*) Posterior diagram and (*B*) dorsal diagram of the skeleton indicate the location of reflective markers on the foot and tibia.

As with the quantitative study of dynamic foot pressure, three-dimensional kinematic analysis of foot motion provides an opportunity to correlate objectively the static evaluation with actual stance phase mechanics. In addition, the mechanical effects of therapeutic interventions, both orthotic and surgical, can be evaluated using this technique.

Biomechanical Evaluation

CHAPTER 8

Evaluation of Overuse Syndromes

Bruce Greenfield, MMSc, PT, OCS
Marie Johanson, MS, PT, OCS

This chapter focuses on major overuse injuries of the lower extremities according to specific anatomic sites and tissues. The pathophysiology of overuse injuries is a local inflammatory response to stress. The causes of overuse injuries are either intrinsic (malalignment syndromes, muscle imbalances) or extrinsic (training error) to the patient. Intrinsic and extrinsic factors are further classified as predisposing, precipitating, or perpetuating factors. A systematic musculoskeletal assessment is therefore necessary to differentiate overuse injuries and to clarify the etiologic factors. Effective treatment is predicated on recognizing and correcting the underlying etiologic factors. Case studies are presented illustrating the problem-solving approach to evaluation and treatment of overuse injuries. Each case delineates and explains predisposing, precipitating, and perpetuating factors related to the overuse injury. Treatment programs that address and correct these factors are presented.

DEFINITION OF OVERUSE INJURIES

Swimming, cycling, and running continue to grow in popularity. A 1985 Gallup poll indicated that 15% of all Americans (approximately 30 million persons) jog regularly.[1] In 1984, more than 100,000 persons completed marathons, and more than 1 million competed in triathalons. The 1984 Ironman triathalon in Hawaii, which combines a 2-mile ocean swim, 112 miles of cycling, and a marathon run, had more than 10,000 applicants for 1000 available entries.[2] Not surprisingly, injuries to the participants of these events are increasing. As far back as 1977, a *Runner's World* poll indicated that two thirds of all joggers suffer injuries to their lower extremities.[3] Marti and associates,[4] in a survey of 4358 male joggers, found that 45.8% had sustained jogging injuries during a 1-year period. Many of the injuries did not result from a single traumatic episode (i.e., a high-velocity force that produced sprain, strain, or fracture of ligaments, muscles, or bones). Instead, most of these injuries occurred insidiously, resulting from overuse of various musculoskeletal tissues. Overuse injuries result from repetitive subtraumatic forces. Breakdown of microscopic tissue occurs faster than the tissue can heal or repair itself. The results are inflammation, degeneration of involved tissues, muscle strain, stress fractures, ligament failure, tendinitis, and tendon ruptures.[5,6]

Inflammatory Response

The essential component in all overuse injuries, regardless of the affected anatomic tissue, is inflammation. The repetitive force of overuse results in tissue microtrauma, which triggers inflammation.

Following injury, initial vasoconstriction and hemostasis is followed within minutes by local vasodilatation and increased intracapillary pressure, which leads to transudation of fluid. Prostaglandins, a group of vasoactive substances, cause vasodilatation and increased vascular permeability. Prolonged capillary permeability results in exudation of fluid, swelling, and pain.[7] The initial medical treatment of overuse is the administration of a nonsteroidal anti-inflammatory agent, which inhibits prostaglandin synthesis.[8]

As inflammation continues, leukocyte cells (neutrophils, monocytes, and eosinophils) migrate to the area. The neutrophil cells initiate degradation of surrounding tissue through activation of proteolytic enzymes contained within their lysosomes. After a few days, neutrophil cells are replaced by monocyte cells, which, in turn, differentiate into macrophage cells. Macrophage cells, which contain proteolytic enzymes, digest cellular debris and connective tissue fragments. Lymphocyte cells are important in chronic inflammation and activate monocyte cells. Monocyte cells, which contain and release proteolytic enzymes, perpetuate the inflammatory response.

Other cells, including endothelial and fibroblast cells, migrate within a few days to the injured area and produce capillary buds and collagen to begin the reparative process. Maturation of collagen is a relatively long-term process, and the patient must modify his or her activities for the next few weeks to rest the injured area. For a runner, activity modification can vary from simply decreasing training distances to being limited to non–weight-bearing activity. An activity level is developed that allows unabated healing and scar maturation.

Most of the symptoms associated with acute inflammation subside within 2 weeks,[9] although subacute symptoms can continue about 1 month after the onset of inflammation. Chronic inflammation is inflammation that persists beyond this period and is characterized by the same signs and symptoms of acute inflammation (redness, heat, edema, and pain) but at a less pronounced level.[10] Histologically, chronic inflammation is characterized by the replacement of leukocytes by macrophages, plasma cells, and lymphocytes at the site of injury.[6]

Chronic inflammation in overuse injuries is perpetuated by one or more mechanical irritants.[10] The tissue response is local proliferation of mononuclear cells.

Macrophages remain in inflamed tissue if an acute inflammation does not resolve, but their role is modified. Macrophages attract fibroblasts, and as the chronic inflammatory state continues, large numbers of fibroblasts invade the area and produce increased quantities of collagen. Often, increased collagen production results in decreased extensibility of a joint or soft tissue structure.

The clinician must recognize that inflammation is a necessary component of healing. Motion applied to the injured area during the initial inflammatory response, however, can lead to chronic inflammation and destruction of surrounding tissues. The goal, therefore, in treating overuse injuries is to minimize chronic inflammation to allow healing.

Tissue Degeneration

Tissue degeneration occurs as a result of cell atrophy. Causes of cell atrophy include chronic inflammation and immobilization.[6] Degenerated tissue is more vulnerable to repetitive stress and can result in mechanical fatigue or failure. Mechanical fatigue or failure of tissue increases the likelihood of recurrent inflammation.[6]

Signs of classic inflammation cannot be found in all overuse injuries.[6,11] The relationship between tissue damage and inflammation is not well understood. Leadbetter[6] suggests that the classic inflammatory response is initiated only after a sufficient degree of structural and microvascular damage occurs.

Because chronic inflammation can result in degeneration of tissue, and degenerated tissue is vulnerable to recurrent inflammation when repetitively stressed, both are likely to occur in overuse injuries.

CAUSES

Factors leading to overuse injuries can be subgrouped as predisposing, precipitating, or perpetuating (Table 8–1). These factors can be further classified as intrinsic and extrinsic.

Predisposing Factors

Predisposing factors are intrinsic to the patient and include malalignment syndromes, leg length discrepancy, and muscle dysfunction of the lower extremity. Several studies have identified malalignment syndrome in overuse injuries.[12–17] James et

TABLE 8–1 Etiologic Factors in Overuse Injuries

Predisposing (Intrinsic)	Precipitating (Extrinsic)	Perpetuating (Intrinsic and Extrinsic)
Malalignment syndromes	Training errors	Combination of intrinsic and extrinsic
Leg length discrepancy	Running surfaces	
Muscle dysfunction	Shoes and equipment	

al,[12] in a series of 180 patients with 232 overuse injuries, identified prolonged or excessive pronation of the ankle and foot in 58% of the patients. Clement,[13] in a retrospective survey of 1650 runners with overuse injuries, found in a majority of these runners anatomic malalignment, including a leg length discrepancy, femoral bone anteversion, and excessive pronation of the ankle and foot. Viitasale and Kvist[14] found a greater prevalence of abnormal subtalar joint pronation in runners with shin splints than in asymptomatic runners. Lutter[15] reviewed 171 overuse injuries to 121 runners and found excessive pronation to be an etiologic factor in approximately 56% of the injuries. Lilletvedt et al[16] found a statistically greater number of malalignment problems (including tibia varum and excessive pronation) in athletes with shin splints than in athletes without shin splints. DeLacerda[17] found that a statistically significant number of patients with excessive pronation developed shin splints after 14 weeks of controlled exercises.[17] Messier and Pittala[18] reported significantly increased velocity and degree of pronation in recreational and competitive runners with shin splints or plantar fasciitis when compared with a control group of uninjured runners. Additionally, they reported a nonsignificant trend toward restricted dorsiflexion in the group of runners with shin splints. In a retrospective study, Buchbinder et al[19] found an abnormal foot position in 77% of 213 runners with knee overuse injuries, abnormal pronation in 43%, and cavus feet in 34%.

Overuse injuries in the lower extremities can result from excessive pronation in the foot and ankle, leg length discrepancy, and muscle dysfunction. The pathomechanical responses in the lower extremities for each of these predisposing factors are discussed next.

ABNORMAL PRONATION

The pathomechanics of excessive pronation can be understood by looking at gait and at the normal foot during heel strike. Ambulation is a series of rotations, starting at the lumbar spine, that propel the body through space. The transverse rotations of the tibia and the femur are transmitted and reduced at the subtalar joint. During the stance phase of gait, the foot does not rotate. The tibia rotates internally at heel strike, and the talus of the ankle follows, resulting in pronation of the subtalar joint, or heel eversion.[20]

Normal mechanics dictate that the tibiofemoral joint extend and the lower extremity rotate externally at midstance. The calcaneus inverts and the talus is pushed by the sustentaculum tali of the calcaneus into a lateral position. The midtarsal joint locks, and the foot becomes a rigid lever for toe-off.[20]

Excessive subtalar joint pronation results in internal rotation of the tibia and delays the external rotation of the lower extremity that accompanies subtalar joint supination. Compensatory internal rotation of the femur may occur, disrupting the normal biomechanics of the lower extremity and altering patellofemoral joint tracking. Excessive pressure between the lateral facet of the patella and the lateral condyle of the femur may result.[21] Excessive pronation fatigues the anterior and posterior tibialis muscles, which are attempting to support the medial border of the foot. Stress is passed upward through the foot to the medial aspect of the knee and hip. This stress may not be significant during the act of walking, but during running increased weight and rotation stresses are produced along the lower extremity. The increased stress can result in tissue fatigue and microtrauma followed by inflammation.

CAVUS FEET

The term "pes cavus" is used to describe deformities of the forefoot and rearfoot in the sagittal and frontal planes. At heel strike, the pes cavus foot tends to maintain the rearfoot in varus,[22] resulting in a reduction of normal subtalar joint pronation. Reduced subtalar joint pronation decreases attenuation of forces at the foot and ankle, thereby increasing forces proximally. At the foot and ankle joint, pes cavus feet are most frequently associated with plantar fasciitis, metatarsalgia, peroneal tendinitis, stress fractures of the fifth metatarsal, and medial longitudinal arch pain.[22,23] More proximally, pes cavus feet are most frequently associated with iliotibial band friction syndrome, lateral knee pain, and, less frequently, chondromalacia patellae.[22]

ABNORMAL TORSIONS

Tibial torsion refers to the rotation of the tibia along its longitudinal axis.[24] Normal tibial torsion is approximately 20° to 25° of external torsion in the adult.[25] Stuberg et al[26] reported that a goniometric measurement of tibial torsion is both reliable and valid when compared with a tomographic measurement (Fig. 8–1). Abnormal pronation is a common secondary problem associated with abnormal external tibial torsion.[27]

"Miserable malalignment" is also associated with overuse injuries.[21] Miserable malalignment, as described by James,[28] is a series of compensatory torsional and frontal plane changes in the lower extremities. Figure 8–2 shows an example of mis-

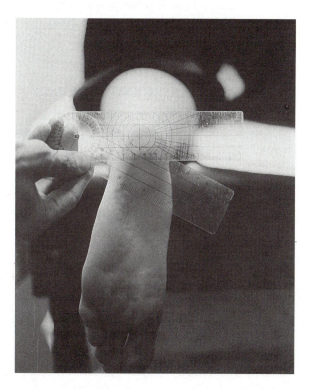

FIGURE 8–1. Tibial torsion is measured with the patient prone, the knee flexed to 90°, and the hip in the approximate neutral position. One arm of the goniometer is aligned with an imaginary line bisecting the medial and lateral malleoli; the other is held perpendicular to a line bisecting the midline of the thigh. The acute angle represents the degrees of tibial external torsion.

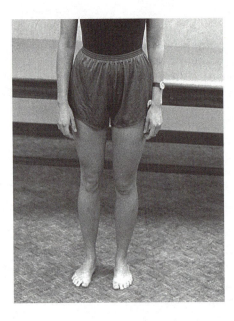

FIGURE 8–2. Miserable malalignment. Femur bone anteversion with squinting patella bone, proximal external tibia bone torsion, tibia bone varum, and subtalar joint pronation.

erable malalignment, illustrating anteversion of the femur, proximal external torsion of the tibia, tibia varum, and subtalar joint pronation. Miserable malalignment with proximal external torsion of the tibia results in an increased Q angle of the extensor mechanism in the knee. An increased Q angle in the knee results in lateral tracking of the patella and predisposes toward chondromalacia patellae.[28] Abnormal pronation may compensate for femoral anteversion and external tibial torsion in individuals with miserable malalignment and may predispose the individual to overuse injuries associated with abnormal pronation.

GENU VARUM AND GENU VALGUM

Genu varum deformities of the knee may result in a functional forefoot varus at heel strike followed by abnormal rapid pronation to allow weight bearing under the medial metatarsal heads. These changes during gait may result in lateral foot pain, Achilles tendinitis, or plantar fasciitis.[29]

Genu valgus deformities are also associated with abnormal pronation in gait,[30] presumably as a result of greater vertical forces medial to the axis of the subtalar joint that increase the degree of calcaneal valgus.

LEG LENGTH DISCREPANCY

Leg length discrepancies have been associated with various musculoskeletal problems. Giles and Taylor[31] found that over twice as many patients with low back pain have a leg length discrepancy of 10 mm or more. Bolz and Davies[32] found that in subjects with a leg length discrepancy of 0.5 cm or more, total leg strength was reduced in the short leg. Subotnick[33] examined 4000 athletes over 6 years and found that 40% had either a functional or anatomic leg length discrepancy. A patient may attempt to equalize a leg length discrepancy by internally rotating the long leg. The resultant subtalar joint pronation functionally shortens the long leg. This posture of excessive pronation, however, produces excessive strain along the medial structures of the ankle and knee, resulting in overuse and pathologic changes of related soft tissues. Environmental functional leg length discrepancies can result from running on transverse grades, which reportedly predispose the runner to excessive supination on the downhill or "long-limb" side and excessive pronation on the uphill or "short-limb" side.[11,18]

MUSCLE DYSFUNCTION

Muscle dysfunctions associated with overuse injuries include imbalances between the quadriceps femoris and hamstring muscles at the knee and the gastrocnemius-soleus and anterior tibialis muscles at the ankle and foot.

Muscle is the best force attenuator in the body.[34] Eccentric or lengthening action of muscle dampens the forces of weight bearing. At heel strike, the lower limb is slowly lowered to the ground. Flexion at the knee is controlled by the eccentric action of the quadriceps femoris muscle. The foot is lowered to the ground by the eccentric contractions of the anterior tibialis, extensor hallucis longus, and extensor digitorum longus muscles. The anterior movement of the tibia over the talus during midstance is controlled by the gastrocnemius-soleus muscle group.[35]

Alterations in muscle function include muscle weakness, poor flexibility, and inadequate endurance for musculoskeletal performance during specific functional activities. Alteration in muscle function results in inadequate or abnormal movement patterns during activities such as running. For example, Elliot and Achland[5] used high-speed cinematography to study the effect of fatigue on the mechanical characteristics of running in highly skilled long distance runners. They found that, toward the end of a race, the runners exhibited less efficient positioning of the foot at foot strike as well as decreased stride length and stride rate. Alteration in muscle function during running can cause bone, ligament, and tendon to be overworked, producing tissue breakdown and pathology.[5]

Hamstring muscle tightness in the presence of quadriceps femoris muscle weakness has been associated with anterior knee pain, including chondromalacia patellae.[28] In the presence of hamstring muscle tightness, patellofemoral joint compressive forces increase during the swing-through phase of gait or recovery phase of running. Quadriceps femoris muscle weakness, especially in the vastus medialis muscle, can result in lateral patellar tracking during knee flexion and extension. The result can be abnormal retropatellar stresses along the lateral facet of the patella with cartilage degeneration. Because the quadriceps femoris muscle controls knee flexion during the stance phase of walking or running, weakness can result in increased shock to the ankle and knee. Such abnormal stresses can lead to hyaline cartilage microtrauma and degeneration. Quadriceps femoris muscle weakness, therefore, places increased stress on the knee and ankle, resulting, with repetitive exercise, in overuse.[28]

Imbalance between gastrocnemius-soleus muscles and weak pretibial muscles, anterior tibialis, extensor hallucis longus, and extensor digitorum longus muscles has been associated with anterior shin splints, especially during repetitive hill running.[36] During uphill running, the pretibial muscles forcefully contract in the recovery phase of running to dorsiflex the ankle, allowing the foot to clear the surface of the ground. Additionally, during downhill running, at heel strike, the pretibial muscles contract eccentrically to control ankle plantar flexion and prevent foot-slap. Overactivation of these muscles can occur in the presence of tight antagonists (the gastrocnemius-soleus muscles). The result may be microtrauma and inflammation of the pretibial muscles, tendons, and bony attachments.[36]

Tightness of the gastrocnemius-soleus muscles may result in compensatory abnormal pronation even in the absence of an intrinsic foot deformity.[37,38] Tight gastrocnemius-soleus muscles may also result in early heel-off in gait resulting in increased stress to the forefoot. Increased stress on the forefoot is a precursor to metatarsalgia.[39] Other potential compensatory changes in response to tight gastrocnemius-soleus muscles include (1) dorsiflexion of the forefoot on the rearfoot, resulting in strain of the midtarsal joints; (2) increased knee flexion, resulting in a functional leg length discrepancy; and (3) hyperextension of the knee, resulting in strain of the posterior knee joint capsule.[39,40]

Precipitating Factors

In contrast to the predisposing factors, which are intrinsic, the precipitating factors in overuse injuries are extrinsic (Table 8–1). According to Cavanaugh,[41] the average runner's pace is 3.83 meters per second, and the foot strikes the ground approximately 5100 times each hour. The ground reaction force at midstance in running is 250% to 300% of body weight.[1] An average runner, therefore, experiences in 1 hour a tremendous amount of force through the lower extremities. Not surprisingly, therefore, according to James et al,[12] training errors are associated with 60% of overuse injuries. Specifically, they found excessive mileage, the intensity of workouts, and a too rapid change in a training routine to be the major training errors. According to Clancy,[42] a series of high-intensity workouts does not allow the tissues in the lower extremity to recover from fatigue and microtrauma.

EXCESSIVE MILEAGE

Excessive mileage may culminate in fatigue of leg muscles. Muscle fatigue is characterized by impaired ability of the muscle to generate normal strength and endurance levels after vigorous exercise. Some of the biomechanical processes that are active in or responsible for the onset of fatigue are neuromuscular and chemical.[43]

Successive days of heavy training deplete glycogen stores in specific muscle fibers, such as the gastrocnemius-soleus muscles, that are used to absorb shock and propel. During midstance phase of running, the gastrocnemius-soleus muscle acts eccentrically to control movement of the tibia over the foot. The gastrocnemius-soleus muscles contract concentrically at toe-off to propel the body. The tensile loading during the contraction, combined with gravitational elongation, is extremely high. When the muscles are depleted of fluid, irritated, and repeatedly contracted, greater stress is placed on tendons, which are undergoing extraordinary stretch.[43] Microtearing of the fascicles of the tendon results in inflammation. Continued running in the presence of microtears and inflammation perpetuates the inflammatory response, thereby creating further tearing and inflammation.

EXCESSIVE SPEED

Increased speed of gait requires the lower extremities to absorb ground reaction forces in a shorter period of time. One gait cycle occurs in 1 second at a 5.0 kilometers per hour (kph) walking speed but occurs in only 0.6 second during 20 kph running.[44] Subtalar joint pronation reaches its maximal level in 0.15 second during walking but in only 0.03 second during running.[8] Generally, joint motion in the sagittal plane increases as speed increases. For example, approximately 10° more of dorsiflexion at the ankle joint is required during midstance and 8° more of plantar flexion is required at toe-off in running as compared with walking.[8,44] Therefore, restricted joint motion is more likely to result in overuse injury during running than walking.

Muscles demonstrate longer relative periods of electrical activity in running as compared with walking. At the ankle joint, the gastrocnemius-soleus muscles are active during the middle 50% of the stance phase during walking, but this increases to the latter 25% of the swing phase through the first 80% of the stance phase during running.[44] Neuromuscular control is often sacrificed to accommodate speed, potentially resulting in greater stress to joints, muscles, and connective tissues.[43] Increased rapidity of movement results in decreased activity of the antagonistic muscle groups and can lead to joint hyperextension as well as overstretching of the musculotendinous unit.[43]

RUNNING SURFACES

Hard, uneven, or sloping surfaces cause increased ground-reactive forces, altering normal biomechanics and producing injury.[42] For example, running along the transverse grade or gutter of a road causes increased pronation of the uphill foot and supination of the downhill foot. The heel of the uphill foot angles into valgus, and the subtalar joint pronates. The excessive or prolonged pronation increases the stress on the foot and ankle structures and produces obligatory internal rotation of the tibia. The prolonged tibial rotation may produce strain of the medial knee structures. Problems similar to those encountered when running along the transverse grade of a road can develop from running on a track. While on the curved portion of the track, the inside foot must pronate and the outside foot must supinate to greater degrees than when running on the straightaways.[23]

As mentioned previously, uphill running requires increased dorsiflexion of the ankle during both the recovery and the support phases. Increased dorsiflexion also occurs at the first metatarsophalangeal (MTP) joint, and increased tension occurs on the plantar fascia and gastrocnemius-soleus muscles. Strain along the plantar fascia results from the windlass effect,[45] which results in tightening of the plantar fascia with hyperextension of the MTP joints. This increased strain can result in microtrauma to the first MTP joint, plantar fasciitis, and Achilles tendinitis.

SHOES AND EQUIPMENT

Improper equipment selection, including inadequate running shoes, also can precipitate an overuse injury. Excessive wear along the outsole, a nonflexible outsole, flared-in shoe last, inadequate heel cushion, and a small toe box have all been implicated as factors in overuse injuries.[42] For example, a nonflexible outsole may reduce the ability of the foot to pronate at the midstance phase of running. A shoe with an inadequate heel cushion reduces the ability of the foot to dissipate ground reaction forces at heel strike. The result of both of these problems is an increase of forces and stress along the heel, ankle, and foot. In addition, excessive wear along the outsole of the shoe may perpetuate excessive pronation during the support phase of running.

The resultant obligatory internal rotation of the leg results in increased stress along the medial structures in the ankle and knee.

The lasting of the shoe is another factor that may precipitate an overuse injury. Straight-lasted shoes are those with symmetry around the long axis of the midsole and toe box. Straight-lasted shoes provide more support to the medial aspect of the shoe. Therefore, they are most ideal for slower runners who excessively pronate.[46] Curve-lasted shoes are designed to provide more support to the lateral portion of the foot and are most ideal for faster runners.

Cleated shoes pose additional considerations. Although long cleats increase traction, danger of locking the foot onto the surfaces increases. Therefore, shoes with a relatively large number of lower, but wider cleats (approximately 9 mm high and 12 mm wide) are recommended.[47]

Perpetuating Factors

Overuse injuries, especially in athletes, are often difficult to treat because the athlete usually resumes the same training pattern (precipitating factors) under the same pathomechanical conditions (predisposing factors) that initially caused the injury. The perpetuating factors of overuse injuries, therefore, are the combination of the precipitating and perpetuating factors already discussed (Table 8–1). To treat overuse injuries successfully, the predisposing and precipitating factors must be eliminated or modified. For each patient, the clinician must evaluate lower extremity biomechanics and muscle flexibility and strength and have a thorough knowledge of the anatomic demands of the sport, the environment in which the athlete is performing, and the equipment and training techniques involved.

CLARIFYING ASSESSMENT OF THE LOWER EXTREMITIES

Evaluation for specific overuse syndromes is addressed in the following section. The clinician, however, should perform a systematic clarifying evaluation of the lower extremities in all cases of overuse. This evaluation includes a comprehensive history of the injury; the patient's occupation, hobbies, and exercise habits; and a thorough biomechanical evaluation of the lower extremities.

History

The initial step in evaluation is history taking. The history provides the clinician with a "road map" for the direction of the remaining clarifying evaluation. The clinician determines whether the injury was traumatic or nontraumatic. Nontraumatic injuries signal overuse and should prompt further questions concerning the patient's work and sports habits. Activities involving repetitive use of the lower extremities are determined. For runners, training methods, shoes, and training surfaces are reviewed.

Questions are asked about the area and nature of pain. The boundaries of pain are delineated, helping the clinician to isolate the involved tissues and anatomic structures. The type of pain—dull, aching, burning, throbbing—is ascertained. Generally a superficial burning pain is a problem with muscle, tendon, or perhaps nerve, whereas a deep ache or dull pain could involve capsule or bone.[48] The patient is questioned about incidences of numbness or tingling, which could indicate compression neuropathy associated with conditions such as tarsal tunnel syndrome of the ankle or Morton's neuroma of the foot.[49] Questions concerning temperature change in the foot and ankle should be asked. Persistent coolness could signal compartment syndrome of the leg.[50]

The nature of the pain over a 24-hour cycle should be ascertained. Knowing what activities precipitate the pain helps the clinician determine the nature of the overuse injury. Activities and previous pain-relieving treatments, such as ice, heat, rest, elevation, or aspirin, provide clues for the clinician about the nature of the injury—acute, subacute, or chronic—so that appropriate and effective treatment can be planned.

Physical Evaluation

An outline of the physical evaluation is presented in Table 8–2. The examination includes the entire lower extremity and is not confined to the area of injury. All intrinsic factors related to overuse are evaluated.

Static postural evaluation is performed from the anterior, posterior, and lateral positions. Anteriorly the alignment of the lower extremities is observed and the degree of torsional or angular malalignment is determined. "Squinting" patellas suggest femoral anteversion and are usually accompanied by an apparent genu varum, proximal external torsion of the tibia, varum of the distal tibia, and compensatory ankle and foot pronation (see Fig. 8–2).[28]

From the side, the clinician looks for genu recurvatum, which indicates a shallow femoral groove that can result in poor patellofemoral joint congruency. Poor congruency results in lateral patellar tracking, which with overuse can lead to anterior knee pain and chondromalacia patellae.

From behind, the pelvic crests, the posterior-superior iliac spines of the pelvis, and the greater trochanters of the femurs are palpated for any asymmetry that might indicate leg length discrepancy or a sacroiliac joint lesion. The leg-to-floor and heel-to-floor angles are measured with a goniometer (Figs. 8–3 and 8–4). These measurements give an indication of the amount of tibial varum and calcaneal eversion during weight bearing. Discussion of these measurements and their significance related to the lower quarter dysfunction is presented in Chapter 7.

The patient is observed walking and, in some instances, running. The mechanics of the subtalar joint are observed during each phase of stance. Generally, at heel strike, the joint should be in the neutral position, followed immediately by rapid pronation toward footflat. From heel-off to toe-off, resupination occurs at the subtalar joint, establishing the foot as a rigid lever for push-off.[20] Pronation beyond footflat is excessive, resulting, as described previously, in prolonged internal rotation of the tibia and femur. Stress is placed along various structures and soft tissues in the foot, ankle, knee, and hip.

The alignment of the extensor mechanism is examined by measuring the Q angle at the knee. The Q angle is measured by placing a goniometer directly over the center of the patella with one arm aimed at the anterior-superior iliac spine of the pelvis and the other in line with the center of the tubercle of the tibia (Fig. 8–5).[28] An excessive Q angle (greater than 15° in women and 10° in men) indicates a propensity for lateral tracking of the patella during range of motion or forceful repetitive contrac-

TABLE 8–2 Physical Evaluation

I. Postural evaluation
   A. Anterior
      1. Miserable malalignment
      2. Leg length discrepancy
   B. Lateral
      1. Genu recurvatum
   C. Posterior
      1. Leg length
      2. Leg-to-floor angle (tibial varum)
      3. Heel-to-floor angle (calcaneal valgus/varum)
II. Dynamic evaluation
   A. Walking or running on treadmill
   B. Observe movement of calcaneus and navicular bone
III. Static evaluation
   A. Q angle
   B. Patellar mobility
      1. Apprehension test
   C. Hip rotation/hip adduction-abduction
      1. Prone (femoral anteversion, femoral retroversion)
      2. Prone knee extension and flexion—adduction/abduction
      3. FABER test, hip capsule tightness/sacroiliac compression
   D. Tibial torsion
   E. Flexibility
      1. Ankle dorsiflexion
         a) Knee straight
         b) Knee flexed 30°
      2. Hamstring muscles
      3. Ober (tensor fascia lata muscle and iliotibial band)
      4. Modified Thomas's test (iliopsoas and rectus femoris muscles)
   F. Strength
      1. Manual
      2. Isokinetic
   G. Functional tests
      1. Hop tests
      2. Proprioceptive tests

tions of the quadricep femoris muscles.[28] The Q angle is often increased in miserable malalignment, owing to external torsion of the proximal tibia, resulting in lateral displacement of the tibial tubercle.

Mobility of the patella is tested with the knee straight and at 30° of flexion. At 30° of knee flexion, the patella is secure in the femoral trochlear groove. Lateral displacement greater than one half the width of the patella indicates hypermobility with potential weakness of the vastus medialis muscle.[28] Patients with a history of a lateral dislocating patella exhibit a positive apprehension sign during forceful lateral glide of the patella (Fig. 8–6).

Hip rotation is tested with the patient prone and with the knees flexed to 90° (Fig. 8–7). Excessive internal rotation suggests femoral anteversion, whereas excessive external rotation suggests femoral retroversion. Either condition may precipitate torsional or frontal plane compensatory changes in the lower extremities. A goniometric measurement can give a numerical estimate of femoral anteversion (Fig. 8–8).[51]

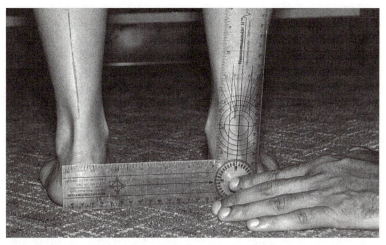

FIGURE 8–3. Leg-floor angle. This angle is formed by a longitudinal line bisecting the distal one third of the lower leg with a horizontal line along the ground. The angle represents the amount of varum in the distal tibia bone.

Tibial torsion can also be measured with the patient in the prone position and the knees flexed to 90° (Fig. 8–1).[26] External tibial torsion less than 20°, indicates internal tibial torsion, whereas external tibial torsion of greater than 25° indicates external tibial torsion.

Flexibility tests include ankle dorsiflexion measured with the knee extended and flexed (Figs. 8–9 and 8–10). Care is taken while passively dorsiflexing the foot to maintain slight inversion. Foot eversion allows pronation to occur at the subtalar and midtarsal joints and gives a false impression of increased dorsiflexion.[52] Other flexi-

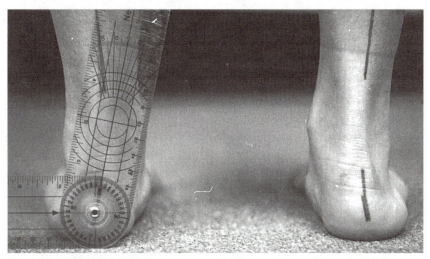

FIGURE 8–4. Heel-floor angle. This angle is found by a longitudinal line bisecting the heel with a horizontal line along the ground. The angle represents the amount of eversion during standing at the subtalar joint.

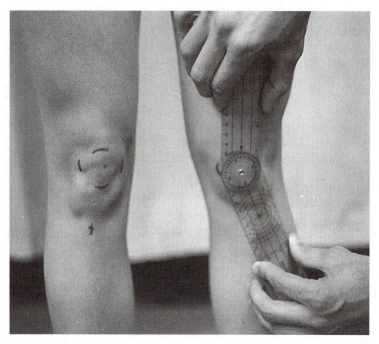

FIGURE 8–5. Q angle. This angle is formed by a line measured between the anterior superior iliac spine (ASIS) of the patella bone to the midpoint of the patella bone, and a line measured between the midpoint of the patella bone and the tibial tubercle of the tibia bone.

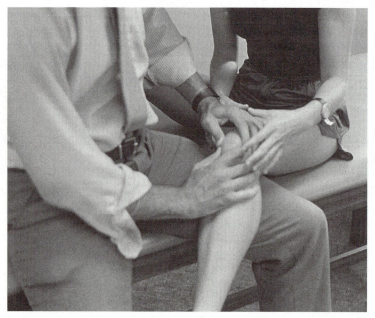

FIGURE 8–6. Apprehension sign for lateral dislocating patella.

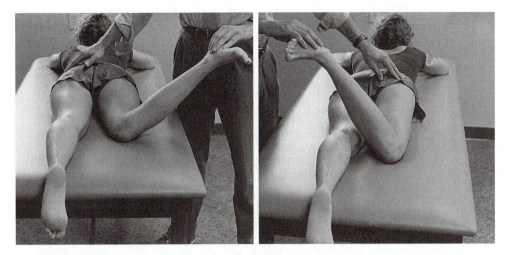

FIGURE 8–7. Hip rotation for femoral anteversion or retroversion tested prone. The hip is maintained in neutral position relative to the pelvis, and the knees are flexed at 90°. Excessive outward rotation of the lower leg indicates femoral anteversion, while excessive inward rotation of the lower leg indicates femoral retroversion.

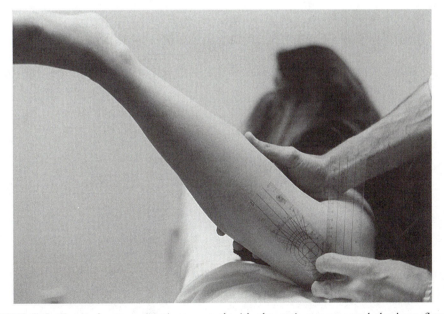

FIGURE 8–8. Femoral anteversion is measured with the patient prone and the knee flexed to 90°. The examiner stands on the contralateral side and palpates the greater trochanter as the hip is internally rotated. At the point of maximal trochanteric prominence, a second examiner aligns one arm of the goniometer along the midshaft of the tibia and the other arm is held in a vertical position.

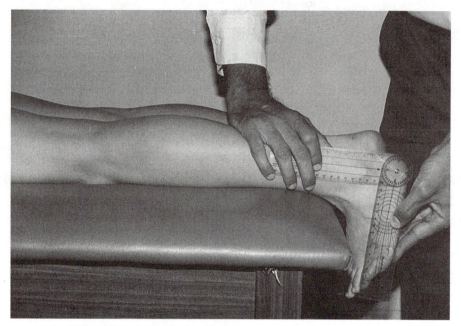

FIGURE 8–9. Ankle dorsiflexion measured with knee straight.

bility tests include the modified Thomas test, hamstring flexibility test, and Ober test (Figs. 8–11 to 8–14). Strength tests, if necessary, are performed using one of the various isokinetic devices on the market. Important agonist-antagonist strength ratios should be ascertained for the ankle dorsiflexors and plantar flexors, the knee extensors and flexors, and the hip abductors and adductors. Normative values for some of these ratios are reported elsewhere.[53]

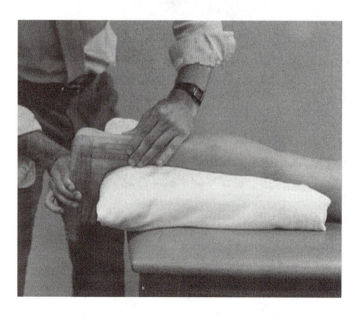

FIGURE 8–10. Ankle dorsiflexion to isolate the soleus muscle measured with knee flexed to approximately 30°.

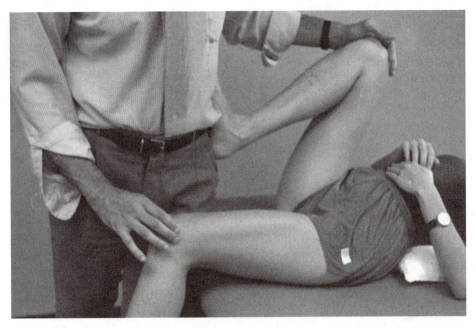

FIGURE 8–11. Modified Thomas test for tightness of the tensor fasciae latae, iliopsoas, and rectus femoris muscles.

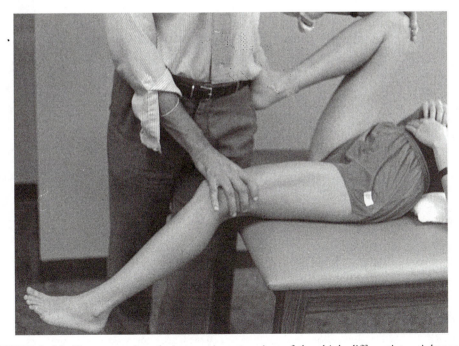

FIGURE 8–12. Knee extension during passive extension of the thigh differentiates tightness of the rectus femoris muscle from iliopsoas muscle.

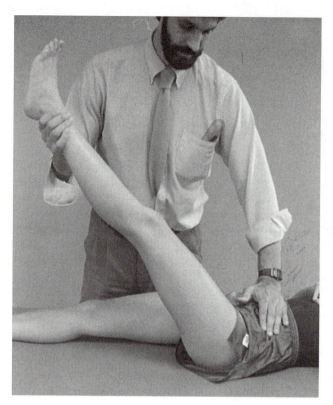

FIGURE 8–13. Hamstring flexibility. Movement of the ipsilateral pelvis and ASIS during straight leg raise indicates end range extensibility of hamstring muscles.

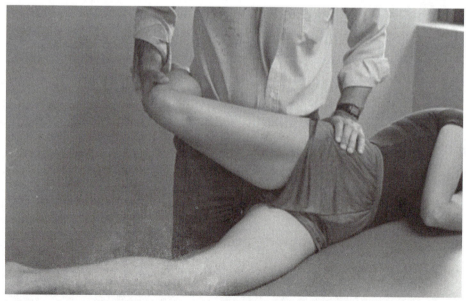

FIGURE 8–14. Demonstration of the Ober test, which tests for tightness of the tensor fascia lata muscle and the iliotibial band (ITB). The hip, with patient sidelying, is abducted and extended. Inability to passively adduct the hip indicates tightness of the tensor fascia lata and ITB.

Functional tests may be included to evaluate strength and proprioceptive ability of the lower extremity during weight-bearing activities. These tests help determine a patient's readiness for return to sporting activities. Functional hop tests as described by Noyes et al[54] include comparison of the involved extremity to the uninvolved extremity in unilateral single hop for distance, unilateral triple hop for distance, unilateral triple crossover hop for distance, and unilateral hopping over 6 meters for time. Voight and Draovitch[55] suggest a series of static stability tests to evaluate proprioceptive ability of the lower extremity before initiation of plyometric activity. The first test consists of unilateral leg stance for 30 seconds with the eyes open followed by 30 seconds with the eyes closed. The second and third tests consist of a unilateral quarter squat and a unilateral half squat each held for 30 seconds with the eyes open and 30 seconds with the eyes closed.

A thorough and systematic evaluation helps the clinician pinpoint the underlying biomechanical factors influencing the overuse injury. Correction of these factors is imperative for successful resolution of the injury and to prevent recurrence. Evaluation and differentiation of specific overuse injuries is presented next.

COMMON OVERUSE INJURIES

Overuse injuries affect different anatomic sites and tissues. A *Runner's World*[3] survey conducted in 1977 cited the most common areas of overuse in runners as the knee (25%), Achilles tendon (18%), shin (15%), ankle (11%), and heel (10%). A survey by Eggold[56] of 146 runners indicated the most common overuse injuries were knee pain (40%), plantar fasciitis (15%), Achilles tendinitis (9%), and shin splints (7%). In Clement's[13] series of 1819 runners, the anatomic areas most affected by overuse were the knee (41.7%), lower leg (27.9%), foot (18.1%), hip (5%), lumbar spine (3.7%), and upper leg (3.6%). Specific syndromes included patellofemoral joint pain syndrome (25.8%), tibia stress syndrome (13.2%), Achilles tendinitis (6%), plantar fasciitis (4.7%), patellar tendinitis (4.5%), iliotibial friction band syndrome (ITFBS, 4.3%), metatarsal fracture (3.2%), and tibial fractures (2.6%). Finally, James' group's[12] survey of 180 runners with overuse injuries listed the following most commonly involved anatomic sites and syndromes: knee (25%), posterior tibial syndrome (13%), Achilles tendinitis (11%), plantar fasciitis (7%), and stress fractures (6%). In the knee pain group, the most common injuries included chondromalacia patella (25%), nonspecific anterior knee pain (20%), ITFBS (17%), and patellar tendinitis (7%).[12]

Based on these surveys, most overuse injuries affect the knee, lower leg, ankle, foot, upper leg, hip, and pelvis. The following case studies illustrate common overuse injuries and their pathomechanics, clinical signs and symptoms, and conservative treatment. The case studies emphasize the problem-solving approach to treatment by identifying, defining, and addressing the predisposing, precipitating, and, hence, perpetuating factors in overuse injuries.

Plantar Fasciitis

According to Bojsen-Møller and Flagsted,[57] the plantar fascia is the most common site of heel pain in runners. The plantar fascia, or aponeurosis, is composed of central, lateral, and medial bands and originates along the medial tubercle of the calcaneus. The plantar fascia courses anteriorly along the arch of the foot, each band attaching to the sides of the proximal phalanx in each toe.[58] According to Hicks,[45] the plantar fascia is responsible for 60% of the stress applied to the foot during footflat. At toe-off, hyperextension of the MTP joints results in tightening of the plantar fascia and assists with resupination of the foot (windlass mechanism). The windlass mechanism of the plantar fascia sustains 1.7 to 3 times body weight.[45]

CASE STUDY

1: Plantar Fasciitis

Subjective. A 27-year-old male recreational basketball and tennis player complained of heel pain that was worse in the morning. The patient reported reduced pain after walking but increased pain during and after basketball or tennis. Pain was unilateral.

Objective. Palpation revealed tenderness along the medial tubercle of the calcaneus. Soft tissue edema was also palpated along the medial aspect of the calcaneus.

Trigger points were palpated along the medial arch, in the muscle of the abductor hallucis brevis. Passive dorsiflexion of the first MTP joint of the foot reproduced pain. Dorsiflexion of the ankle with the knee straight was limited to the neutral position (90°).

Forefoot varus deformities were measured at 12° in the involved foot and 10° in the uninvolved foot. Valgus of the calcaneus bones during standing was observed in both subtalar joints.

Assessment. Plantar fasciitis secondary to overstretching of the plantar fascia from its medial attachment along the calcaneus.

Predisposing Factors. Excessive pronation of the subtalar joint causes the calcaneus to move into eversion to compensate for the forefoot varus deformity, producing a stretching of the plantar fascia.

According to Lutter,[59] a majority of patients with plantar fasciitis present with either a pronated or a cavus foot. Excessive pronation of the subtalar joint results in abnormal and prolonged eversion of the calcaneus. Prolonged eversion of the calcaneus bone during footflat results in stretching of the plantar fascia. If the foot fails to resupinate at toe-off, increased strain is placed on the plantar fascia owing to the windlass effect. Conversely a cavus foot occurs in the presence of limited subtalar joint eversion. Plantar fasciitis may develop because of the intrinsic inability of the cavus foot to dissipate the weight-bearing forces, particularly from heel strike to midstance. As a result, in either a pronated or a cavus foot, during repetitive exercise such as running, microtears occur at the insertion of the plantar fascia on the medial tubercle of the calcaneus, resulting in localized inflammation.[59]

Achilles tendon tightness results in compensatory, increased dorsiflexion of the first MTP joint during the stance phase of gait or running. Dorsiflexion of the first MTP joint via the windlass effect stretches the plantar fascia at its insertion along the medial tubercle of the calcaneus.[60]

Precipitating Factors. Basketball and tennis: The patient averaged 2 hours of play daily, 5 days a week.

Perpetuating Factors. The aforementioned activities combined with intrinsic problems delineated as the predisposing factors to perpetuate the injury. Perpetuating factors are always a combination of predisposing and precipating factors and therefore are not delineated in subsequent case studies.

Treatment. Ice and iontophoresis with 10% hydrocortisone were applied for 30 minutes to the inflamed area. Foot orthoses were fabricated using medial forefoot and rearfoot posts of 5 to 7 mm to allow the subtalar joint to function close to neutral position. Stretching exercises, by lengthening the gastrocnemius-soleus muscles of the ankle and foot, rebalance muscle flexibility in the ankle and foot during the stance phase of walking and running.

Achilles Tendinitis

Seen more often in men than women, Achilles tendinitis, with or without peritendinitis is often associated with repetitive or high-impact sports, such as running, basketball, or volleyball.[37]

CASE STUDY

2: Achilles Tendinitis

Subjective: A 40-year-old man who jogs approximately 30 miles per week reported insidious onset of pain and stiffness along the posterior aspect of the ankle. Pain occurred primarily during running and subsided with rest. The patient jogged regularly along hilly terrain.

Objective. Tenderness and mild swelling were palpated along the Achilles tendon proximal to its insertion at the calcaneus. Passive dorsiflexion of the ankle with the knee straight reproduced pain. Resisted plantar flexion of the gastrocnemius-soleus muscle group was strong and slightly painful.

Structurally the patient demonstrated bilateral forefoot varus deformities of 10°. Subtalar joint mobility was within normal limits. Static evaluation indicated bilateral eversion of 10°. During walking and running, the patient exhibited early and excessive pronation.

Flexibility tests indicated that dorsiflexion of the ankle with the knee straight was limited to 90° (neutral). With the knee flexed to 30°, dorsiflexion of the ankle increased to 95°.

Assessment. Achilles tendinitis.

Predisposing Factors. Clement et al[37] found 56% of 109 runners with Achilles tendinitis displayed *excessive pronation.* Angiographic studies indicated an area of hypovascularity approximately 2 to 6 cm proximal to the Achilles tendon insertion along the posterior aspect of the calcaneus.[61] Increased and excessive internal rotation of the tibia during pronation draws the Achilles tendon mediad. During running, a whipping action is created along the Achilles tendon. This action "wrings out" the hypovascular area of the tendon, resulting in microtears and inflammation.

Poor flexibility of the Achilles tendon also has been implicated in Achilles tendinitis. The gastrocnemius-soleus muscle group performs eccentrically during midstance of running to control anterior movement of the tibia over the talus. Poor flexibility of these muscles, especially during hill running, increases strain on the Achilles tendon, resulting in microtrauma. Additionally the gastrocnemius-soleus muscles contract concentrically during push-off to propel the foot. Weakness of these muscles increases stress on the Achilles tendon and, during repetitive running, can result in microtears and local inflammation.

Precipitating Factors. Repetitive uphill running results in increased ankle dorsiflexion to allow the foot to clear the ground. Increased strain along the Achilles tendon results from poor flexibility of the gastrocnemius-soleus muscles. These muscles contract eccentrically at midstance to control the forward momentum of the tibia. Increased speed of the tibia at midstance, during downhill running, results in increased eccentric contraction force in the gastrocnemius-soleus muscles. Forceful repetitive eccentric contractions result in breakdown of the connective tissue component of muscle, including tendon.

Treatment. The initial treatment of acute Achilles tendinitis includes ice and rest from the activity that precipitated the problem. Iontophoresis with 10% hydrocortisone is effective in reducing inflammation. An oral anti-inflammatory, such as phenylbutazone, also reduces the inflammatory reaction. After the acute symptoms subside, a gradual stretching or lengthening and strengthening program for the gastrocnemius-soleus muscles should be performed. Stretching should be gentle, using a low-load, 10-second hold. Usually 10 to 20 repetitions twice daily should be satisfactory. Strengthening can be performed non–weight bearing (open kinetic chain exercise) using Theraband or, if indicated, isokinetic exercises. Basic tenets of isokinetics, including initial submaximal contractions, progressing, as tolerated, to maximal contractions, should be followed.[53]

Because Achilles tendinitis can result in gradual degeneration of the tendon leading to complete spontaneous rupture of the tendon,[62] specific exercises for strengthening of the tendon are essential after inflammation has resolved. The progressive resistive exercise program outlined by Curwin and Stanish[63] varies both the resistance and the velocity of eccentric contractions, to increase tendon strength gradually. Eccentric muscle contractions produce greater musculotendinous tension levels than concentric contractions, and, in contrast to concentric contractions, the tension level rises with increases in angular joint velocity.[64]

Strengthening exercises performed in weight bearing (or closed kinetic chain exercise) better simulate functional activities that require specific recruitment patterns of different muscles as well as proprioceptive responses than do open kinetic chain strengthening exercises.[65] Therefore, closed kinetic chain exercises should be introduced in the final phases of rehabilitation to prepare the patient for a return to jogging. Some examples of closed kinetic chain strengthening exercises for the gastrocnemius-soleus muscles include calf raises, squats, and step-ups.

Correction of underlying ankle and foot biomechanics includes an orthotic to control excessive pronation. Orthotics were fabricated with 5-mm forefoot and rearfoot posts. Clement and Taunton[37] treated with orthotics the excessive pronators in 109 patients with Achilles tendinitis. In the majority of cases, the results were good to excellent.

Correction of training errors involves reducing mileage and hill running and improving footwear. Footwear should include a flexible sole, such as a strip-last shoe, which provides flexibility in the midsole area and reduces stress on the Achilles tendon. The heel of the shoe should be well-padded to provide a lift for the Achilles tendon as well as shock absorption. The heel lifts, according to Clement and Taunton,[37] should be between 12 and 15 mm of thickness.

Shin Splints

According to Slocum,[66] shin splints are a common recognizable clinical entity characterized by nonsterile mechanical inflammation of the muscle and tendon and are brought about by overexertion of the muscles to the lower part of the leg during weight bearing.[67] Slocum lists the following criteria for differentiating shin splints from other disorders of the lower leg or ankle: (1) the lesion must lie at the origin, belly, or muscle-tendon junction of the ankle plantar flexors or dorsiflexors; (2) pain must be related to rhythmic, repetitive exercises; (3) classic signs of inflammation—heat, redness, swelling, tenderness—should be present at the site of the lesion; and (4) conditions resulting from direct trauma or disease must be excluded.

Therefore, shin splints may be narrowly defined as a nonsterile mechanical inflammation of the muscles and related soft tissues of the lower leg, excluding stress fractures and compartment syndromes. Depending on the affected muscles, shin splints can be anterolateral or posteromedial.[67] Anterolateral shin splits involve the pretibial muscles, including tibialis anterior, extensor hallucis longus, and extensor digitorum longus. These muscles are active during several phases of gait and running. At heel strike, the pretibial muscles act eccentrically to lower the foot and ankle and thus can become inflamed if the running shoe has a hard heel or running takes place on a hard surface. Conversely, during the swing phase, the pretibial muscles contract concentrically to dorsiflex the ankle and clear the foot from the ground or running surface. A muscle imbalance between a weak pretibial muscle group and tight gastrocnemius-soleus muscles results in overactivation of the pretibial muscles during swing phase and at heel strike. The necessity for increased ankle dorsiflexion while running hills increases the strain along the pretibial muscles. The resultant strain on the pretibial muscles can result in microtears and local inflammation.

Posterolateral shin splints are associated with nonsterile, mechanical inflammation of the posterior tibial, flexor digitorum longus, and flexor hallucis longus muscles and related muscle-tendon junctions. These muscles are active after heel strike, eccentrically contracting to lower the arch and assist in pronation. At push-off, in conjunction with the gastrocnemius-soleus complex, these muscles contract concentrically, propelling the foot and leg. When excessive pronation is present after heel strike, eccentric overactivation of the muscles attempts to support the medial arch and navicular bone of the foot, resulting in strain and microtears. Research has shown a strong positive correlation between excessive pronation and posteromedial shin splints.[14]

In cases in which only active resisted plantar flexion is painful, one should suspect periostitis at the attachment of the medial half of the soleus muscle to the posteromedial tibia. The soleus muscle syndrome was identified as a cause of postero-medial shin splints through cadaver electromyographic (EMG) and open biopsy analysis by Michael and Holder.[68]

CASE STUDY

3: Posteromedial Shin Splints

Subjective. A 21-year-old woman complained of pain along the inside of her lower legs after aerobic-type exercises. She performed high-impact aerobics 2 hours daily, 7 days a week. She wore dancing slippers rather than an aerobic-type tennis shoe or well-padded running shoe. The pain was relieved by rest and application of ice.

Objective. Active range of motion of the involved ankle was within normal limits. Passive eversion was slightly painful; significant pain was reproduced during passive dorsiflexion of the ankle. Passive dorsiflexion of the ankle remained painful with the knee flexed to 30°. Heel raises also reproduced pain along the posteromedial aspect of the lower leg. Manual palpation of the pos-teromedial distal tibia reproduced the pain.

Foot evaluation using a goniometer demonstrated forefoot varus of 15° in the involved extremity and 10° in the uninvolved extremity. Range of motion of the subtalar joint was measured using a goniometer at 10° eversion and 20° of inversion in both feet. Postural evaluation in standing indicated a valgus posi-tion from the neutral position of both calcaneus bones.

Gait assessment revealed excessive pronation of the foot during the stance phase of gait. Instability of the foot occurred during push-off. Excessive move-ment (pronation) during midstance occurred at the midtarsal joint.

Assessment. Posteromedial shin splints with pain during resisted plantar flexion (heel raises) of the ankle and stretch into dorsiflexion (knee flexed), prob-ably a result of soleus muscle syndrome.

Predisposing Factors. Excessive pronation with eversion of the calcaneus in the foot during standing and jumping resulting in traction on the posteromedi-al fibrous attachments of the soleus muscle along the tibia.

Precipitating Factors. Repetitive jumping (2 hours daily) during aerobic exer-cises increased stress at the attachment of the soleus muscle along the tibia, resulting in microtears and local inflammation. Inadequate rest—performing aerobic exercises daily—precluded soft tissue repair and healing of the soleus muscle.

Inadequate footwear—using dancing slippers—provided poor arch support and accentuated excessive pronation.

Treatment. Early treatment included rest from aerobic exercise, ice, and ion-tophoresis with 10% hydrocortisone along the posteromedial aspect of the tibia bone. Treatment time was 30 minutes. Gentle stretching, as described previous-ly, with the knee flexed at 30° was performed daily to the soleus muscle.

Foot orthotics with 8-mm forefoot and rearfoot posts on the involved side and 5-mm forefoot and rearfoot posts on the uninvolved side were fabricated. The posts should correct 60% of the forefoot varus abnormality and allow the calcaneus to function close to the neutral position of the subtalar joint. The patient was instructed to purchase an aerobic shoe with a flexible, well-padded insole. A firm, wide heel counter provides good medial and lateral support to the heel.

A progressive resistive exercise program initially used elastic for open kinetic chain strengthening of the ankle joint plantar flexors and invertors. As symptoms decreased, the program was progressed to bilateral calf raises and then to unilateral calf raises.

Exercise modification included performing aerobic exercise only 1 hour daily, three to four times per week. This schedule precludes overstressing of tissues in the lower leg and allows for tissue recovery and repair.

Stress Fractures of the Tibia

Stress fractures are frequently seen as a cause of pain in the distal third of the posteromedial tibia.[69,70] Persistent overuse of bone that is unaccustomed to stress causes rapid focal, circumferential periosteal resorption of bone with a small cortical cavity. Not all stress fractures progress to the point of actual disruption of bone cortex. Simple cortical hypertrophy along the posteromedial cortex of the tibia may be the only sign seen on radiographic examination.[70]

CAUSES

Stress fractures result from overuse or overtraining (or both). Sullivan et al[71] correlated various training factors in 51 runners with stress fractures. The most common sites were the tibia, fibula, metatarsals, and pelvic bones, in that order. The majority of the runners ran more than 20 miles per week and ran on hard surfaces. Thirty-one changed training methods before injury; the majority increased their weekly mileage dramatically. Nineteen of the 51 runners exhibited excessive pronation. In most cases, radiographic changes showed an area of localized cortical bone thickening with periosteal and endosteal reactions. The results suggest that for many runners there is a maximum, and that to exceed it places the runner at risk for soft tissue breakdown. Additionally, malalignment of the lower extremity associated with excessive pronation is a predisposing factor.

TREATMENT

Treatment is rest from the activity that is causing the pain. Oral anti-inflammatory medicines help to reduce the inflammation. As symptoms subside, an alternative exercise program, such as cycle-ergometer or swimming, can help maintain cardiovascular fitness. Orthotics are used to correct excessive pronation of the foot. Training begins gradually, usually on a level track that has a softer surface than pavement. Running should not be resumed until symptoms resolve and radiographic evidence indicates no cortical bone defect. Serial radiographs, every 2 weeks after pain onsets, are useful for diagnosis and to monitor progression of fractures. Absence of radiographic presentation (at least during initial examination), even in the presence of stress fractures, is not uncommon. Diagnostic accuracy is therefore initially enhanced by the use of a bone scan.

Compartment Syndromes

Compartment syndromes in the lower leg result when increased tissue fluid pressure in a closed fascial compartment encroaches on the circulation to nerves and muscles within that compartment. The anterior, posterior, deep posterior, and lateral compartments of the lower leg may be affected.[72,73]

SIGNS AND SYMPTOMS

Pain over the involved compartment, paresthesia over the distribution of the involved nerve, muscle weakness, and positive stretch signs of the involved muscles develop as compartment pressures become abnormally elevated.[73]

TREATMENT

Treatment includes discontinuation or modification of the activity that precipitated the problem. Acute compartment syndrome is a medical emergency necessitating immediate decompression of the involved fascial compartment. Subacute or chronic compartment syndromes may be helped with soft tissue work, including massage to promote circulation and stretch to the investing fascia. A chronic problem, however, may require a permanent modification of activity, such as reducing the weekly mileage of a runner.

Chondromalacia Patellae

Softening or fissuring of the hyaline cartilage covering the posterior surface of the patella is known as chondromalacia patellae. The cartilage breakdown results from abnormal pressure or load between the retropatellar surface and the corresponding trochlear groove of the femur. Abnormal pressure results in either too much load or too little load between the opposing articular forces. In either case, diffusion of synovial fluid through the layers of hyaline cartilage is compromised, resulting in inadequate nutrition of chondrocytes and subsequent cell death and loss of ground substance. Softening and fibrillation of hyaline cartilage increases stress along the underlying subchondral bone, which is richly innervated with pain fibers.

CASE STUDY

4: Chondromalacia Patellae

Subjective. A 16-year-old high school cheerleader presented with anterior knee pain made worse by exercise, especially running. She reportedly jogged 20 miles weekly along a flat, well-contoured macadam street in her neighborhood. The patient reported insidious onset of pain and no history of microtrauma. Squatting activities and stair climbing were painful. The patient reported reduced pain along her anterior knee after rest and application of ice.

Objective. There was tenderness to palpation along the lateral facet of the patella and the lateral condyle of the femur. Active range of motion of the involved knee was within normal limits when compared with that in the uninvolved knee. Patellofemoral joint crepitus was audible during knee extension and flexion. Excessive lateral glide of the patella with the knee flexed 30° elicited a positive apprehension sign. Conversely the lateral retinaculum of the vastus lateralis muscle was tight to passive stretch. Significant atrophy was palpated in the vastus medialis obliquis muscle. Straight leg raising was limited bilaterally by tightness of the hamstrings.

Structurally the patient demonstrated miserable malalignment, with femoral anteversion, proximal external tibial torsion, tibia varum, and subtalar joint pronation. The result was an increased Q angle of 25° in the involved knee. The femoral anteversion was confirmed with excessive internal rotations in the hip joints, and tibial torsion measured 30° bilaterally (see Fig. 8–1). The patient also demonstrated significant recurvatum in both knees.

Evaluation of the foot indicated forefoot varus of 10° on the involved side, as compared with 8° on the uninvolved side.

Assessment. Chondromalacia of the lateral patella and lateral condyle of the femur.

Predisposing Factors. Miserable malalignment with proximal external tibial torsion resulted in an increased Q angle and lateral patellar tracking.

Excessive pronation in the stance or support phase of running and walking with obligatory internal rotation of the tibia and femur resulted in increased compression between the lateral patellar facet and the lateral trochlear groove of the femur.

Atrophy of the vastus medialis obliquis resulted in poor medial dynamic stabilization of the patella.

Tight lateral retinaculum of the vastus lateralis muscle exacerbated lateral tracking of the patella.

The quadriceps femoris muscle contracts during forward swing in the recovery phase of running to extend the knee at heel strike. Increased quadriceps femoris muscle force may produce tight or inextensible hamstring muscles when the leg swings forward. The result is increased compressive force between the patella and the trochlear groove of the femur during running.

Loss of eccentric quadriceps femoris muscle strength during weight-bearing activities may result in altered patellofemoral joint reaction forces and potential microtrauma to the retropatellar hyaline cartilage.[74,75] Eccentric muscle contraction of the quadriceps femoris muscle group at heel strike controls knee joint flexion during the early stance phase of running. Knee joint flexion in early stance assists with attenuation of ground reaction forces.[41,44]

Precipitating Factors. Jogging 20 miles weekly along a macadam road, a relatively soft, yielding surface, is not, in this author's opinion, a training error. The patient did perform squatting maneuvers during cheerleading, however, that increased the patellofemoral joint compression forces.

Treatment. Treatment is designed to reduce patellofemoral joint compression forces, improve patellar tracking and control during knee flexion and increase quadriceps femoris muscle eccentric strength. Patellofemoral joint compression forces increase during increasing amounts of knee flexion. The patient is advised, therefore, to avoid activities such as stair climbing, cycling, or getting in or out of a low chair, which require repetitive knee flexion or squatting.

Quadriceps muscle strengthening is the most essential component of nonoperative management of patellofemoral pain. Quadriceps femoris wasting and weakness are almost constant accompaniments of chondromalacia patellae. Improved quadriceps femoris muscle strength, particularly the vastus medialis obliquis, helps maintain the central position of the patella during knee movement in the trochlear groove of the femur. Straight leg raising or short-arc exercises performed in the final 30° of extension minimize patellofemoral joint compression forces. Straight leg raising exercises should be performed 100 times daily. Initially, no weight is applied to the quadriceps femoris muscle. The patient should gradually increase weight resistance to the quadriceps femoris in 1-pound increments, to a maximum of 10 to 15 pounds.

Closed kinetic chain strengthening of the quadriceps femoris muscles is included in the strengthening program to simulate more closely the functional activities of the patient. Examples of closed kinetic chain exercises include leg press, stair-climbing machines, squats, wall slides, and step-ups. The range of motion for these exercises should be limited from full extension to 30° to 45° of flexion to strengthen the quadriceps femoris muscle while avoiding excessive patellofemoral joint compression forces[75,76].

Hamstring stretching was performed daily. In addition, the patient was instructed to glide the patella medially with the knee extended. Gliding the patella medially lengthens the soft tissue structures, including the lateral retinaculum of the vastus lateralis along the lateral border of the patella.

The patient was fitted with a patellofemoral joint brace made of neoprene with a doughnut-shaped cut-out for the patella. A lateral wedge was used to buttress the lateral aspect of the patella and prevent lateral tracking or subluxation.

Orthotics were used to correct excessive pronation and correct associated rotational changes in the lower extremities. The orthotics were fabricated, posting the forefoot varus abnormalities in both feet, with medial forefoot and rearfoot posts. The girth of both posts was 5 mm.

The patient was instructed to avoid activities involving repetitive squatting and knee flexion. Her cheerleading routines were modified accordingly to avoid such harmful positions. Conservative treatment is generally effective in relieving signs and symptoms associated with chondromalacia patellae. In a prospective study of chondromalacia patellae in athletes, DeHaven et al[77] showed nonoperative measures were successful in 82% of 100 cases. In the same study, 66% of conservatively treated patients were able to return to unrestricted athletic activities. Gruber suggested that conservative treatment should be abandoned if no improvement is shown after 3 months.[78]

Iliotibial Band Friction Syndrome

The iliotibial band is a thick band of fascia that forms part of the insertion of the tensor fasciae latae and gluteus maximus muscles. It continues distally along the lateral aspect of the thigh in continuity with the lateral intermuscular septum and inserts into Gerdy's tubercle along the anterolateral aspect of the tibia bone.[58] During knee flexion greater than 30°, the iliotibial band lies on or behind the lateral condyle of the femur, whereas with the knee extended, the iliotibial band lies anterior to the lateral femoral condyle.[79] Therefore, flexion and extension movements of the knee under stress produce irritation and subsequent inflammatory reaction in the iliotibial band.[79-81]

ITBFS is associated with overuse syndrome resulting from friction during flexion and extension of the knee between the iliotibial band and the lateral epicondyle of the femur. The condition is usually found in runners and cyclists.[82,83]

CASE STUDY

5: Iliotibial Band Friction Syndrome

Subjective. A 30-year-old male long-distance runner (50 miles weekly) complained of a few months' history of lateral knee pain that was worse during running. Walking with the knee extended afforded relief. The patient frequently ran along the crown of the road with his involved leg on the low side.

Objective. Evaluation of the hip indicated inextensibility of the iliotibial band to passive stretch, secondary to a positive Ober's sign. Palpation of the femoral epicondyle reproduced the patient's pain. Active range of motion of the knee reproduced the patient's pain within a given painful arc, at approximately 30° of flexion. This point in the range brings the iliotibial band into contact with the prominence of the lateral condyle of the femur.[81] Lower extremity malalignment and leg-heel and heel-forefoot relationships were normal.

Assessment. ITFBS.

Predisposing Factors. Tight tensor fascia latae muscle and associated iliotibial band increased friction stress of the iliotibial band along the bony prominence of the lateral epicondyle of the femur.[80,81]

Precipitating Factors. Lindenberg et al[82] found that runners with ITBFS tended to run with the involved leg along the low part of the road crown. Running in that position restricts pronation, thereby prolonging external tibial rotation and promoting genu varum. The result was increased stretch of the iliotibial band along the lateral epicondyle. Lindenberg's group also found that 67% of 36 long distance runners with ITBFS had recently switched to inflexible running shoes, which restrict subtalar joint pronation.[82] The authors treated many of these runners with flexible running shoes and a lateral heel wedge to promote pronation.

Treatment. Ice and ultrasound (10/watts cm^2) plus 10% hydrocortisone were applied to the inflamed area for 10 minutes. Stretching of the iliotibial band, as demonstrated in Figure 8–14, was performed by the clinician with the patient's leg passively adducted. The patient was instructed to run along a level surface instead of the crown of the road.

SUMMARY

Major overuse syndromes can involve the foot, ankle, knee, and hip. They present a diagnostic challenge for the clinician. Effective treatment of the overuse injuries includes evaluation of predisposing (intrinsic) factors and precipitating (extrinsic) factors relative to the individual patient. Predisposing factors such as malalignment syndromes and muscle dysfunction result in pathomechanics that alter normal forces and stresses along various musculoskeletal tissues. Incorrect training methods and conditions precipitate tissue breakdown and injury.

The case studies presented illustrate the problem-solving approach to treatment of common overuse syndromes. Correction of the predisposing and precipitating factors is emphasized. Without correction of these factors, therapeutic modalities are ineffective and superfluous.

REFERENCES

1. Mann, RA: Biomechanics of running. In Mack, RP (ed): American Academy of Orthopedic Surgeons Symposium on the Foot and Leg in Running Sports. CV Mosby, St. Louis, 1982.
2. Murphy, P: Ultrasports are in, in spite of injuries. Physician Sports Med 14:180, 1986.
3. Henderson, J: First aid for the injured runner. Runners World 12:32, 1977.
4. Marti, B, Vader, JP, Minder, CE, and Abelin, T: On the epidemiology of running injuries: The 1984 Bern grand-prix study. Am J Sports Med 16:285, 1988.
5. Elliot, B and Achland, T: Biomechanical effects of fatigue on 10,000 meter running techniques. Res Quart Ex Sports 52:160, 1981.
6. Leadbetter, WB: An introduction to sports-induced soft-tissue inflammation. In Leadbetter, WB, Buckwalter, JA, and Gordon, SL (eds): Sports-Induced Inflammation: Clinical and Basic Science Concepts. American Academy of Orthopaedic Surgeons, Park Ridge, IL, 1990, pp 3–23.
7. Arthritis Foundation: Primer on the rheumatic diseases. JAMA 224:19, 1973.
8. Herring, SA and Nilson, KL: Introduction to overuse injuries. Clin Sports Med 6:225, 1987.
9. Kloth, LC and Miller, KH: The inflammatory response to wounding. In Kloth, LC, McCulloch, JM, and Feedar, JA (eds): Wound Healing: Alternatives in Management. FA Davis, Philadelphia, 1990, pp 3–13.
10. Cummings, GS, Crutchfield, CA, and Barnes, MR: Soft Tissue Changes in Contractures, vol 1. Stokesville Publishing, Atlanta, GA, 1983.
11. Clancy, WG: Tendinitis and plantar fasciitis in runners. In D'Ambrosia, R and Drez, D (eds): Prevention and Treatment of Running Injuries. Charles B. Slack, Thorofare, NJ, 1982.
12. James, SL, Bates, BT, and Ostering, LR: Injuries to runners. Am J Sports Med 6:40, 1978.
13. Clement, DB: A survey of overuse running injuries. Physician Sports Med 9:47, 1981.
14. Viitasale, JT and Kvist, M: Some biomechanical aspects of the foot and ankle in athletes with and without shin splints. Am J Sports Med 11:125, 1983.
15. Lutter, L: Injuries in the runner and jogger. Minnesota Med 63:45, 1980.
16. Litlevedt, J, Kreighbaum, E, and Philips, LR: Analysis of selected alignment of the lower extremity related to the shin splint syndrome. J Am Podiatr Assoc 69:211, 1979.
17. DeLacerda, FG: A study of anatomical factors involved in shin splints. J Orthop Sports Phys Ther 2:55, 1980.
18. Messier, SP and Pittala, KA: Etiologic factors associated with selected running injuries. Med Sci Sports Exerc 20:501, 1988.
19. Buchbinder, MR, Napora, NJ, and Biggs, EW: The relationship of abnormal pronation to chondromalacia of the patella in distance runners. J Am Podiatr Assoc 69:159, 1979.
20. Inman, VT, Rolston, HJ, and Todd, F: Human Walking. Williams & Wilkins, Baltimore, 1981, pp 1–21.
21. Tiberio, D: The effect of excessive subtalar joint pronation on patellofemoral mechanics: A theoretical model. J Orthop Sports Phys Ther 9:160, 1987.
22. Lutter, LD: Cavus foot in runners. Foot Ankle 1:225, 1981.
23. Smith, WB: Environmental factors in running. Am J Sports Med 8:138, 1980.
24. Staehli, LT: Rotational problems of the lower extremities. Orthop Clin North Am 18:503, 1987.
25. Wright, DG, Desai, SM, and Henderson, WH: Action of the subtalar and ankle-joint complex during the stance phase of walking. J Bone Joint Surg [Am] 46:361, 1964.
26. Stuberg, W, Temme, J, Kaplan, P, et al: Measurement of tibial torsion and thigh-foot angle using goniometry and computed tomography. Clin Orthop 272:208, 1991.
27. Root, ML, Orien, WP, and Weed, JN: Clinical Biomechanics, vol II: Normal and Abnormal Function of the Foot. Clinical Biomechanics, Los Angeles, 1977.
28. James, SL: Chondromalacia of the patella in the adolescent. In Kennedy JC (ed): The Injured Adolescent Knee. Williams & Wilkins, Baltimore, 1979, pp 214–218.
29. Mann, RA, Baxter, DE, and Lutter, LD: Running symposium. Foot Ankle 1:190, 1981.

30. Smidt, GL: Gait in musculoskeletal abnormalities. In Smidt, GL (ed): Gait in Rehabilitation. Churchill Livingstone, New York, 1990, pp 199–252.
31. Giles, LGF and Taylor, JR: Low back pain associates with leg length inequality. Spine 6:510, 1981.
32. Bolz, S and Davies, G: Leg length differences and correlations with total leg strength. J Orthop Sports Phys Ther 6:123, 1984.
33. Subotnick, SI: Limb length discrepancy of the lower extremity (the short leg syndrome). J Orthop Sports Phys Ther 3:11, 1981.
34. Basmajian, JV: Muscles Alive: Their Function Revealed by Electromyography, ed 4. Baltimore, Williams & Wilkins, 1979.
35. James, SL and Brubaker, CE: Biomechanics of running. Orthop Clin North Am 4:605, 1973.
36. Subotnick, SI: The shin splints syndrome of the lower extremity. Podiatr Sports Med 66:43, 1976.
37. Clement, DB, Taunton, JE, and Smart, GW: Achilles tendinitis and peritendinitis: Etiology and treatment. Am J Sports Med 12:179, 1984.
38. Kibler, WB, Goldberg, C, and Chandler, TJ: Functional biomechanical deficits in running athletes with plantar fasciitis. Am J Sports Med 19:66, 1991.
39. Subotnick, SI: Equinus deformity as it affects the forefoot. J Am Podiatr Assoc 61:423, 1971.
40. Perry, J: Contractures: A historical perspective. Clin Orthop 219:8, 1987.
41. Cavanaugh, PR: The biomechanics of lower extremity action in distance running. Foot Ankle 7:197, 1987.
42. Clancy, WG: Runner's injuries. Am J Sports Med 8:137, 1980.
43. Solomonow, M and D'Ambrosia, R: Biomechanics of muscle overuse injuries: A theoretical approach. Clin Sports Med 6:253, 1987.
44. Mann, RA: Biomechanics of walking, running, and sprinting. Am J Sports Med 8:345, 1980.
45. Hicks, JH: The mechanics of the foot. II. The plantar aponeurosis. J Anat 80:25, 1954.
46. Kulund, DW: The Injured Athlete, 2nd ed. JB Lippincott, Philadelphia, 1988.
47. Roy, S and Irwin, R: Sports medicine: Prevention, education, management, and rehabilitation. Prentice-Hall, Englewood Cliffs, NJ, 1983.
48. Cyriax, J: Textbook of Orthopaedic Medicine, vol 1, Diagnosis of Soft Tissue Lesions, ed 6. Cassell, London, 1979, pp 64–103.
49. Kopell, HP and Thompson, WAL: Peripheral Entrapment Neuropathies, ed 2. Robert E. Krieger, 1976.
50. Leach, RE, Hammond, G, and Stryker, WS: Anterior tibial compartment syndrome, acute and chronic. J Bone Joint Surg 49A:451, 1967.
51. Ruwe, PA, Gage, JR, Ozonoff, MB, and DeLuca, PA: Clinical determination of femoral anteversion. J Bone Joint Surg [Am] 74A:820, 1992.
52. Tiberio, D, Bohannon, RW, and Zito, MA: Effect of subtalar joint position on the measurement of maximum ankle dorsiflexion. Clin Biomech 4:189, 1989.
53. Davies, GJ: A Compendium of Isokinetics in Clinical Usage, ed 3. S & S, Wisconsin, 1987.
54. Noyes, FR, Barber, SD, and Mangine, RE: Abnormal lower limb symmetry determined by function hop tests after anterior cruciate ligament rupture. Am J Sports Med 19:513, 1991.
55. Voight, ML and Draovitch, P: Plyometrics. In Albert, M (ed): Eccentric Muscle Training in Sports and Orthopaedics. Churchill Livingstone, New York, 1991.
56. Eggold, JF: Orthotics in the prevention of runner's overuse injuries. Physician Sports Med 9:125, 1981.
57. Bojsen-Møller, F and Flagsted, KE: Plantar aponeurosis and integral architecture of the ball of the foot. Anat 121:599, 1976.
58. Warwick, R and Williams PL (eds): Gray's Anatomy, British ed 35. WB Saunders, Philadelphia, 1973.
59. Lutter, LD: Running athletes in office practice. Foot Ankle 3:153, 1982.
60. Marshall, RN: Foot mechanics and joggers injuries. N Z Med J 88:288, 1978.
61. Lagergren, C and Lindholm, A: Vascular distribution in the achilles tendon—an angiographic and microangiographic study. Acta Chir Scand 116:491, 1958.
62. Ralston, EL and Schmidt, ER: Repair of the ruptured Achilles tendon. J Trauma 11:15, 1971.
63. Curwin, S and Stanish, WD: Tendinitis: Its Etiology and Treatment. DC Heath & Company, Lexington, MA, 1984.
64. Albert, M: Physiologic and clinical principles of eccentrics. In Albert, M (ed): Eccentric Muscle Training in Sports and Orthopaedics. Churchill Livingstone, New York, 1991.
65. Greenfield, BH and Tovin, BJ: The application of open and closed kinematic chain exercises in rehabilitation of the lower extremity. J Back Musculoskel Rehabil 2:38, 1992.
66. Slocum, DB: The shin splint syndrome: Medical aspects and differential diagnosis. Am J Surg 114:875, 1967.
67. Andrews, JR: Overuse syndromes of the lower extremity. Clin Sports Med 2:139, 1983.
68. Michael, RH and Holder, LE: The soleus syndrome: A cause of medial tibial stress (shin splints). Am J Sports Med 13:87, 1985.
69. Jackson, DW and Bailey, D: Shin splints in the young athlete: A nonspecific diagnosis. Phys Sports Med 3:45, 1975.
70. Devas, MB: Stress fractures of the tibia in athletes or "shin soreness." J Bone Joint Surg 40B:227, 1958.

71. Sullivan, D, Warren, RF, Pavlou, H, and Kelman, G: Stress fractures in 51 runners. Clin Orthop 187:188, 1984.
72. Reneman, RS: The anterior and lateral compartment syndrome of the leg due to intensive use of muscles. Clin Orthop 113:69, 1975.
73. Wiley, JP, Clement, DB, Doyle, DL, and Taunton, JE: A primary care perspective of chronic compartment syndrome of the leg. Physician Sports Med 15:111, 1987.
74. Bennett, JG and Stauber, WT: Evaluation and treatment of anterior knee pain using eccentric exercise. Med Sci Sports Exerc 18:526, 1986.
75. Steinkamp, LA, Dillingham, MF, Markel, MD, et al: Biomechanical considerations in patellofemoral joint rehabilitation. Am J Sports Med 21:438, 1993.
76. Hungerford, DS and Barry, M: Biomechanics of the patellofemoral joint. Clin Orthop 144:9, 1979.
77. DeHaven, DE, Dolan, WA, and Mayer, PJ: Chondromalacia patellae in athletes: Clinical presentation and conservative management. Am J Sports Med 7:5, 1979.
78. Gruber, MA: The conservative treatment of chondromalacia patellae. Orthop Clin North Am 10:105, 1979.
79. Renne, JW: The iliotibial band friction syndrome. J Bone Joint Surg 57A:110, 1975.
80. Noble, CA: Iliotibial band friction syndrome in runners. Am J Sports Med 8:232, 1980.
81. Noble, HB, Hajek, MR, and Porter, M: Diagnosis and treatment of iliotibial band tightness in runners. Physician Sports Med 10:67, 1982.
82. Lindenberg, G, Pinshaw, R, and Noakes, TD: Iliotibial band friction syndrome in runners. Physician Sports Med 12:118, 1984.
83. Holmes, JC, Pruitt, AL, and Whalen, NJ: Iliotibial band syndrome in cyclists. Am J Sports Med 21:419, 1993.

CHAPTER 9

The Diabetic Foot

Jennifer M. Bottomley, MS, PT
Nathan Schwartz, DPM

Diabetes and foot problems come close to being synonymous terms and present a difficult management scenario for healthcare professionals. The pathologic processes of neuropathy and macrovascular and microvascular disease are common to the lower extremity of the diabetic patient. These processes may occur exclusively or together, placing the patient at increased risk for ulceration, gangrene, and infection.[1] The metabolic effects of diabetes are profound and insidious, affecting all parts of the body. The nervous system deteriorates, leading to diminished sensation and peripheral neuropathy, and the peripheral vascular system commonly develops arteriosclerosis obliterans.[2] The diabetic is usually more susceptible to infection and has associated avascularity, atrophy of tissue, neuropathic changes, and the general lack of concern for foot health that creates an "endemic situation."[3] This situation necessitates constant monitoring and prophylactic care.

This chapter presents epidemiologic and economic facts related to diabetic foot problems; metabolic and nutritional components that have an impact on care of the diabetic foot; the pertinent anatomy, physiology, and pathomechanical considerations necessary for comprehensive treatment of diabetic foot problems; and resources available to enhance the care of the diabetic individual. Special emphasis is placed on preventive and rehabilitative measures that can be employed to minimize the devastating effects of foot ulceration and the complications that follow.

EPIDEMIOLOGY AND ECONOMIC FACTS OF DIABETIC FOOT PROBLEMS

Approximately 12 million people in the United States have diabetes, a disorder whose acute and chronic complications cost an estimated $20 billion annually.[4] Diabetes is associated with more than 50% of the 120,000 lower limb amputations performed annually in the United States for indications other than trauma. The overall risk for amputation is increased in diabetics 17-fold beyond that for people without diabetes.[5] This probably reflects, in part, the prevalence of potent pathophysiologic risk factors for amputation, including peripheral neuropathy and severe arteriosclerosis obliterans. Additional risk factors in diabetic individuals involve more complex pathology (i.e., failure of cutaneous wound healing and gangrene) or predisposing environmental events (i.e., mechanical trauma resulting from ill-fitting shoes causing skin ulceration).

Diabetes is the third leading cause of death among blacks, and more than 50% of adult Hispanics and Native Americans have diabetes.[6] The incidence of diabetes increases exponentially with age and is most prevalent in the elderly population.[7] Diabetes in the diagnosed population aged 65 years and older affected 3.3 million people in 1990 and is projected to increase to 4.1 million in 2010 and to 6.8 million by 2030. The sum of the direct and indirect costs for medical care, morbidity, disability, and mortality associated with diabetes was $20.4 billion in 1987.[7]

Diabetes results in 35,000 major amputations annually in the United States.[8] In many cases, loss of the second limb is inevitable within a few years, and death is imminent a few years later.[9] About $1.2 billion is spent yearly on medical expenses for diabetic individuals undergoing amputation.[10] Each year, approximately 12,000 to 15,000 elderly individuals suffer amputation of part or all of their lower extremities resulting from wounds that could possibly have been prevented through patient education and proper orthotic and shoe gear interventions.[9] Demographic studies indicate that the Medicare costs of acute, subacute, and chronic care following hospitalization for severe ulceration or amputation range from $6,000 to $30,000 per elderly diabetic individual and that, within 3 years, more than half of older diabetics sustaining amputation die from complications, incurring the greatest medical expenses during the end stages of their lives.[7]

These epidemiologic and economic figures clearly make prophylactic diabetic foot care an imperative. A therapeutic shoe or orthotic is less costly than hospitalization for ulcer care, surgical and postsurgical expenses, rehabilitation, the purchase of a prosthesis, and the qualitative costs of psychosociologic disabilities resulting from amputation (i.e., severely compromised activities of daily living and a diminished quality of life).

EVALUATIVE FINDINGS IN DIABETIC FOOT PROBLEMS

The best time to gather as much information as possible is when a patient is first seen. The patient's medical, family, and social history; habits; present illness; and detailed analysis of the diabetic state are crucial for appropriate intervention. One must ascertain what kind of treatment has been rendered and what results were obtained. One of the most important parts of the initial evaluation is to listen to the patient, not only what is said, but also how it is said, because these patients may suffer from emotional problems associated with their disease. As time passes and the clinician becomes more involved with the patient's treatment, there is a tendency for the clinician to lose objectivity and feel responsible for treatment failure, when, in reality, patient compliance is the problem. There is no doubt that seasoned clinicians have gained most of their knowledge from patients by having open minds and being good listeners.

To be effective, clinicians must be extremely thorough in their physical assessment. The patient should take off both shoes, and the examiner should assess the involved and the uninvolved sides to make a proper comparison. Foot inspection as well as shoe wear patterns are important in the initial assessment of the diabetic patient. Subtleties in diabetics can be extremely revealing when recognized. In contrast to healthy patients who respond to injury and infection with inflammation, swelling, and redness, diabetics do not necessarily respond because of attenuated humoral and vascular responses. Accordingly, a diabetic with a foot that shows minimal changes and a break in the skin can be in a dangerous situation.

PATHOPHYSIOLOGY OF DIABETIC FOOT PROBLEMS

Three principal pathophysiologic factors are responsible for foot ulcers and lower extremity amputations in diabetes: neuropathy, ischemia, and infection.[11,12] The mechanisms of injury can include direct trauma and repetitive stress to the insensitive and poorly vascularized diabetic foot.[13]

Peripheral Neuropathy

Neuropathy occurs commonly in diabetic patients, increasing in incidence linearly with the duration of the disease.[14,15] Peripheral sensory loss predisposes the foot to injuries from minor trauma. Repetitive pressure to prominent areas of the insensate foot, commonly from poorly fitting shoes, may produce cumulative minor trauma with eventual ischemic necrosis and skin breakdown.[13] The resulting skin ulcerations often are complicated by delayed healing. Because of sensory loss, early foot ulcers may be neglected and present only after extensive infection is established.

Diabetes interferes with appropriate cellular and humoral responses to infection. The principal pathologic condition that leads to ulceration and infection, however, is the loss of the protective cutaneous sensory barrier in the diabetic foot. Protective sensation defined by Nawoczenski and Birke[16] is 5.07 g of pressure using Semmes-Weinstein monofilaments. Specific evaluation of the entire plantar surface of the foot determines areas of sensory loss that are vulnerable for breakdown.

Vibratory and temperature sense are diminished early in the disease process, compromising proprioception, kinesthesia, and awareness of temperature gradients. During normal walking, the foot is constantly protected from abnormal subluxatory motion by proprioceptors. The pathomechanical changes that occur in diabetes represent joint subluxation due to muscle weakness. Without proper innervation to signal this altered joint position, the foot becomes more vulnerable to injury. The inability of the diabetic patient to perceive pain and trauma because of altered sensation causes damage in the form of microfractures at the joint surfaces. Over a period of time, repeated trauma may cause complete dislocation and destruction of the joint resulting in Charcot changes (Fig. 9–1).

Muscular strength is decreased owing to poor nerve conductivity, decreased energy utilization by muscle cells, altered and inefficient biomechanical gait patterns,

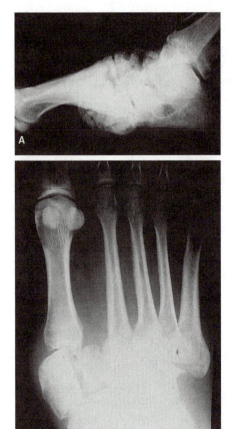

FIGURE 9–1. Examples of Charcot changes: (*A*) Severe disorganization of the tarsus and lesser tarsus. (*B*) Dislocation of the tarsometatarsal and the first and second cuneiforms.

and inactivity. Neuropathy affecting the motor nerves of the intrinsic foot muscles can cause changes in gait, alterations in pressure distribution, and foot deformities such as the classic diabetic "claw toe."[17] These processes may be synergistic with sensory loss increasing the probability of skin breakdown.

The skin of the diabetic is often either dry, scaly, and fissured or excessively moist, further increasing susceptibility to breakdown. Autonomic neuropathy may occur, leading to abnormalities in skin hydration (anhidrosis or hyperhidrosis) and alterations in the distribution of blood flow by arteriovenous shunting away from the nutritive capillary bed.[18] Anhidrosis causes dry skin, cracks, and fissures. Fissures are difficult to treat and often occur about the heel, an area with poor circulation and thus prone to bacterial infections. Hyperhidrosis is characterized by excessive perspiration. This problem makes the diabetic individual more prone to fungal and yeast infections.[19] Such infections can be extremely serious, especially if they occur between the toes, where the potential for a break in the skin and subsequent infection is great. To avoid this occurrence, all diabetics must keep their feet as dry as possible, especially between the toes.

The plantar surface of the foot has the thickest skin on the body to protect the metatarsal heads and neurovascular structures during weight bearing. The skin on the plantar aspect of the foot can withstand extremely high pressures, up to 500 pounds per square inch (psi)[20]; however, if the nervous system is not informing the brain about pain, pressure, and position, the structures in the foot may be subjected to irreversible damage. Even light pressure (5 psi) can cause necrosis over an extended period of time.[13]

Paresthesia is a form of insensitivity that can be perceived as a tingling or burning sensation.[21] Diabetics often describe their "numbness" as painful. The degree to which this problem is disabling cannot be appreciated without experiencing this state of altered sensation. Currently, paresthesias are treated with medications that have many side effects, and the results are variable. In podiatry, the use of posterior tibial nerve blocks has been popular. A nerve block appears to be beneficial in treating paresthesia by paralyzing the sympathetic and sensory fibers to the posterior tibial artery. This intervention causes increased blood flow and breaks the pain cycle. From a physical therapy perspective, the loss of innervation to active muscles has its obvious negative consequences. In research currently underway, preliminary results indicate that Buerger-Allen exercises (see section on treatment suggestions) are effective in enhancing circulation in the lower extremities and diminishing, if not eliminating, paresthetic pain in diabetics, in addition to improving muscle function through active foot and ankle pumping.[22]

Evaluating Sensation and Neurologic Involvement

The neurologic examination requires a reflex hammer, tuning fork (128 cps), and Semmes-Weinstein monofilaments. Testing for vibratory, proprioceptive, temperature, and protective sensation should be done with the patient's eyes closed. The boundaries of any hyperesthesias or hypoesthesias must be distinguished, and it must be determined if these patterns are symmetric or assymmetric. The absence or presence of sweating should be noted. Reflexes to be tested include the patellar reflex and the ankle jerk. As the ankle jerk is increasingly difficult to elicit with increasing age, it may appear to be absent. To aid this reflex, the foot should be gently pronated and dorsiflexed to put tension on the Achilles and the tendon is gently tapped. The clinician should test for the Babinski reflex to determine if there is a superficial plantar response. To determine if there is clonus, forcibly dorsiflex the foot at the ankle. To test for balance loss, the clinician should have the individual stand with eyes closed and feet close together and compare this with the same stance with the eyes open (Romberg's sign).

Muscle strength should be tested in all lower extremity muscles using a graded manual muscle test. Again, symmetry should be noted. Gait evaluation is a helpful adjunct to muscular evaluation to determine unsteady gait patterns, footdrops, or the presence of a "steppage" gait. Range of motion and joint mobility should be evaluated, and any deformities (e.g., Charcot joints; hammer, claw, or mallet toes; hallux abductus valgus) should be noted because these abnormalities are usually indicative of intrinsic foot muscle weakness. Trophic nail changes should also be evaluated.

The Semmes-Weinstein monofilaments are a reproducible, accurate mode for testing sensation and reliable in predicting those individuals at risk for ulceration owing to loss of protective sensation.[23,24] The Carville group[23] measured protective sensation using the Semmes-Weinstein monofilaments and found that those individuals who could not feel the 5.07 monofilament were at greater risk for skin breakdown than those who could feel this level of stimulation. They demonstrated that 5.07 monofilament was the protective sensation threshold. Standardizing of sensory testing is crucial in the evaluation so that adequate protective measures can be taken to prevent feet at risk from developing ulcers.

Vascular Involvement in Diabetes

Limb ischemia in diabetes may be caused by arteriosclerosis obliterans or other conditions that lead to cutaneous ischemia. Cutaneous ischemia may be a critical factor in delayed wound repair and can result in failure to eradicate infection.[25] This ischemia results not only from peripheral arterial disease, but also from alterations of the small cutaneous vessels or potentially correctable local conditions, such as tissue edema. Abnormalities in cutaneous capillary flow and nutrient delivery are well documented in diabetes. These abnormalities have been attributed not only to arteriovenous shunting caused by autonomic neuropathy,[18] but also to occlusive pressure from interstitial edema.[9]

Vasodilation and vasoconstriction can result from autonomic nerve dysfunction in diabetes. Vasoconstriction is more common and, to some extent, is treatable. Vasoconstriction greatly compromises blood flow in the small vessels of the foot. In the interdigital area, thrombosis of the digital vessels and platelet aggregation can occur and can result in the subsequent loss of the digit (Fig. 9–2).

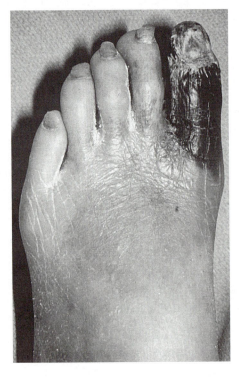

FIGURE 9–2. Dry gangrene of the first toe caused by complete stoppage of the arterial flow to the digit.

Vascular Testing

Vascular evaluation should include the palpation and grading of the femoral, popliteal, dorsalis pedis, and posterior tibial pulses and the observation of other clinical signs and symptoms indicating vascular compromise to the lower extremities. These include intermittent claudication, foot temperature (i.e., cold feet), nocturnal pain, rest pain, nocturnal and rest pain relieved by dependency, blanching on elevation, delayed venous filling time after elevation, dependent rubor, atrophic skin, absence of hair growth, and presence of gangrene. Any lesions, areas of hyperkeratosis, or discoloration should be observed.

Palpating for the pedal pulses can yield a qualitative measure of the dorsalis pedalis or posterior tibial artery circulation, but the examiner must realize that there can be a substantial decrease in flow to the extremity even though arterial ankle pulses are good. Arterial pressures taken at the ankle level and compared with systolic pressures at the antecubital fossa can also be deceptive. False normal pressure can be recorded if there is calcification of the arterial wall. Either the Doppler ultrasonic flow detector or the pneumoplethysmograph can show a pulse waveform that can illustrate the arteries' relative elasticity. The ultrasonic flow detector is an inexpensive instrument that detects the flow of blood through the arteries by producing an audible signal.[26] By virtue of the sound produced, the relative condition of the vessel can be determined. Similarly, the pneumoplethysmograph measures the arterial elasticity but by a different method; this instrument measures subtle changes in the volume or size of the part measured. A graph of the arterial pulsations is then produced. This instrument is more accurate than ultrasound but is expensive and difficult to use. Capillary filling time is measured with the foot elevated as pressure is applied to a toe to prevent blood flow temporarily. The return of color should not take more than 3 to 6 seconds once the pressure is released. This test may produce some false-negative results.

Skin temperature measurements are useful if the circulatory problem is assymmetrical, although test results may be variable because of ambient temperature.

To differentiate an organic disorder, such as blockage of the lumen of the vessel, from a vasospastic condition, temporary dilation of the vessel in question is a useful vascular test. This approach is accomplished by using an arterial tourniquet for 3 minutes and then releasing it. The perfusion distal to the tourniquet should increase if the condition is due to vasospasm.

Observation of blanching and filling times is accomplished through the use of Buerger-Allen vascular assessment. A stopwatch is used to determine the time the veins on the dorsum of the foot require to fill with blood after they have been drained when the leg is elevated. Basically, this approach appraises the general circulation in the foot by measuring the time for blood to enter and fill the veins that have been emptied by elevation. The arterial blood being pumped into the dependent leg diffuses into the arterioles, the capillaries, the venules, and the veins of the foot. The time of venous filling is subject to several variables: the arterial blood pressure, the caliber of the arteries, the volume of blood reaching the capillary bed of the foot with each thrust of the heart, and the rate of venous return. A filling time up to 20 seconds indicates reasonably good collateral circulation. A venous filling time greater than 20 seconds is indicative of a compromised peripheral vascular system and venous insufficiency.

The rubor of the skin should be noted. Dependent rubor is the reddish blue color of the toes and forefoot caused by reduced blood flow in the capillaries. When there is diminished arterial flow, peripheral resistance drops with arteriocapillary dilatation and maximum oxygen extraction by the tissues. With dependency, these parameters become exaggerated. The actual degree of rubor can be noted when measuring venous filling time. Maximum rubor is usually evident in 2 to 3 minutes and manifests as a dusky red color when severe ischemia is present.[27]

In the presence of foot lesions, the lesion should be graded for objective monitoring. Wagner's classification[28] grades vascular dysfunction in grades of 0 to 5 as follows:

Grade 0 foot: The skin is without ulceration. No open lesions are present, but potentially ulcerating deformities, such as bunions, hammer toes, and Charcot's deformity, may be present. Healed partial foot amputations may also be included in this group.

Grade 1 foot: A full-thickness superficial skin loss is present. The lesion does not extend to bone. No abscess is present.

Grade 2 foot: An open ulceration is noted deeper than grade 1 and may penetrate to tendon or joint capsule.

Grade 3 foot: The lesion penetrates to bone, and osteomyelitis is present. Joint infection or plantar fascial plane abscess may also be noted.

Grade 4 foot: Gangrene is noted in the forefoot.

Grade 5 foot: Gangrene involving the entire foot is noted. The foot is not salvageable with local procedures.

In the presence of an ulceration, objective documentation of wound size is best accomplished by tracing the wound on sterilized x-ray film or through photographs on a line-graphed film. This procedure is helpful in monitoring improvement or decline in wound status.

Infection in the Patient with Diabetes

There are many reasons why patients with diabetes can develop infection leading to morbidity. To eliminate the infection successfully and prevent its recurrence, the clinician must be aware of all aspects of the disease. The predisposing conditions, the physiology, and the mechanics of the infection must be examined.

To recognize the mechanics of infection effectively, the physiology of inflammation secondary to trauma must first be understood. In the diabetic patient, trauma usually predisposes the patient to infection. Brand[29] has done numerous experiments with the foot pads of rats. He applied 20 pressure stimulating events, 10,000 times a day, simulating ordinary walking. The foot pads showed only a small rise in temperature and some swelling after the first day. When this test was repeated daily, however, ulcers and necrosis had developed by the end of a week. The repeated stress caused a gradual buildup of inflammatory cells, and with diapedesis, these cells leaked into the interstitial spaces. The final necrosis began in the deeper tissues and gave the appearance of autolysis. When the repetitions were decreased to 8000 a day and the rats were given "weekends off," there was only mild inflammation. At the end of 6 weeks, the foot pads actually looked better than at the beginning of the test.

Pathomechanics in the Diabetic Foot

Friction and pressure forces combine as shear force during dynamic walking. At heel contact, there is a direct downward force of the body weight through the heel or an upward ground reactive force into the heel. The foot contacts the ground in supination and during the first 25% of stance pronates with the leg and thigh internally rotating. The foot is fixed on the ground by the body weight pushing downward and ground reactive forces pushing upward. Shear force results from parts of the body sliding relative to each other in a direction parallel to their plane of contact. Shear force is most responsible for tissue breakdown in the insensitive foot.[30]

The diabetic foot is special because of concurrent neurologic and circulatory involvement. Alterations of sensory impulses are evidenced by absent vibratory, pin-prick, and pressure sensation. Motor involvement accompanies sensory involvement with muscular atrophy and weakness, leading to toe deformities, prominent metatarsal heads, intrinsic muscle wasting, equinus deformity, varus position of the hindfoot, and proximal malalignment. The intrinsic muscles function to stabilize the metatarsophalangeal joints during midstance immediately before push-off. The extensor hallucis longus muscle weakness allows hammering of the hallux by the overriding pull of the long flexors.

The plantar aspect of the foot is protected by fat pads, which act to dissipate weight-bearing forces in all directions, protecting and acting as shock absorbers. Atrophy or distal displacement of the protective subcutaneous fat pad leads to soft tissue trauma and breakdown under the metatarsal heads. Preexisting deformity and abnormal foot function are accentuated, leading to tissue ulceration. For example, if the toes are contracted at the metatarsophalangeal joint, a distal positioning of the fat padding occurs, leaving the plantar surfaces of the metatarsal bones unprotected. Hyperextension at the metatarsophalangeal joints in combination with the pull of the extensor muscles produces a retrograde force that plantar flexes the metatarsal producing excessive pressure at the heads of the metatarsals during weight bearing (Fig. 9–3).

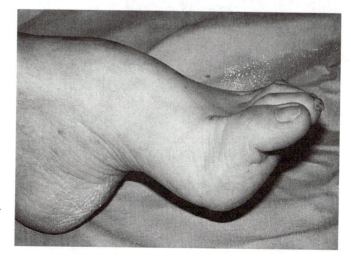

FIGURE 9–3. Pes cavus deformity. Demonstrates the retrograde force of the proximal phalanx on the metatarsal and the anterior positioning of the plantar fat pad to the metatarsal head.

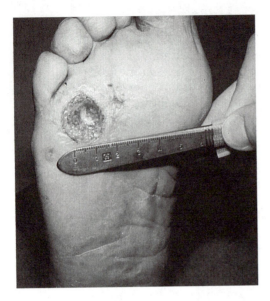

FIGURE 9–4. Mal perforans ulceration under the fourth metatarsal head.

In a study by Boulton et al,[31] diabetic patients with foot neuropathy demonstrated abnormally high pressures beneath the metatarsal heads that were not found in patients with diabetes who did not have peripheral neuropathy. The increased pressure psi and the inability to perceive the trauma cause the neuropathic ulcer called mal perforans (Figs. 9–4 and 9–5). Additionally, Brand's research[29] clearly indicates that owing to repetitive trauma at a site that the patient cannot feel, the skin eventually breaks down. Semmes-Weinstein monofilament testing along with vibratory test-

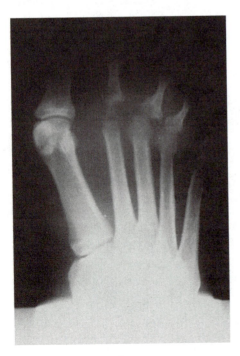

FIGURE 9–5. Osteomyelitis of the second, third, and fourth metatarsal-phalangeal joints secondary to mal perforans.

ing is an essential part of the diabetic foot evaluation for determination of impaired pressure/pain and protective sensation.

Foot lesions account for 20% of all diabetic hospitalizations and 50% to 70% of all nontraumatic amputations performed yearly.[32] Removal of one of the lesser toes because of irreversible soft tissue and bony destruction has moderate effects on the posture and function of the foot. Ablation of the hallux and metatarsal head has a dramatic effect on function of the foot in gait. As the weight-bearing surface area beneath the foot decreases, the pressure on the remaining weight-bearing surface area increases. Identical pressure on a diminished surface area can cause rapid soft tissue breakdown. With amputation of the hallux, the forces at push-off are transmitted laterally to the lesser digits through the long flexor tendons, causing hammering or clawing of the toes. Ulceration at previous ulcer sites is unfortunately all too common an occurrence in the diabetic individual.

TREATMENT SUGGESTIONS IN DIABETIC FOOT PROBLEMS

The major objective of treating the diabetic foot is to prevent tissue ulceration, which can best be accomplished through patient education regarding adequate nutrition, skin care, and safety tips. For instance, an elderly patient with diabetes should use a thermometer or ask a relative or friend without diabetes to measure water temperature in a bath before immersing the feet in water that may be too tepid. Checking the feet nightly for reddened areas should be done with a mirror under the plantar surface or help from another person. Establishment of a full-time podiatry clinic enabled Grady Memorial Hospital in Atlanta to reduce the amputation rate by 24% in its diabetic population within the first year of operation.[33]

The major objectives in treating the diabetic foot are to protect the plantar surface of the foot from repetitive microtrauma and accommodate deformities that could be traumatized by excessive shoe pressures resulting in ulceration and amputation. Total contact full foot orthotics using soft shock absorbing materials help to distribute weight-bearing pressures over the entire plantar surface of the foot away from the vulnerable bony prominences. A Thermold (P.W. Minor, Batabia, NY) leather shoe is recommended for the insensitive diabetic foot.

The provision of orthotics and shoes in the management of foot problems in the diabetic is only one facet of physical therapy intervention. Numerous forms of treatment are available that supplement and enhance the overall outcomes of treatment. These interventions include manual therapies, such as joint and soft tissue mobilization, Buerger-Allen exercise, therapeutic exercise, muscle strengthening, stretching, range of motion, and massage. Modalities such as high galvanic electrical stimulation have been shown to enhance wound healing. In addition, gait training, graded walking programs, and patient education are vital components to comprehensive treatment programs for foot problems in the individual with diabetes.

Treatment of Infection

Infection may be regarded as a war. There is a battle between the host and the invading parasitic microorganisms, and other factors are involved as well. Without help, the patient with diabetes may lose the battle against infection. With help and adequate circulation, the battle can definitely be won. In many instances, it may take a long time to win and the effort of a team of dedicated and trained clinicians and therapists. The patient must be able to tolerate emotionally protracted and sometimes painful therapeutic regimens. There is no doubt that this aspect may be the most difficult part of the battle. Another aspect of this battle against infection has to be considered: The cost is high. The expense of a 3- to 6-week hospital stay may range from $15,000 to more than $20,000. This reality produces an additional challenge, especially today, when there are so many pressures for cost containment. Consequently, this war may have to be fought for the most part at home or in an extended care facility, with professional treatment and supervision. The goals are to eliminate infected and necrotic tissue, establish drainage, and promote growth of granulation tissue.

Treating infections in the diabetic foot is difficult because of the inability of parenteral antibiotics to diffuse into the infected area owing to the diseased state of the small vessels.[34] Additionally the control of the diabetic state is extremely important, and the presence of infection makes control increasingly more difficult.

Peripheral vascular disease in diabetic patients is often thought both to promote infection and to impair effective antibiotic delivery to infected tissues. Some studies indicate that bacterial killing may be impaired below critical levels of partial pressure oxygen.[34,35]

An abscess, the most common type of active infection in the diabetic foot, insulates itself from treatment by producing a protective fortress or barrier. This walling off of the infected site coupled with small vessel disease renders parenteral antibiotics ineffective. Local care—violating the barrier and gaining entry to the abscess, cleaning out the infected tissue, and establishing drainage—is necessary to eradicate the abscess. In some instances, opening the abscess is performed inadequately. There are several spaces in the foot that can become infected independently of each other. Even if a huge incision is made on the plantar aspect of the foot, an abscess can flourish on the dorsal aspect. Therefore, these feet must be assessed constantly, and if there is a cessation or regression of healing, a careful evaluation of the current therapy must be undertaken and changed accordingly.

In addition, the control of the diabetic state is important to enhance the host's ability to provide some defense against the invading bacteria and perform all of the repair. When the blood glucose level is out of control, these functions are greatly impaired. To make things worse, in the presence of infection, control of the diabetic state is extremely difficult, and it is usually not until the infection is under control that the blood glucose level is successfully brought back within satisfactory limits.

Total Contact Casting

Brand[36] advocates the use of a total contact short leg cast for chronic ulcers. This method allows the patient to ambulate with protection from external stress and trauma. In addition, because the cast is well molded and minimal padding is applied, pressure is distributed evenly and is maintained as long as the cast is worn. This total contact cast also counteracts lymphatic congestion, which compromises the healing process.

Modifying Pressure Distribution in the Insensate Foot

Accommodative devices are insoles that are placed in shoes to balance the feet, allowing pressures to be evenly distributed and permitting support and shock absorption of the foot. An orthotic, in contrast, supports and controls the foot by neutralizing pronatory forces. Fabrication of orthotics and principles of orthotic management are discussed in detail in Chapter 10.

Accommodating shoe gear should be used by patients with diabetes, and walking barefoot should be prohibited. The shoe's upper should be soft, so as not to irritate any prominence or developing deformity. The accommodative insole that is used should be able to adapt to changes as well. A combination of an expanded polyethylene such as Plastazote (Alimed, Inc., Dedham, MA) which can be heat molded to provide total contact, mounted on a shock absorbing material such as PPT or covered with a neoprene such Spenco that is soft and retains its shape makes an excellent accommodative insole. This type of accommodative orthotic has saved many insensitive feet, by protecting the foot from trauma to prominent areas and redistributing the forces to provide even weight bearing through total contact on the plantar surface.

In some instance, when there is an existing imbalance of the weight-bearing surface owing to fixed deformities, additional Plastazote or Aliplast can be added to distribute weight-bearing forces evenly. The concept here is to put additional material in areas that are not bearing excessive weight (Figs. 9–6 to 9–9), thereby bringing the ground up to meet the foot and accommodate the deformity.

Because of the thickness of the orthotic, the shoe must have adequate depth to accommodate it. Extra-depth shoes, such as the P.W. Minor Thermold shoes, allow not only the room needed for the accommodative insole, but also allow for modification of the upper through heat molding to accommodate lesser toe deformities (Fig. 9–10). The Medicare Diabetic Shoe Bill, which went into effect in May 1993, allows for coverage of two pairs of prescription shoes and custom-molded orthotics each year for high-risk diabetic patients who are eligible for Medicare Part B benefits.[37]

Many advocate the use of a rigid-sole rocker-bottom shoe, which lessens pressures under the metatarsal heads during push-off. The apex of the rocker is posi-

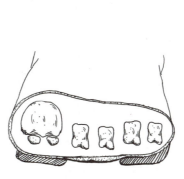
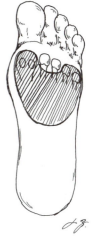

FIGURE 9–6. Accommodative padding to protect the second and third metatarsal heads.

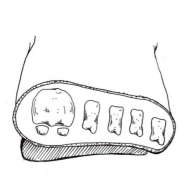
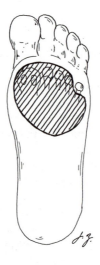

FIGURE 9–7. Accommodative padding to protect the fifth metatarsal head.

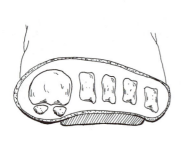
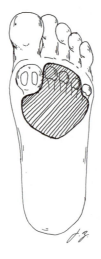

FIGURE 9–8. Accommodative padding to protect the first and fifth metatarsal heads.

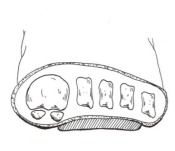
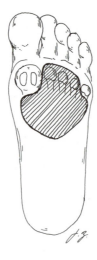

FIGURE 9–9. Accommodative padding to protect the first metatarsal head.

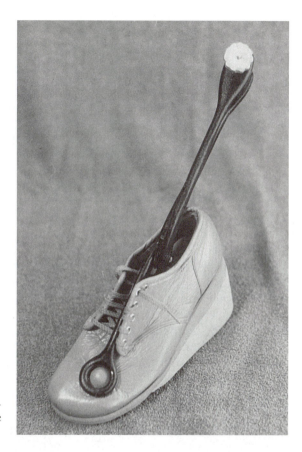

FIGURE 9–10. Modification of Thermold shoe to accommodate lesser toe deformities.

tioned just proximal to the metatarsal heads, allowing for the shoe itself to provide for forward propulsion of the foot.

The hyperkeratotic tissue that forms as a response to increased pressure and friction should be periodically debrided because this tissue increases the pressure, alters the mechanical properties, and causes the deeper layers of skin to retain water and become macerated. The viability of the tissue is decreased, thus predisposing the area to breakdown.

Buerger-Allen Exercises

The incidence of peripheral vascular disease is high in patients with diabetes mellitus owing to the vascular involvement imposed by the neurologic and metabolic state of the disease.[38] The importance of treating diabetic patients with arterial insufficiency is threefold: to enhance peripheral circulation, to prevent limb loss, and to permit healing of wounds. The aim of Buerger-Allen exercises in the treatment of occlusive arterial disease is to improve circulation in a noninvasive therapeutic way.

Buerger-Allen exercises are postural exercises that hypothetically increase local collateral circulation through postural changes, thereby enhancing circulation.[39] The addition of active muscle contraction during each positional change also appears to improve circulation by stimulating blood flow to the working muscles to increase oxygenation and by the "milking" of the contracting muscles around the vascular structures. The theory on which Buerger-Allen exercises are based is that the alternating emptying and filling of blood vessels increases the efficiency of transporting blood by stimulating the peripheral vascular system.[40] To date, there is no hard evidence in support of the benefits of these exercises; however, research currently underway clearly indicates that there are physiologic improvements observed that enhance circulation, facilitate wound healing, and decrease hypersensitivity and pain in the lower extremities of diabetic patients with peripheral vascular involvement.[22]

Buerger-Allen exercises are performed according to the protocol displayed in Figures 9–11 through 9–13. The individual lies supine with the legs elevated at an angle of 45° until blanching occurs or for a maximum time of 3 minutes (Fig. 9–11). Active pumping and circling of the feet and isometric quadriceps and gluteal contractions are performed for the first minute or more in the elevated position. Once the blanching has occurred, the patient sits up and hangs the lower leg over the edge of the bed (Fig. 9–12). While in this position, the individual is encouraged actively to plantar flex, dorsiflex, and circle the feet. This position is maintained for a minimum of 3 minutes or until rubor has occurred. Lastly the individual lies supine with the lower extremities flat for 3 minutes (Fig. 9–13). Again, active muscle contraction of the leg muscles is performed for at least 1 minute in this position. *One note of caution:* In the presence of severe physiologic compromise in the cardiovascular system, the authors recommend assuming the flat/supine position between the elevation and dependent phases to prevent the consequences of orthostatic hypotension. The entire sequence is repeated three times in each exercise session. Buerger-Allen exercises should be per-

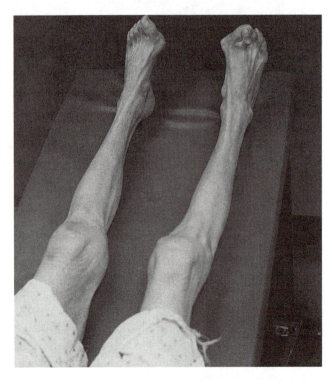

FIGURE 9–11. Buerger-Allen exercises: legs elevated at an angle of 45° in the supine position.

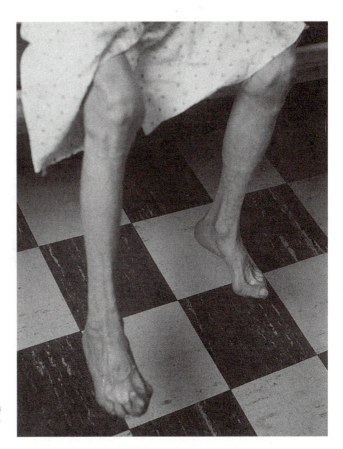

FIGURE 9–12. Buerger-Allen exercises: legs in dependent position when sitting.

formed twice each day for maximum benefit. If peripheral neuropathy is present and active muscle contraction is not possible, the clinician can passively plantar flex and dorsiflex the foot in each of the respective positions to increase blood flow facilitated by the pumping action of the surrounding musculature. The authors have successfully employed high-frequency electrical stimulation to elicit threshold muscle contractions in the lower extremities of the diabetic patient with peripheral neuropathy.

Electrical Stimulation and Blood Flow

With peripheral neuropathy in diabetes, often an active muscle contraction is not possible. Muscle contraction is responsible for increasing blood flow not only through its increasing oxidative demand, but also by its pumping action. Direct current may be necessary to facilitate muscle contraction when neuropathy exists to increase oxygenation of the working muscle. The externally stimulated muscles contract through depolarization of the sarcolemma as initiated by the depolarization of the innervating nerve. Blood flow increases to the area to increase the oxygen delivered and to remove the metabolites that working muscles produce.

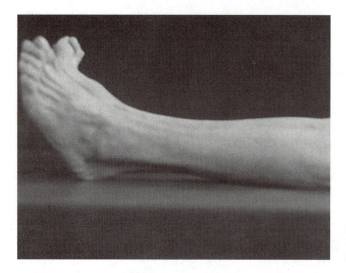

FIGURE 9–13. Buerger-Allen exercises: legs flat in the supine position.

High Galvanic Electrical Stimulation in Wound Healing

The rationale for the use of electrical stimulation for promoting circulation and affecting wound healing includes the effect of the electrical stimulus on microorganisms, the type of injury, and the tissue repair process. Results from studies show that the use of low amplitudes of direct current (high galvanic) provide the most effective means for promoting wound healing.[41–46] A cathodal current affects microorganism growth in both in vivo and in vitro models with a noted decrease in *Escherichia coli* B growth rate[47,48] and a decrease in infected wounds of *Pseudomonas aeruginosa*.[48] Additionally a negative polarity decreases the growth rate of *Staphylococcus aureus*.[49] Two mechanisms are proposed for the decrease in the growth rate of the microorganisms. First, continuous electrical stimulation of the single-celled organism disrupts its homeostatic mechanism to the point of death. Second, negative current disrupts intracellular activity causing an irreversible disruption of enzyme processes or regulatory mechanisms involved in transport across the cell membrane.[50] Research findings support the use of negative direct current for retarding the growth rate of microorganisms.

Tissue damage causes disruption of cell membranes and alteration of cellular constituents. This produces an electrical potential difference between injured and intact tissues called an "injury potential."[51] Initially the injury potential is positive, but as the wound heals and infection subsides, the potential becomes negative. This change would indicate that there is a naturally occurring polarity associated with the repair process.

There is also blood cell migration that occurs with the use of electrical stimulation that has a beneficial influence in wound healing. Under the positive pole, a clumping of leukocytes and a thrombosing in small vessels have been found.[52] This change indicates a migration of waste products toward the cathode. Under the negative pole, there is dermal cell movement with a migration of epithelial cells toward the anode, which would aid in the healing process. Low-frequency stimulation also has been shown to significantly increase the rate of protein and DNA synthesis under the negative pole.[41,42]

Clinical experience reveals that approximately 2.5 months are required for a diabetic ulcer in the foot to heal, a finding substantiated by other researchers.[43-45] Negative polarity helps to move fluid from the area, increase blood flow, and facilitate wound healing. A positive polarity has germicidal effects and a sedative effect on the nerve. The benefits of high galvanic electrical stimulation in the treatment of both nonsurgical and surgical wounds in the diabetic have been repeatedly observed.

Patient Education

Once a foot ulcer has been healed, preventing recurrence is paramount. The foot has been compromised by the trauma of infection, and scar tissue has formed, limiting circulation and mobility of the tissues. The foot will never be as healthy as it was before the infection (Fig. 9–14) and becomes more prone to trauma and injury. Patients must constantly monitor the condition of their feet, and if a problem occurs, immediate action must be taken. Rest and proper therapy should be instituted at the first sign of a problem.

Diabetic patients should be instructed in the examination and care of their feet. They should look for area of redness, dry skin, overhydration, and hyperkeratotic developments, such as corns and calluses. They should look for any areas of pressure that may be the result of shoe pressure or wrinkles and seams in their socks. Patients

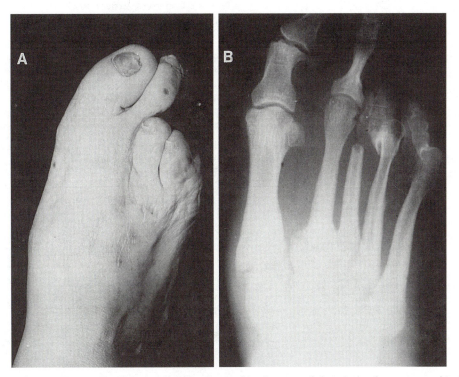

FIGURE 9–14. (*A*) The clinical and (*B*) radiographic changes of the repeated surgery to this diabetic foot in an effort to eliminate infection.

need to be advised as to the type of sock to be worn (heavy cotton or wool) and how to purchase shoes properly. Guidelines for exercise need to be individually tailored for each patient. The individual should be instructed to have toenails and hyperkeratotic areas periodically trimmed and debrided by a podiatrist. The diabetic should not attempt to clip his or her own nails or file calluses. Advice should be provided regarding temperature of bath water and the avoidance of soaking the feet for extended periods of time. Foot protection needs to be encouraged, and the individual should avoid walking barefoot, even for short distances within the home.

There are many resources for educating the diabetic in self-monitoring and care of the feet. These resources are provided in Table 9–1. Appropriate materials should

TABLE 9–1 Patient Educational Resources

Krames Communications
312 90th Street
Daly City, CA 94015-1898
Pamphlets
  The Foot Book (#1078)
  Foot Owner's Manual (#1005)
  Ankle Owner's Manual (#1073)
  Foot Surgery (#1119)
  Laser Foot Surgery (#1321)
  Walking for Fitness (#1263)
  Running (#1117)
  Diabetes and Your Feet (#1372)

Thermal-Moldable Shoes, Inc.
100 DeVille
Williamsville, NY 14221-4408
Pamphlets
  For Diabetics on the Go
  For Arthritics on the Go
  Thermold Shoes

P.W. Minor and Son, Inc.
3 Treadeasy Avenue
PO Box 678
Batavia, NY 14021-0678
Extra depth shoes

The Langer Foundation
1011 Grand Boulevard
Deer Park, NY 11729
Pamphlets
  Walking as an Exercise
  Facts for Runners and Other Athletes
  When Your Feet Hurt You Hurt All Over

Channing L. Bete Co. Inc.
Scriptographic Booklet
South Deerfield, MA 01373
Pamphlets
  About Foot Care
  Fun, Fitness and Your Feet

The Arthritis Foundation
Massachusetts Chapter
Parker Building
124 Watertown, MA 02172
Pamphlets
  Arthritis Surgery Information to Consider
  Arthritis Basic Facts
  Arthritis—Exercise and Your Arthritis
  Arthritis—A Serious Look at the Facts

Fund for Podiatry Education and Research
9312 Old Georgetown Road
Bethesda, Maryland 20814
Newsletter
  Foot News

U.S. Department of Health, Education, and Welfare
U.S. Government Printing Office
Washington, DC 20402
Pamphlet
  Feet First—A Booklet About Foot Care

Pal Health Technologies, Inc.
293 Herman Street
Perkin, IL 61554
Pamphlets
  Maybe You Need Orthotics
  What Is Pronation?
  Oh My Aching Feet!
  Foot Surgery
  Walking—Make it Easy on Yourself
  Running . . . and Jogging
  Skiing—Your Feet . . .
  Ice Skating/Roller Skating

Department of Public Health
Center for Health Promotion
150 Tremont Street
Boston, MA 02111
Pamphlet
  Walking—A Lifetime Activity

be given to each patient on an individual basis. Educating patients in the prevention of foot problems is probably the single most important component of intervention.

Surgery

Surgical intervention to eliminate osseous deformity and modify pressure may be necessary to prevent ulceration and potential infection. Operating on patients with diabetes has been shown to have good results in healing, provided that circulation is adequate. Healing of a sterile surgical wound that is closed is easier than healing of one that is open and infected; however, the surgical sites of these patients must be watched carefully. In the presence of neurologic involvement, the diabetic individual is more prone to injury after surgery and may not notice that anything is amiss.

GENERAL CONSIDERATIONS IN DIABETES

Pathophysiology in Diabetes Mellitus

Diabetes mellitus is a chronic disease that affects approximately 12 million people in the United States.[53] Insulin is needed for glucose to be transferred from the blood to the muscle and fat cells.[54] People who suffer from diabetes cannot produce enough insulin (type I) or cannot properly use the insulin they do produce (type II), causing hyperglycemia.[55]

The complex nature of diabetes creates a broad spectrum of physical complications and reactions, which can make the condition extremely dangerous. Diabetes is the leading cause of blindness and can cause glaucoma and cataracts, which have a direct impact on ambulatory status. Diabetics are twice as likely to have heart attacks and strokes, 5 times more prone to foot ulceration with the development of gangrene, and 17 times more prone to kidney disease when compared with the general population.[54] All of these problems affect function by influencing endurance and weight-bearing capabilities leading to inactivity. Complications of diabetes also affect the mouth, reproductive system, nervous and vascular systems, the muscular system, and skin and reduce an individual's defense mechanisms in the presence of infection.

Approximately 18% of the population between the ages of 65 and 74 years has diabetes mellitus.[56] In general, elderly individuals tend to have an impaired glucose tolerance compared with younger individuals. Data suggest that only about 10% of the variance in total serum glucose response to an oral glucose load is attributable to age.[57] Body weight and the level of physical activity appear to have a more important role in the pathogenesis of hyperglycemia. The major factors involved in hyperglycemia and the development of type II diabetes mellitus include poor second-phase insulin secretion, failure to inhibit glucose production, a defect in the insulin receptor and postreceptor sites, obesity, and lack of physical activity. Regardless of the cause of diabetes mellitus in the elderly, evidence reveals that control of glucose levels improves the quality of life and decreases morbidity and mortality rates.

Although no clear understanding of the cause of diabetes has been found, and there is no cure, the disease has been found to be controllable by achieving and maintaining normal blood glucose levels.[58] This accomplishment requires a carefully balanced utilization of four critical components: diet, exercise, education for self-monitoring, and drug therapy.

Nutrition and Diabetes Mellitus

By its nature, diabetes is a condition in which food is improperly metabolized producing too much glucose. Therefore, diet control is critical to diabetes control, especially in type II diabetes.[58] Patients with diabetes should be encouraged to consume fewer calories and to eat less fat and simple sugars.

There are a number of effects on vitamin and mineral status in diabetes mellitus.[59] Diabetes mellitus is associated with decreased zinc absorption and hyperzincuria.[60] Zinc deficiencies are associated with poor wound healing, poor immune function, immune dysfunction, and anorexia.[61] Supplementary zinc administration has been shown to improve immune function[62] and facilitate wound healing[63] in patients with zinc deficiencies.

Chromium plays a role in normal glucose homeostasis. Deficiency of chromium has been implicated in glucose intolerance.[64] Copper levels are elevated in type II diabetes mellitus.[65] The clinical significance of this is not clearly known; however, Klevay[65] demonstrated that experimentally induced copper deficiency resulted in elevation of cholesterol levels. Thiamine is essential for the transport of metabolized glucose into the Krebs cycle. In type II diabetes mellitus, erythrocyte transketolase activity, an indirect measure of thiamine status, is elevated. This finding may be related to poor availability of intracellular glucose. Diabetes mellitus is also associated with pernicious anemia. Vitamin B_{12} deficiency is common in the diabetic and associated with posterior column neuropathy and dementia.

Exercise and Diabetes Mellitus

The second area of control in diabetes is exercise. Exercise improves blood glucose control, improves circulation, reduces cardiovascular risk, and keeps the patient fit.[66,67] Daily exercise increases the tissue sensitivity to insulin for 2 to 3 days following the exercise, thereby decreasing the need for insulin injection.[67]

Impaired glucose tolerance has been shown in cross-sectional studies to be related to the level of physical activity and fitness.[68] In a prospective trial of the effects of exercise on glucose tolerance, Seals et al[69] found that although glucose levels did not change, both insulin and C peptide levels decreased. In addition, high-density lipoprotein cholesterol levels increased and triglyceride levels decreased. In patients with type II diabetes mellitus, short-term exercise programs do not show a major advantage over dietary control of glucose intake[70]; however, long-term exercise programs did result in improvements of glucose tolerance.[71,72] In combination with dietary control, the possible benefits of exercise on glucose tolerance are evident. Besides the possible beneficial effects of exercise on glucose tolerance, exercise training may also improve cardiovascular fitness, lipid profiles, hypertension, osteopenia, and psychological function in diabetic patients. Risks of exercise in diabetics include hypoglycemia, ketosis, dehydration, myocardial ischemia, arrhythmias, acceleration of proliferative retinopathy, increased proteinuria, and trauma (particularly in patients with neuropathy). The National Institutes of Health consensus panel concluded that the effects of exercise on metabolic control in noninsulin-dependent diabetes mellitus are often variable and of small magnitude.[73] Pacini et al[74] demonstrated that normal weight, physically active older subjects have normal insulin-binding capacity, insulin sensitivity, and insulin secretory capacity in response to glucose stimulation. Helmrich et al[75] showed that increased activity levels actually decreased the incidence of diabetes mellitus. Studies of long-term exercise programs need to be undertaken before a formal recommendation for an exercise prescription can be given; however, the benefits of exercise for cardiovascular conditioning and the potential for modifying glucose intolerance in the diabetic clearly outweigh the risks.

Education and Diabetes Mellitus

Patients with diabetes should receive a thorough education about the disease, its complications, and the specific steps that must be taken to control it. Self-monitoring involves a routine check of glucose levels, either by checking the urine or blood. Blood glucose monitoring is the method of choice because it is a more accurate measurement of glucose levels. In addition, self-monitoring of skin condition, especially in the lower extremities, is a vital component of diabetic education.

Drug Therapy for Diabetes

Drug therapy for diabetes consists of oral agents (type II only) and insulin. Insulin is obtained from animal sources, such as cows and pigs, or from a biosynthesis process that results in insulin products that are the same as human insulin.[55] The synthesized insulin has gained popularity because fewer insulin antibodies are formed and there are fewer allergic reactions. Insulin requirements may change in patients who become ill, especially with vomiting or fever. Signs of hyperglycemia may be caused by a missed insulin dose, overeating, not following the diabetic diet, or if a patient has a fever or infection. Signs include excessive thirst or urination (or both), dry mouth, drowsiness, flushed dry skin, fruitlike breath odor, stomachache, nausea, vomiting, and difficulty breathing. Signs of hypoglycemia may be caused by too much insulin, missing a snack or meal, sickness, too much exercise, drinking alcoholic beverages, or taking medications that contain alcohol. Signs include anxiety, chills, cold sweats, cool pale skin, confusion, drowsiness, excessive hunger, headache, nausea, nervousness, shakiness, vision changes, and unusual tiredness or fatigue. The consumption of a sugar-containing food (e.g., orange juice, honey) should reverse the signs.

Resources Available to the Patient with Diabetes

The best source for information on diabetes is the American Diabetes Association (ADA) (2 Park Avenue, New York, NY 10016; 1-212-683-7444). Members of ADA include physicians, research scientists, and dietitians as well as diabetics and their families. The association sponsors educational lectures, film presentations, and diabetes screening clinics nationally.

There are numerous organizations that provide patient educational materials.

Shoe manufacturers and orthotic material suppliers provide shoes and orthotics specific to the needs of the diabetic. Some of these resources are listed in Table 9–1.

CASE STUDY

A 78-year-old white woman was admitted to a nursing home for rehabilitation following acute hospitalization for 3 days with primary diagnosis of type II diabetes mellitus presenting with a grade II plantar ulceration under metatarsal heads II and III of the right lower extremity. Confounding diagnoses include history of myocardial infarct, peripheral vascular disease, obesity, and diminished visual acuity secondary to cataracts. There is no history of falls, although patient reports "dizziness" on standing.

Initial Evaluative Findings

Patient is insulin dependent. Functional activity level decreased; requires assistance in all instrumental activities of daily living and self-care activities (basic activities of daily living); requires supervision in toileting and transfer activities. Feeds, bathes, and dresses self. Independently ambulates functional distances within home environment without assistive devices (50 to 100 feet). Requires minimal assistance without assistive devices in ambulation outside of home with frequent rest periods (600 to 800 feet). Lives in own home with husband who is 80 and in relatively good health. Daughter lives two blocks away and assists patient in necessary activities of daily living on a daily basis.

Patient presents with grade II ulceration metatarsal heads II and III on plantar surface of right foot. Yellow drainage, which is odorous. Redness surrounding ulceration. Patient with hallux abductus valgus (HAV) bilaterally, Hammer toes digits II bilaterally, claw toes III–V bilaterally. Severe dense keratosis under metatarsal heads II and III on left. Trophic nail changes both great toes with involution bilaterally. Skin dry with deep fissures and flaking both feet.

Radiograph findings: No evidence of osteomyelitis.

Sensory and neurologic assessment reveal absence of vibratory sensation both lower extremities in a socklike pattern distally and diminished vibratory sensation upper extremities in a glovelike pattern distally. Absence of protective sensation both plantar surfaces with response level exceeding 5.07 g as per Semmes-Weinstein monofilament testing. Inability to distinguish between hot and cold all four extremities. Absence of ankle jerk bilaterally. Diminished patellar reflex right greater than left. Babinski sign absent bilaterally. Positive Romberg sign in standing.

Muscle strength generally within the 4/5 range throughout with the following exceptions 2/5 anterior tibialis and 3/5 posterior tibialis bilaterally.

Gait pattern: Slow, shuffling gait with increased double stance time. No heel strike or push-off. Absence of any distinct vertical pathway of either foot. Minimal toe clearance. Marked lateral sway right greater than left without vertical rise. Twenty degrees of foot abduction on right, 8° of foot abduction on left. Absence of arm swing. Decrease in hip and knee excursion.

Range of motion and joint mobility within normal limits with the following exceptions: −3° dorsiflexion right ankle without tibial-fibular splay; 0° dorsiflexion on left.

Ankle and foot edema bilaterally +3 pitting. 1+ posterior tibialis and dorsal pedalis pulses bilaterally; all else 2+ in lower extremities. Greater than 1 minute blanching and filling times both lower extremities to Buerger-Allen testing. Marked dependent rubor bilaterally with dusky red coloration right foot.

Transfers require supervision secondary to orthostatic hypotension. Ambulation independent within room (50 to 100 feet), requires supervision and occasional contact guard for longer distances without assistive devices.

Treatment Approach

1. Podiatric debridement of ulceration under metatarsal heads II and III of right foot and hyperkeratotic area under metatarsal heads II and III of left foot. Nails trimmed and filed. Debridement of involuted nails bilaterally.
2. Total contact full foot orthotics with accommodative pressure relief padding under metatarsal heads II and III bilaterally. Materials: Plastazote #2 with PPT padding.
3. Fitted for extradepth Thermold shoes. Stretching of toe box to accommodate lesser toe deformities and HAV bilaterally. Rocker-bottom sole provided to facilitate push-off without undue forefoot stresses.
4. Grade II joint mobilization both proximal and distal tibial-fibular articulations, talar rocking, and calcaneal distraction.
5. High galvanic electrical stimulation with positive polarity first four treatments (until laboratory values negative for bacterial growth) modified to negative polarity at 200 mV surged pulse with 120 pps for 60 minutes daily until wound healing complete (68 days).
6. Buerger-Allen exercises twice a day, three cycles.
7. Lower extremity and trunk strengthening exercises daily.
8. Gait and transfer training.
9. Cardiovascular reconditioning/weight reduction walking program.

Note: Patient also seen by nutritionist for dietary consultation and weight reduction program and by occupational therapist for activities of daily living.

Length of stay in long-term care facility: 92 days

Upon Discharge
1. Instructed patient, husband, and daughter in muscle strengthening exercises and stretching for foot and lower extremities. Written instructions provided.
2. Instructed patient, husband, and daughter in Buerger-Allen exercises to be done once a day. Written instructions provided.
3. Instructed patient, husband, and daughter in proper foot and nail care and inspection in conjunction with nursing and podiatry.
4. Reviewed safe transfer and ambulation techniques with patient and husband and instructed patient, husband, and daughter in cardiovascular reconditioning walking program, monitoring, and progression.

Results

On discharge from long-term care facility, patient independent in all basic activities of daily living. Requires supervision and occasional assistance with instrumental activities of daily living. Ambulating independently within home without assistive devices (200 to 300 feet). Requires supervision only for distances greater than 1000 feet.

Ulceration of right foot: Complete healing obtained at 62 days (high galvanic electrical stimulation treatment continued for an additional 6 days).

Sensory and neurologic assessment reveals diminished vibratory sensation all four extremities. No change in reflexes from initial evaluation.

Muscle strength 4/5 throughout.

Gait pattern: Safe ambulation with good foot clearance. Swing-stance time with decrease in double stance. Heel strike present bilaterally. Push-off assisted by rocker-bottom sole. Good toe clearance. No significant lateral sway. No assymmetry right to left. Eight degrees of foot abduction right, 4° of foot abduction left. Arm swing intact. Good hip and knee excursion.

Joint range of motion and joint mobility within functional limitations throughout.

Ankle and foot edema bilaterally +1 pitting. 2+ femoral, popliteal, posterior tibialis, and dorsal pedalis pulses bilaterally. Blanching time 0.75 minute. Filling time 1.00 minute. Moderate dependent rubor bilaterally.

Patient reports an increased feeling of well-being and an overall improvement in functional capabilities.

Assessment

Wound completely healed. Patient with improvement in activities of daily living both basic and instrumental, improvement in ambulatory distance and safety in addition to observed increase in stability of gait pattern, and improvement in transfer capabilities. Sensory and vascular improvement noted. Increase in range of motion and strength of both lower extremities noted. Observed and reported improvement in the quality of life.

SUMMARY

Understanding as much as possible about diabetes allows an appreciation of the disease and how it may produce dramatic changes in human anatomy and physiology. Although understanding of the disease has increased, there are still many areas for investigation and improvement that could evolve into treatment approaches.

An excellent example of preventive intervention is to strive to maintain "optimal health" in the diabetic individual. This goal involves not only foot care, but also attention to control of the disease via nutrition and drugs, implementation of physical fitness programs, and education of the patient in self-care and monitoring.

Sensory loss in the lower extremities resulting from diabetes mellitus often predisposes individuals to ulceration of the foot. An ill-fitting shoe or a wrinkle in the sock may go unnoticed and lead to friction, skin breakdown, and a resulting foot ulcer. If undetected, even the smallest ulcer may lead to amputation of a lower extremity. Screening of the foot during evaluation can prevent this devastating loss. Intervention could include education of the aged individual in foot inspection (or education of a family member or friend if the elderly diabetic individual's eyesight is compromised), proper shoe fitting, and techniques for dealing with sensory loss (i.e., as temperature sensation diminishes, the individual needs to test bath water temperature with a thermometer or have someone else test the water before putting his or her insensitive feet into a steamy bath). With proper skin care and professional (podiatric) care of the nails and calloused, injury is less likely to occur. The cost of a therapeutic diabetic shoe (e.g., the P.W. Minor Thermold shoe) is $160 to $190 per pair and provides protection and ample room for the forefoot and accommodative orthotics. Compared to the cost of ulcer care, which at a minimum is $6000, and the cost of hospitalization and preventive rehabilitation for amputation, which averages $30,000,[4] this option is inexpensive. The principle of obtaining relative "optimal health" in the diabetic patient is not only cost-effective, but also clearly would lead to an overall improvement in the quality of life.

REFERENCES

1. Spencer, F, Sage, R, and Graner, J: Incidence of foot pathology in the diabetic population. J Am Podiatr Med Assoc 75:590–592, 1985.
2. Kozak, GP and Rowbotham, JL: Diabetic foot disease. In Kozak, GP, Hoar, CS, Rowbotham, JL, et al (eds): Management of Diabetic Foot Problems. WB Saunders, Philadelphia, 1984, pp 1–8.
3. Helfand, AE: Podiatric management of the diabetic foot in the elderly. In Helfand, AE (ed): Clinical Podogeriatrics. Williams & Wilkins, Baltimore, 1981, pp 106–121.
4. American Diabetes Association: Direct and Indirect Costs of Diabetes in the United States in 1987. American Diabetes Association, Alexandria, VA, 1988.
5. Gerard, K, et al: The cost of diabetes. Diabetic Med 6:164–170, 1989.
6. Government Relations Update: Bustamante offers bill focused on Diabetes Prevention Programs. American Diabetes Association Newsletter, August 1989.
7. Gleis, L: Financing the care of diabetes mellitus in the 1990s. Diab Care 13:1021–1023, 1990.
8. Nemchik, R: From research to practice: Saving the diabetic foot. Diabetes Spectrum 1:153–155, 1990.
9. Pecoraro, RE, Reiber, GE, and Burgess, EM: Pathways to diabetic limb amputation: Basis for prevention. Diab Care 13:513–521, 1990.
10. Levin, ME and O'Neal, LW (eds): The Diabetic Foot, 4th ed. CV Mosby, St. Louis, 1988.
11. Boulton, A: The diabetic foot. Ann Acad Med Singapore 7:359–363, 1978.
12. Edmonds, M: The diabetic foot: Pathophysiology and treatment. Clin Endocrinol Metab 15:889–916, 1986.
13. Brand, P: Repetitive stress in the development of diabetic foot ulcers. In Levin, M and O'Neal, L (eds): The Diabetic Foot. CV Mosby, St Louis, 1988, pp 83–90.
14. Pirat, J: Diabetes mellitus and its degenerative complications: A prospective study of 4400 patients observed between 1947 and 1973 (part I). Diab Care 1:168–188, 1978.
15. Kannel, W and McGee, D: Diabetes and cardiovascular disease: The Framingham study. JAMA 241:2035–2038, 1979.
16. Nawoczenski, D, Birke, J, Graham, S et al: The neuropathic foot—a management scheme. Phys Ther 69:287–291, 1989.
17. Sims, DS, Cavanagh, P, and Ulbrecht, J: Risk factors in the diabetic foot, recognition and management, Phys Ther 68:1887–1902, 1988.
18. Edmonds, M, Roberts, V, and Watkins, P: Blood flow in the diabetic neuropathic foot. Diabetologia 22:9–15, 1982.
19. Jurado, R and Walker, HK: Diabetic autonomic neuropathy. In Davidson, J (ed): Clinical Diabetes Mellitus: A Problem-Oriented Approach. Georg Thieme Verlag, New York, 1986, pp 426–449.
20. Brand, PW: Patient monitoring. In Trautman, JR (ed): The Effects of Pressure in Human Tissues. Northwestern University Publishers, Carville, LA, 1977, pp 50–51.
21. Walker, K: Peripheral neuropathy. In Davidson, J (ed): Clinical Diabetes Mellitus: A Problem-Oriented Approach. Georg Thieme Verlag, New York, 1986, pp 416–425.
22. Bottomley, JM: A comparison of the effects of Buerger-Allen exercises and high galvanic electrical stimulation on lower extremity blood flow in diabetic patients. Publication pending. Diabetic Med 2:96.

23. Birke, JA and Sims, DS: Plantar sensory threshold in the ulcerative foot. Leprosy Review 57:261–267, 1986.
24. Dorairaj, A, Reddy, R, and Jesudasan, K: An evaluation of the Semmes-Weinstein 6.10 monofilament as compared with 6 nylon in leprosy patients. Ind J Leprosy 60:413–417, 1988.
25. Niinikoski, J: Cellular and nutritional interactions in wound healing. Med Biol 58:303–309, 1980.
26. Baker, JD: Postrest Doppler ankle pressures. Arch Surg 113:1171, 1978.
27. Rowbotham, JL, Gibbons, GW, and Kozak, GP: Guidelines in examination of the diabetic leg and foot. In Kozak, GP, Hoar, CS, Rowbotham, JL, et al (eds): Management of Diabetic Foot Problems. WB Saunders, Philadelphia, 1984, pp. 9–16.
28. Wagner, FW: The dysvascular foot: A system for diagnosis and treatment. Foot Ankle 2:64–69, 1981.
29. Brand PW: The diabetic foot. In Davidson, J (ed): Clinical Diabetes Mellitus: A Problem-Oriented Approach. Georg Thieme Verlag, New York, 1986, pp 376–382.
30. Habershaw, G and Donovan, J: Biomechanical considerations of the diabetic foot. In Kozar, GP, Hoar, CS, Rowbotham, JL, et al (eds): Management of Diabetic Foot Problems. WB Saunders, Philadelphia, 1984, pp 32–44.
31. Boulton, AJM, Hardisty, CA, Betts, RP, et al: Dynamic foot pressures and other studies as diagnostic and management aids in the diabetic neuropathy. Diab Care 6:25, 1983.
32. Bailey, TS, Yu, HM, and Rayfield, EJ: Patterns of foot examination in a diabetes clinic. Am J Med 78:371–374, 1985.
33. Canter, K: Podiatric health planning for the aging veteran. J Am Podiatr Med Assoc 76:47–51, 1986.
34. Knighton, D, Halliday, B, and Hunt, T: Oxygen as an antibiotic: The effect of inspired oxygen on infection. Arch Surg 119:199–204, 1984.
35. Hunt, T, Linsey, M, Grilis, H, et al: The effect of differing ambient oxygen tensions on wound infection. Ann Surg 181:35–39, 1975.
36. Brand, PW: The insensitive foot (including leprosy). In Jahss, MH (ed): Disorders of the Foot, vol 2. WB Saunders, Philadelphia, 1982, pp 1266–1286.
37. Black, E: Diabetic shoe legislation. Podiatry Today p 79, April 1993.
38. Minaker, KL: Aging and diabetes mellitus as risk factors for vascular disease. Am J Med 82 (suppl 1B):47–53, 1987.
39. Ebel, A and Kim, D: Exercise in peripheral vascular disease. In Basmajian, JV and Wolf, S (eds): Therapeutic Exercise, 4th ed. Williams & Wilkins, Baltimore, 1990, pp 371–386.
40. Wisham, MB, Lawrence, H, Abramson, MD, et al: Value of exercise in peripheral arterial diseases. JAMA 153:10–12, 1953.
41. Bourguignon, GJ and Bourguignon, LYW: Electric stimulation of protein and DNA synthesis in human fibroblasts. FASEB J 1:398, 1987.
42. Bourguignon, LYW, Wenche, J, Majercik, MH, and Bourguignon, GJ: Lymphocyte activation and capping of hormone receptors. J Cell Biochem 37:131–138, 1988.
43. Akers, TK and Gabrielson, AL: The effect of high voltage galvanic stimulation on the rate of healing of decubitus ulcers. In Wachtel, H (ed): Biomedical Sciences Instrumentation. Instrument Society of America, Research Triangle Park, NC, 1984, pp 99–100.
44. Alon, G, Azaria, M, and Stein, H: Diabetic ulcer healing using high voltage current. Phys Ther 66:775–782, 1986.
45. Feeder, JA and Kloth, LC: Acceleration of wound healing with pulsing direct current. Phys Ther 65:741–749, 1985.
46. Ross, CR and Segal, D: High voltage galvanic stimulation—an aid to post-operative healing. Current Podiatry 19:26–31 May 1981.
47. Rowley, BA: Electrical current effects on E. coli growth rates. Proc Soc Exp Biol Med 139:929–934, 1972.
48. Rowley, BA, McKenna, JM, and Chase, GR: The influence of electrical current on an infecting microorganism in wounds. Ann NY Acad Sci 238:543–548, 1974.
49. Barranco, SD, Spadero, JA, and Berger, TJ: In vitro effect of weak direct current on Staphylococcus aureus. Clin Orthop Rel Res 100:250, 1974.
50. Wheeler, P, Wolcott, L, Morris, J, et al: Neural considerations in the healing of ulcerated tissue by clinical electrotherapeutic application of weak direct current: Findings and theory. In Reynolds, DV and Sjoberg, AE (eds): Neuroelectric Research. Charles C Thomas, Springfield, IL, 1971, pp 83–96.
51. Burr, HA, Taffel, M, and Harvey, WC: An electrometric study of the healing wound in man. Yale J Biol Med 12:483–491, 1940.
52. Harrington, DB, Meyer, R, and Klein, RM: Effects of small amounts of electric current at the cellular level. Ann NY Acad Sci 238:300, 1974.
53. American Diabetes Association: Position statement: Office guide to diagnosis and classification of diabetes mellitus and other categories of glucose intolerance. Diab Care 15(suppl 2):4, 1992.
54. Gambert, SR: Diabetes Mellitus in the Elderly: A Practical Guide. Raven Press, New York, 1990.
55. Jackson, RA: Mechanisms of age-related glucose intolerance. Diab Care 13(suppl 2):9–19, 1990.
56. Harris, MI, Hadden, WC, Knowler, WC, et al: Prevalence of diabetes and impaired glucose tolerance and plasma glucose levels in U.S. population aged 20–74 years. Diabetes 4:523–534, 1987.

57. Zavaroni, I, Dall'Aglio, E, and Bruschi, F: Effect of age and environmental factors on glucose tolerance and insulin secretion in a worker population. J Am Geriatr Soc 34:271–278, 1986.
58. Bergman, M: Principles of Diabetes Management. Medical Examination Publishing, New York, 1987.
59. Mooradin, AD and Morley, JE: Micronutrient status in diabetes mellitus. Am J Clin Nutr 45:877–895, 1987.
60. Kinlaw, WB, Levine, AS, Morley, JE, et al: Abnormal zinc metabolism in type II diabetes mellitus. Am J Med 75:273–277, 1983.
61. Morley, JE: Nutritional status of the elderly. Am J Med 81:679–695, 1986.
62. Niewoehner, CB, Allen, JI, Boosalis, M, et al: The role of zinc supplementation in type II diabetes mellitus. Am J Med 81:63–68, 1986.
63. Hallbook, T and Lanner, E: Serum-zinc and healing of venous leg ulcers. Lancet 2:780–782, 1972.
64. Wallach, S: Clinical and biochemical aspects of chromium deficiency. J Am Coll Nutr 4:107–120, 1985.
65. Klevay, LM: Hypercholesterolemia produced by an increase in the ratio of zinc to copper ingested. Am J Clin Nutr 26:1060–1065, 1978.
66. Jette, DU: Physiological effects of exercise in the diabetic. Phy Ther 64:3:339–342, 1984.
67. Kohl, HW, Villegas, JA, Gordon, NF, and Blair, SN: Cardiorespiratory fitness, glycemic status, and mortality risk in men. Diab Care 15:184–192, 1992.
68. Rosenthal, MJ, Hartnell, JM, Morley, JE, et al: UCLA geriatric rounds: Diabetes in the elderly. J Am Geriatr Soc 35:435–447, 1987.
69. Seals, DR, Hagberg, JM, Hurley, BF, et al: Effects of endurance training on glucose tolerance and plasma lipid levels in older men and women. JAMA 252:645–649, 1984.
70. Krotkiewski, M, Lonnroth, P, Mandroukas, K, et al: The effects of physical training on glucose metabolism in obesity in type II diabetes mellitus. Diabetologia 28:881–890, 1985.
71. Saltin, B, Lindgarde, F, Houston, M, et al: Physical training and glucose tolerance in middle-aged men with chemical diabetes. Diabetes 28(suppl):30–32, 1979.
72. Bogardus, C, Ravussin, E, Robbins, DC, et al: Effects of physical training and diet therapy on carbohydrate metabolism in patients with glucose intolerance and non-insulin dependent diabetes mellitus. Diabetes 33:311–318, 1984.
73. Karam, JH: Therapeutic dilemmas in type II diabetes mellitus: Improving and maintaining B-cell and insulin sensitivity. West J Med 148:685–690, 1988.
74. Pacini, G, Valerio, A, Beccaro, R, et al: Insulin sensitivity and beta-cell responsivity are not decreased in elderly subjects with normal OGTT. J Am Geriatr Soc 36:317–323, 1988.
75. Helmrich, SP, Ragland, DR, Leung, RW, et al: Physical activity and reduced occurence of non-insulin-dependent diabetes mellitus. N Engl J Med 325:147–152, 1991.

SECTION **III**

Treatment Approaches to Restore Normal Movement

CHAPTER 10

Biomechanical Orthotics

Robert A. Donatelli, PhD, PT, OCS
Michael J. Wooden, MS, PT, OCS

The foot functions as an important part of the lower kinetic chain and is designed to distribute and dissipate kinetic forces during the stance phase of gait. Foot orthotics are recognized as an important adjunct to the treatment of lower extremity dysfunction related to poor mechanics and alignment. The term "foot orthotics" includes many different types of orthotics—flexible, semirigid, rigid, biomechanical, sand splint, sorbothotics, functional, power soles, University of California Biomechanical Laboratory (UCBL) device, Helfet orthotics, Whitman, Roberts, Roberts-Whitman, Thomas heel, Schaffer plate, and accommodative orthotics.[1–18] For the clinician, deciding what kind of foot orthotic to prescribe can be confusing and frustrating.

For the purposes of this chapter, foot orthotics are divided into three categories: biomechanical or functional, accommodative, and pediatric. A biomechanical foot orthotic assists the lower kinetic chain in force attenuation by controlling excessive movement in the foot and ankle. Accommodative orthotics were discussed in Chapter 9. This chapter focuses on the indications, prescription, and techniques for biomechanical orthotics. A brief discussion of pediatric orthotics is also provided.

BIOMECHANICAL ORTHOTICS

The role of the functional, biomechanical orthotic is to control abnormal and potentially harmful movement of the subtalar joint (STJ) and midtarsal joint. Such an orthotic device should meet the following criteria: be comfortable; conform to the contours of the foot; support the STJ as close to its neutral position as is practical, thereby reducing compensations that result in excessive pronation or supination; allow a normal sequence of STJ and midtarsal joint motion during stance; and be adjustable according to the patient's response.

Until recently, there have been few studies demonstrating how orthotics control excessive motion.[19–22] Studies employing motion analysis demonstrated the effectiveness of orthotics on controlling excessive rearfoot and midfoot pronation. The excessive pronation was defined by the measurement of the forefoot varus deformity and the calcaneal valgus position in standing. The forefoot deformity was measured to be 6° or greater, and the standing calcaneal valgus was 3° or greater.[23–27] All the studies using motion analysis on subjects exhibiting excessive pronation displayed a significant reduction in the degree of pronation during the stance phase of gait. McCulloch et al[25] indicated that the reduction in pronation was significant during running and walking. When walking with the orthotic, there was a significant increase in the duration of stance time as measured from heel strike to heel rise.

Johanson et al[23] determined the orthotic prescription by the measurement of the forefoot varus deformity. For example, if the forefoot varus deformity was measured to be 10°, 60% of the 10° was used for the forefoot varus post (6 mm), and 50% of the 10° was used for the rearfoot varus post (5 mm). A maximum of 7° varus post was used in the forefoot and 6° varus post in the rearfoot. The different combinations of forefoot and rearfoot posting demonstrated that the combined forefoot and rearfoot post reduced motion of the calcaneus in the frontal plane the greatest.[23] Eng and Pierrynowski[26] used a maximum of 6° varus post in the forefoot and 4° in the rearfoot. The aforementioned forefoot and rearfoot varus posting reduced the frontal and transverse plane movements of the talocrural/subtalar joint. In addition, the frontal plane motion at the knee during contact and midstance phases of running was also reduced. Relief of pain and the ability to return to previous levels of activity are major factors in determining success with orthotic therapy.[28]

There is no evidence to indicate that the use of foot orthotics can structurally change a flatfoot deformity in adults; however, Bordelon,[29] Mereday et al,[30] and Bleck and Berzins[31] demonstrated roentgenographic changes in children treated with foot orthotics. In the pediatric studies, orthotics were used to correct hypermobile flatfoot.

A biomechanical foot orthotic has two important components, a forefoot and a rearfoot post. The post is a wedge on the medial or lateral side of the orthotic designed to support or control movement, primarily in the frontal plane.

Rearfoot Posting

The effect of a rearfoot post on the biomechanics of the STJ and midtarsal joint is not fully understood. A varus post (medial wedge) is thought to limit or control eversion of the calcaneus and internal rotation of the tibia directly after heel strike.[9] Smith et al[6] and Johanson et al[23] reported that semirigid orthotics reduced the amount and rate of calcaneal eversion during running. The results of studies relating orthotic use to rearfoot movement are conflicting. Johanson et al,[23] Nigg et al,[32] Cavanagh,[33] and Clarke et al,[34] have shown that rearfoot varus posts significantly decrease maximum eversion, whereas Bates et al[35] found no change in maximum eversion. Brown et al[24] reported that both prescription orthotics and "off the shelf" shoe inserts decreased maximum eversion, but there was no significant difference between the two. Taunton et al[36] reported significant decreases in total eversion during the support phase of running, but no changes in tibial rotation were found.

Root et al[37] believe that rearfoot posting should position the STJ in the neutral position and that a minimum of 4° normal pronation is necessary immediately after heel strike to allow shock absorption and transverse plane rotation of the lower extremity. Therefore, an orthotic rearfoot post should control but not eliminate motion from heel strike to foot flat.

In the authors' experience, it is often not possible to reposition the STJ fully to neutral. Extreme excessive pronation, sometimes associated with a forefoot varus of as much as 20°, would require corresponding degrees of posting, which would not fit comfortably in shoes. Even though the STJ may be pronated 10° to 15° early in stance, the maximum tolerable corrective rearfoot post is 5° or 6°. How much posting can be comfortably used depends on a thorough evaluation and, where possible, the patient's response to a trial of temporary posting.

Forefoot Posting

There is even less understanding of how forefoot posts affect the biomechanics of the midfoot and rearfoot. Shaw[38] believes the purpose of a forefoot post is to act as a crutch. The crutch holds the abnormal forefoot in a normal or near-normal relationship to the rearfoot and the supporting surface (Fig. 10–1). The forefoot posts are prescribed for one of two deformities: Forefoot varus is supported with a medial wedge, with a forefoot valgus using a lateral post.

Supporting the forefoot abnormalities reduces the need for rearfoot compensation. For example, as previously described in Chapter 2, forefoot varus is compensated for by rearfoot STJ pronation. Forefoot varus, by itself, is not destructive to the foot. At the STJ, however, compensatory pronation results in an "unlocking" of the foot, creating hypermobility and loss of a rigid lever from midstance through push-off. This abnormal pronation of the STJ allows the inverted (varus) forefoot to contact the ground for weight bearing, but the amount of pronation is excessive, and the resultant hypermobility can be destructive to the foot and to the rest of the lower kinetic chain during propulsion.

Forefoot posting reduces the need for compensatory STJ pronation by bringing the ground surface up to the weight-bearing aspects of the metatarsal heads (Fig. 10–2). The STJ does not have to pronate as much to allow the medial aspect of the foot to contact the ground. Full correction of the forefoot abnormality is not always necessary. A review of 80 patient charts indicated that the average forefoot varus post corrected 62% of the abnormality. For example, the average forefoot varus abnormality was 8.5°, so the average forefoot varus post corrected 62% of the 8.5°, or a 5° forefoot varus post was prescribed. If forefoot varus was 10°, a 6° forefoot post was used. Conversely, with forefoot varus abnormalities of 6° or less, the forefoot post corrected 90% to 100% of the abnormality. The size of the forefoot post is limited by the tolerance of the patient and the constraints of the shoe.

Summary of Posting Principles

The rearfoot post is designed to alter the position of the STJ from heel strike to footflat. If the calcaneus is excessively everted at heel strike, the STJ is in excessive pronation. A rearfoot varus post inverts the calcaneus closer to its neutral position to allow the STJ to pronate normally from heel strike to footflat. Conversely, if the calcaneus and the subtalar joint are excessively inverted and supinated at heel strike, a

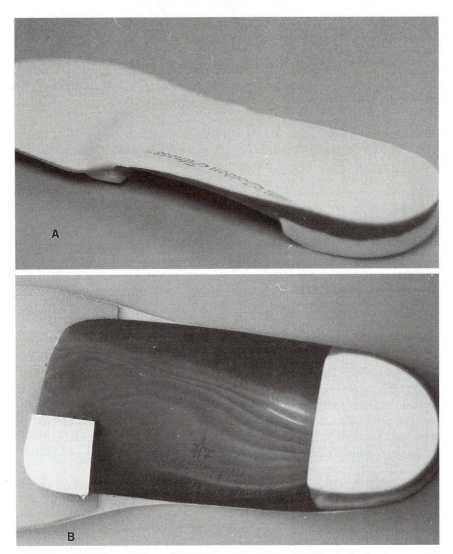

FIGURE 10–1. (*A*) Plastic laboratory-fabricated orthotic. (*B*) Extrinsic forefoot and rearfoot posts added.

rearfoot valgus (lateral) post everts the STJ closer to its neutral position. The rearfoot post must be dynamic; that is, it must control but not eliminate STJ movement. The maximum amount of rearfoot posting is usually 5° to 6°. Any more posting may cause the heel to ride up and out of the shoe.

The forefoot post supports the forefoot deformity by bringing the ground closer to the metatarsals, thereby reducing the need for rearfoot compensation. The forefoot post is indicated when the forefoot deformity is creating problems during the propulsive phase of stance. Generally the maximum forefoot post that fits comfortably in a shoe is 6° to 8°.

In painful foot lesions, particularly those involving the metatarsal heads, posting is often not tolerated; softer materials, metatarsal pads, or relief cut-outs may have to

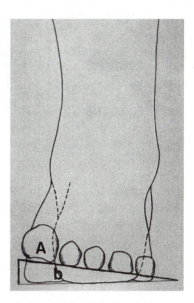

FIGURE 10–2. Forefoot post. (*A*) First metatarsal head. (*B*) Forefoot varus (medial) post.

be substituted. Posting is contraindicated in the insensitive foot, in which excessive forces on plantar structures are not perceived by the patient. These forces can create lesions with resultant serious complications.

Heel Lifts

Forefoot and rearfoot posts are frontal plane corrections, whereas a heel lift (or heel platform) is a sagittal plane correction for ankle joint equinus. Whether the limitation in ankle joint dorsiflexion is caused by bony, soft tissue or postural factors, the STJ often compensates for this limitation by pronating excessively, especially from heel rise through push-off. Adding a heel lift to the orthotic reduces the need for compensatory pronation. The maximum amount tolerated comfortably is 5 to 6 mm.

In-Office Orthotic Fabrication

Several systems exist to allow for the fabrication of foot orthotics in the clinician's office. The advantages to these systems are (1) the orthotic is ready for the patient to use immediately, and (2) the orthotic can be adjusted by the clinician without having to return it to a laboratory. Keeping in mind the requirements for a functional orthotic already listed, several factors should be considered when purchasing an in-house system. The clinician should be able to individualize the orthotics with a wide variety of sizes, rigidities, and densities and should be able to post forefoot and rearfoot, first temporarily as patient response is gauged, then permanently with effective bonding.

In the authors' experience, the Biothotic system (Orthofeet, Inc., Hillsdale, NJ). In addition to posting, the Biothotic allows for the application of heel lifts and metatarsal, scaphoid, and arch pads. Relief cut-outs can be incorporated into the orthotic, and a variety of top covers can be used.

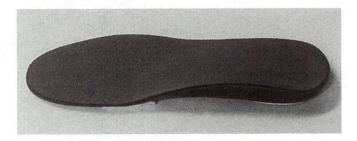

FIGURE 10–3. Full length biothotic.

Figures 10–3 through 10–9 illustrate some of steps in fabricating the Biothotic. The case studies presented later in this chapter give examples of how to determine appropriate posting.

Laboratory Orthotics

Most patients with biomechanical or accommodative problems respond well to the in-office Biothotic. For some, however, a laboratory-fabricated orthotic, made from a cast of the foot, is the treatment of choice. This fact is particularly true for the obese patient or one whose activities demand a more durable, plastic orthotic. Children with hypermobile feet also require casting for a more rigid plastic device. These orthotics can be made from casts or impressions taken in non–weight-bearing, semi–weight-bearing, or full weight-bearing positions, often without benefit of measurements or posting prescriptions. Because the clinician's evaluation is concerned with determining compensations that result in deviations from the ideal neutral posi-

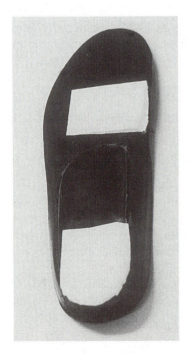

FIGURE 10–4. Forefoot and rearfoot varus posts added to plantar aspect of orthotic.

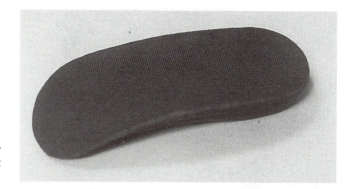

FIGURE 10–5. Three-quarter length orthotic, trimmed to fit dress shoes.

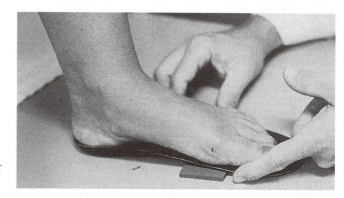

FIGURE 10–6. Placement of forefoot varus post.

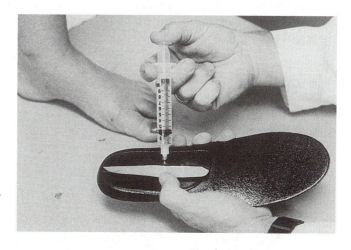

FIGURE 10–7. Activation of biothotic by injecting water into arch cell.

tion, the most biomechanically sound method is to cast the foot in a non–weight-bearing position, with the STJ held in neutral. This position captures the position of the forefoot before compensation and allows the clinician to request from the laboratory the required amount of posting and lifting that reduces the amount of compensation needed. Figures 10–10 through 10–13 demonstrate the neutral casting procedure with the patient in the prone non–weight-bearing position.

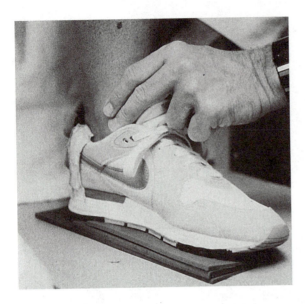

FIGURE 10–8. Patient stands on medial wedges to maintain subtalar neutral as orthotic forms in shoe.

Figure 10–14 shows a generic prescription form that lists the most important information required by orthotics laboratories. The case studies presented later in the chapter give examples of how to complete the form.

PEDIATRIC FOOT ORTHOTICS

Treatment of hypermobile flatfoot in children remains controversial. A review of the literature reveals conflicting opinions, ranging from no treatment to treatment by rigid foot orthotic devices.[38–50]

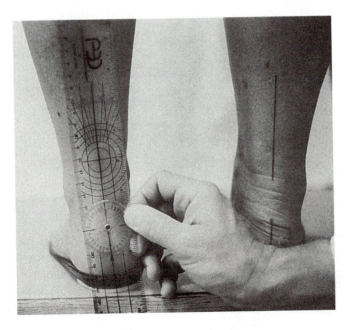

FIGURE 10–9. Finished orthotic; subtalar joint is now nearly neutral.

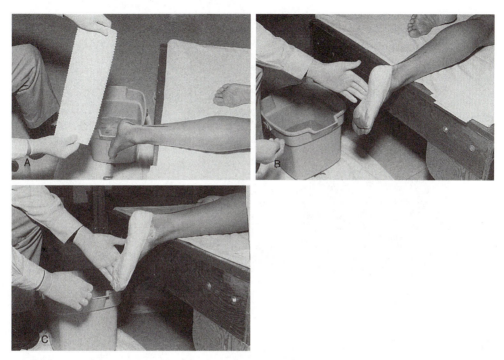

FIGURE 10–10. (A) Two double-thickness, extra fast setting plaster splints, measuring 5 inches by 30 inches are used. (B) The first splints are placed posteriorly from the heel. (C) The second splint is placed anteriorly from the toes.

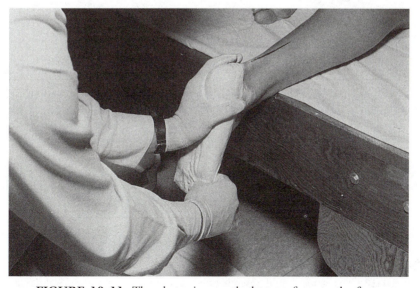

FIGURE 10–11. The plaster is smoothed to conform to the foot.

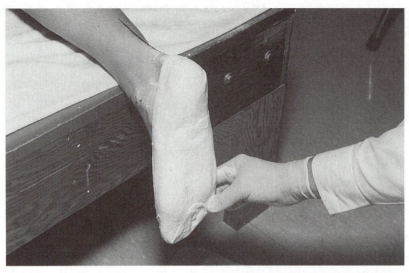

FIGURE 10–12. As the plaster sets, the subtalar joint is held in neutral by gently distracting downward on the fifth toe. Note: To avoid misshaping the cast, do not grasp the metatarsals.

Research

There has been an increase in data concerning the conservative care of hypermobile flatfoot in children. Penneau[45] evaluated ten children radiographically. The radiographs were taken with the patient barefoot and wearing a Thomas heel, over-the-counter inserts, and two molded plastic orthotics called University of California Biomechanical Laboratory (UCBL) devices. No significant radiographic changes in

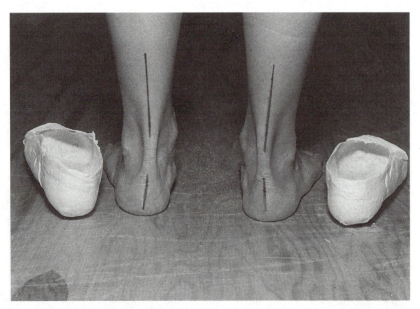

FIGURE 10–13. The casts should resemble the deformity—in this case, calcaneus valgus or pronation.

LABORATORY ORTHOTIC PRESCRIPTION

Therapist Info: **Patient Info:**

    Name _____   Name _____

    Address _____   Address _____

                                              Occupation/Activity _____

                                            Age _____ Height _____ Weight _____

Orthotic Type: Shoe Size _____ Sex _____

    _____ Rohadur

    _____ Sports

    _____ Semi-rigid

    _____ Accommodative

    _____ Children (gait plate, Roberts Whitman, etc.)

Posting Instructions

    Forefoot: _____ Extrinsic   _____ Intrinsic

       Left   _____ °varus   _____ °valgus

       Right   _____ °varus   _____ °valgus

    Rearfoot:

       Left   _____ °varus   _____ °valgus

       Right   _____ °varus   _____ °valgus

    Heel Lift:

       Left   _____ inch

       Right   _____ inch

Covers/extensions:

    _____ Spenco

    _____ Leather

    _____ PPT

    _____ Vinyl

Special Instructions:

FIGURE 10–14. A generic prescription form for casted orthotics. Format will vary depending on the laboratory used.

these children's feet were seen with the use of any of these foot orthotics. Bleck and Berzins[31] reported on 71 children, mean age 4.7 years, who used the Helfet heel seat and the UCBL device. They found the rate of improvement, measured by radiographs, was approximately 1° for every 2 months of wear. The mean duration of orthotic use was 14.5 months. Mereday et al[30] studied the effects of the UCBL device on ten children for 2 years. The children's ages ranged from 3 to 12 years. Results indicated relief from pain and improvement in gait while wearing the orthotics. There was no indication, however, that structural changes resulted from the use of the inserts. Finally, Bordelon[29] treated 50 children from 3 to 9 years of age with a custom-molded insert. The results of Bordelon's study indicated that bony deformities could be corrected by 80% with the initial fitting. The correction of bone alignment averaged 5° per year. Radiographs were taken initially and after each child had worn the orthotics for 3 years. Six children were evaluated after removal of the orthotics. The radiographs demonstrated that only one child showed significant loss of correction. The average time out of the orthotics was 25 months.

Kirby[46] demonstrated a new method of foot orthosis modification that enhances the control of rearfoot pronation. The medial heel skive technique involves selectively removing small amounts of the medial segment of the plantar heel of the positive cast of the foot to create a varus wedging effect within the heel cup of the foot orthosis. The varus wedge results in an increased supination moment across the STJ axis of the foot. Clinically the varus wedge enhances the pronation control on pediatric flexible flatfeet and other types of excessively pronated feet.[46] Schoenhaus[47] reported an orthotic device, used to prevent hyperpronation of the foot, that incorporates a deep heel seat to cup the calcaneus.

Aharonson et al[48] described a foot-ground pressure pattern of flexible flatfeet in boys and girls, aged 4 to 6 years. Standing at ease, the children exerted most of their ground pressure through the posterior weight-bearing area. The remaining ground forces were distributed between the middle and anterior segments of the foot. The middle area exerted as much as 30% of the total foot-ground pressure in extreme cases of flexible flatfeet. Correcting the valgus inclination of the calcaneus to neutral by inserting a medial leather wedge to the heel restored the longitudinal arch and the normal distribution of the foot-ground pressure of the standing child.[48]

Wenger et al[49] performed a prospective study to determine the effectiveness of corrective shoes or inserts on flexible flatfoot in children. A total of 129 children diagnosed with flexible flatfeet using radiographic findings were randomly assigned to one of four groups: group I, controls; group II, treatment with corrective orthopedic shoes; group III, treatment with Helfet heel-cup; or group IV, treatment with a custom-molded plastic insert. Ninety-eight patients completed the 3-year study. Analysis of radiographs before and after treatment demonstrated a significant improvement in all groups ($P < 0.01$), including the controls. The conclusion was that wearing corrective shoes or inserts for 3 years does not influence the course of flexible flatfeet in children.[49]

Gould et al[50] monitored the development of the longitudinal arch of the foot and determined the influence of arch support footwear on the development of a neutral arch in toddlers 11 to 14 months of age until 5 years. A total of 125 beginner walkers were obtained during a period of 1.5 years and divided into four groups wearing different footwear. After 4 years, the group was evaluated by physical examination, radiograph films, and pedotopography. At the initial examination, all the toddlers demonstrated pes planus by all the above-mentioned measurements. The results of the study indicated that the longitudinal arch developed regardless of the footwear worn. The group wearing the arch support footwear, however, manifested a more rapid development of the longitudinal arch during the first 2 years and continued until 5 years of age.

Orthotic Devices

The feet of children are malleable and can be easily molded to most orthotics. The pediatric orthotic attempts to alleviate structural deformities that may lead to abnormal compensations in the foot and protects the foot during its growth period.

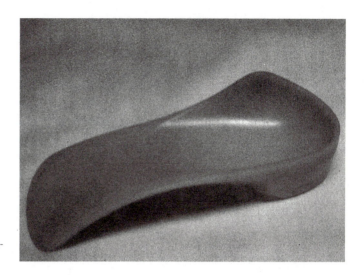

FIGURE 10–15. Whitman-Roberts foot orthotics.

Several types of pediatric foot orthotics are made from rigid (fiberglass and Rohadur) or flexible (Plastizote, rubber, sponge) materials. Polypropylene, cork, and leather are intermediary materials that are neither rigid nor flexible. Orthotics commonly used for children include Whitman-Roberts orthotic, Shaffer plates, heel stabilizers, out-toe gait plates, and functional posted orthotics.[17]

The Whitman-Roberts orthotic (Fig. 10–15) is a combination of the Roberts and the Whitman orthotics. This orthotic controls or maintains a rectus heel and stimulates supination. A high medial flange is used to limit medial rotation of the talus, and a high lateral flange controls calcaneal eversion. The Whitman-Roberts device is useful in children over 9 years of age.[17]

The Shaffer plate orthotic (Fig. 10–16) has a medial flange to support the foot and is used in older children or adolescents. The Shaffer plate does not control excessive

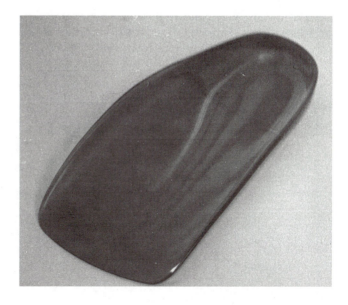

FIGURE 10–16. Shaffer plate.

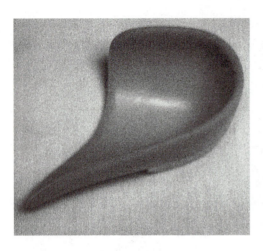

FIGURE 10–17. Type A heel stabilizer (top view).

calcaneal eversion and should not be used in severe structural collapse of the pediatric foot.

Heel stabilizers can be tolerated until 8 to 10 years of age. The heel stabilizers control the foot better than any other form of orthotic device. A type A heel stabilizer (Fig. 10–17) limits inversion and eversion of the calcaneus by confining the heel. There is no control of the forefoot and minimal arch support. Types A and C are designed to control the heel and midfoot maximally. Type A is used for a mild to moderately pronated foot. The medial and lateral flanges are used to support and control the rearfoot, midfoot, and forefoot. Type C differs from type B in that the medial and lateral flange extend to the first and fifth metatarsophalangeal joints.

The type D heel stabilizer (Fig. 10–18) promotes abduction of the forefoot. The lateral plantar flange extends beyond the fourth and fifth metatarsophalangeal joints to limit dorsiflexion of these joints. Therefore, the foot must roll inward, allowing dorsiflexion at the three medial metatarsophalangeal joints. The result is abduction of the forefoot, reducing a toe-in gait.

The out-toe gait plate (Fig. 10–19) functions like the type D heel stabilizer. The out-toe plate is most frequently used in children who demonstrate an in-out toe deformity and who are older than 8 to 10 years.

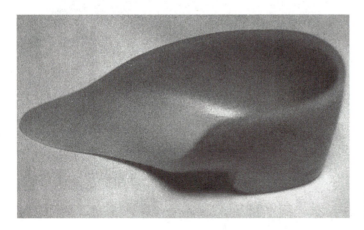

FIGURE 10–18. Type D heel stabilizer.

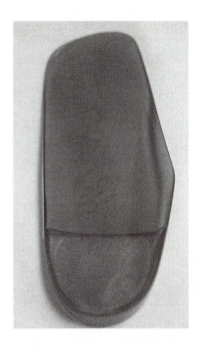

FIGURE 10–19. Out-toe gait plate (top view).

Functional type orthotics (Fig. 10–20) should be used for older children or adolescents. This orthotic does not confine the young foot sufficiently to reduce medial and lateral instabilities. Furthermore, it may be detrimental, forcing the child's foot into a posted varus or valgus position. A rectus position of the forefoot occurs when the metatarsal heads are parallel to the horizontal plane. The rectus position of the forefoot is more desirable in attempting to correct varus and valgus deformities. Rearfoot posting is more common in pediatric orthotics to position the STJ in neutral.

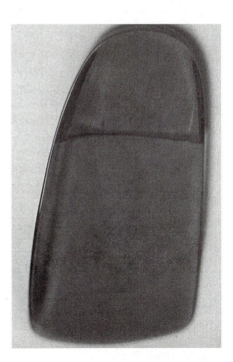

FIGURE 10–20. Functional orthotic with an intrinsic forefoot post and an extrinsic rearfoot post. Rodahur translucent plastic material (top view).

Summary of Pediatric Orthotic Principles

The pediatric orthotic is prescribed to control excessive rearfoot movement in the stance phase of gait. Rigid materials are more commonly used to control movement. A medial flange and a lateral flange may be prescribed in severe hypermobile flatfoot deformities.

Studies indicate that the use of a medial rearfoot wedge in the pediatric patient is effective in reducing excessive foot pronation, increasing rate of medial longitudinal arch development, and improving distribution of weight-bearing force to the foot.[46-50]

CASE STUDIES

This section reviews cases requiring orthotic prescription in the adult and pediatric patient.

1: Congenital Flatfoot with a Diagnosis of Talipes Calcanel Valgus

A 5-year-old patient reported medial arch pain on impact of jumping. Radiographic evaluation demonstrated a vertical talus and a decreased inclination angle of the calcaneus.

On physical evaluation, ligament laxity of several joints in the lower extremities was observed. The range of motion of the STJ was 35° inversion and 15° eversion. Dorsiflexion of the ankle bilaterally was measured in the non–weight-bearing position at 20°. In the standing position, the calcaneus was noted to be in excessive eversion. During ambulation, when excessive weight-bearing occurred along the medial aspect of the foot, excessive rearfoot mobility and abnormality in the weight-bearing position were noted. Figure 10–21 lists the findings of the static evaluation.

Maximum control of the rearfoot is necessary to allow the STJ to function from its neutral position. If the rearfoot is stabilized, forefoot and midfoot breakdown can be avoided. The orthotic affording the most control and support to the rearfoot, midfoot, and forefoot is the type C heel stabilizer.

This patient should be reevaluated every 6 months, to determine growth and structural changes. A possible progression of foot orthotics may occur over the next 8 to 10 years, ranging from the heel stabilizer (maximum control), to the Whitman-Roberts (moderate control), and, finally, the Shaffer plate (minimal calcaneal eversion control).

2: Plantar Fasciitis of the Right Heel and a Neuroma of the Left Forefoot, Secondary to Late Pronation During Push-off

A 42-year-old man complained of right medial heel pain that was worst in the morning during the step taken after arising. The patient is an intense runner, averaging 60 to 70 miles per week. When running at the end of the day, the first 2 to 3 miles were always very painful. There was no history of knee or foot pain.

EVALUATION WORKSHEET

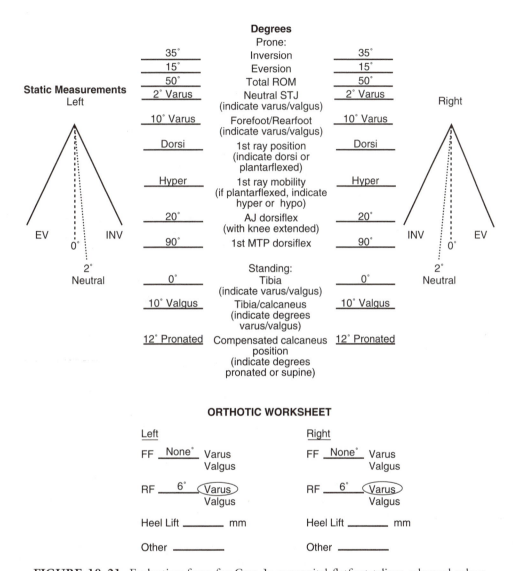

FIGURE 10–21. Evaluation form for Case 1: congenital flatfoot talipes calcaneal valgus.

Evaluation revealed a normal medial arch in the weight-bearing position, with the right foot abducted secondary to external rotation of the lower limb. No toe deformities were noted. Figure 10–22 lists the findings of the initial static evaluation. In the non–weight-bearing position, with the rearfoot in neutral position, a forefoot varus of 6° was noted with a hypermobile first ray. Range of motion of the calcaneus was 10° of eversion and 20° of inversion. The left foot showed a rectus forefoot (perpendicular to the rearfoot): No varus or valgus was noted. The calcaneus range of motion was the same as on the right. Radiographic evaluation revealed a heel spur on the right calcaneal area at the inser-

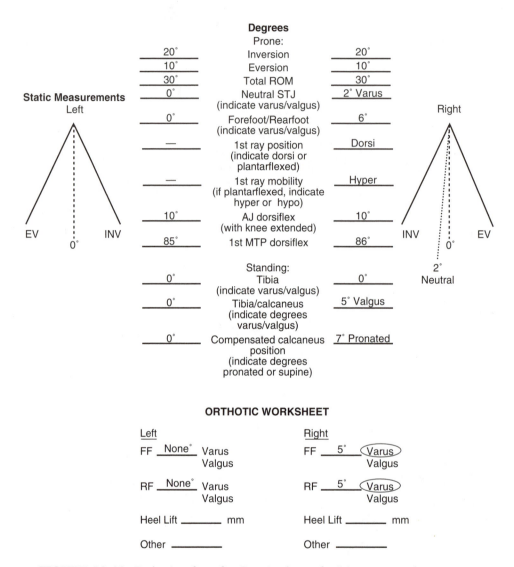

FIGURE 10–22. Evaluation form for Case 2: plantar fasciitis, neuroma, late pronator.

tion of the plantar fasciae. Palpation of the medial aspect of the calcaneus was tender.

Gait Assessment

An instability of the right foot was observed during push-off. The instability was seen at push-off because the patient showed a heel whip at that time. The unstable first ray caused overstretching of the plantar fascia. The right foot abducted during push-off to avoid dorsiflexion of the first metatarsophalangeal joint and overstretching of the plantar fascia.

An orthotic with a forefoot post of 5° on the right and a 5° rearfoot post was prescribed. The left orthotic was not posted because deformities were not present. The patient ran for 1.5 years without pain, during which time he set a new personal record that was 5 minutes faster than his previous marathon races.

After 1.5 years the patient returned, complaining of left heel pain and numbness in the lateral border of the right foot. In addition, a neuroma was present between the second and third metatarsals, and it reproduced paresthesia between the second and third toe web spaces when palpated. A forefoot varus on the left and 9° of forefoot varus on the right were measured when the patient was evaluated. Hypermobility of the first ray was noted on the right. The medial border of the left heel was also tender and painful when palpated.

The patient had obviously overextended himself during the previous 18 months. The increased running velocity produced excessive forces on the forefoot, causing further breakdown. The semirigid orthotics were unable to assist the foot in attenuation of the increased forces for longer than 18 months. The neuroma developed because of the increased shear forces between the metatarsals.

A new pair of orthotics was fabricated with a forefoot varus post of 7° on the right and 5° on the left. A rearfoot varus post of 6° was prescribed bilaterally, with 4° of motion. After running for 2 weeks with the new pair of orthotics, numbness and paresthesia were completely relieved on the right and 50% of the left foot heel pain was relieved.

3: Plantar Fasciitis and Heel Pain

A 38-year-old laboratory technician and part-time graduate student had experienced several months of right Achilles tendon pain as well as pain on the plantar aspect of the right heel. Pain had developed insidiously as the patient became more active at work and school. The patient was diagnosed as having Achilles tendinitis and plantar fasciitis. A series of ultrasound treatments, injections, and oral anti-inflammatory medication had been given, without success.

Assessment revealed moderate tenderness of the Achilles tendon just above its insertion into the calcaneus. Tenderness of the plantar fascia at its origin on the calcaneus was noted. Figure 10–23 shows the static evaluation measurements of the foot and ankle.

On gait analysis, abnormal supination throughout the stance phase of gait was observed. There was no evidence of STJ or midtarsal joint pronation from heel strike to footflat; the foot remained supinated through push-off.

These findings indicated probable loss of shock absorption because of the abnormal supination. Temporary posting with 4° forefoot valgus posts was constructed. Additionally, heel lifts of about 5 mm were added, to take some tension off the Achilles tendon. A 2° rearfoot valgus post was added to help promote normal pronation from heel strike to footflat.

The patient's response to the temporary posting was excellent: She reported better than 75% reduction of pain while using the orthotics. Therefore the posts were glued permanently to the Biothotics. In addition to promoting normal pronation, the orthotics provided cushioning at heel strike. At the 1-month follow-up visit, the patient reported continued relief of symptoms and was advised to continue using the orthotics indefinitely.

EVALUATION WORKSHEET

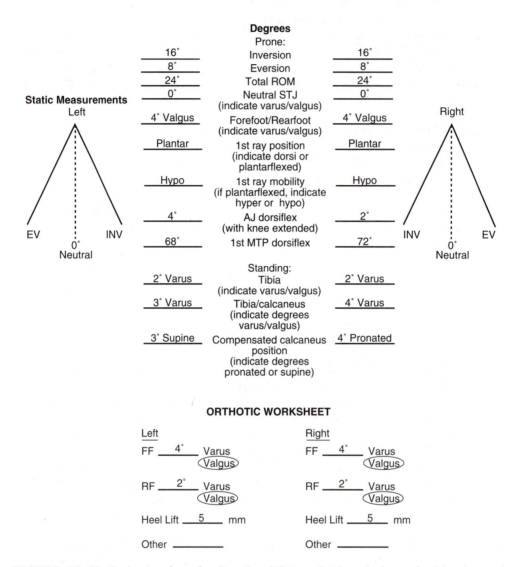

Degrees

Static Measurements Left		Prone:	Right	
16°		Inversion	16°	
8°		Eversion	8°	
24°		Total ROM	24°	
0°		Neutral STJ (indicate varus/valgus)	0°	
4° Valgus		Forefoot/Rearfoot (indicate varus/valgus)	4° Valgus	
Plantar		1st ray position (indicate dorsi or plantarflexed)	Plantar	
Hypo		1st ray mobility (if plantarflexed, indicate hyper or hypo)	Hypo	
4°		AJ dorsiflex (with knee extended)	2°	
68°		1st MTP dorsiflex	72°	

Standing:

2° Varus	Tibia (indicate varus/valgus)	2° Varus
3° Varus	Tibia/calcaneus (indicate degrees varus/valgus)	4° Varus
3° Supine	Compensated calcaneus position (indicate degrees pronated or supine)	4° Pronated

ORTHOTIC WORKSHEET

Left		Right	
FF __4°__ Varus ~~(Valgus)~~		FF __4°__ Varus ~~(Valgus)~~	
RF __2°__ Varus ~~(Valgus)~~		RF __2°__ Varus ~~(Valgus)~~	
Heel Lift __5__ mm		Heel Lift __5__ mm	
Other _____		Other _____	

FIGURE 10–23. Evaluation form for Case 3: achilles tendinitis and plantar fasciitis; abnormal supination.

4: Medial Knee Pain Associated with Jogging and Leg Length Discrepancy

A 30-year-old recreation therapist presented with a 3-month history of right medial knee pain associated with jogging. The patient denied any direct injury, stating that pain developed after she increased her jogging mileage from 15 miles to about 25 miles per week. The pain did not respond to several weeks of rest and anti-inflammatory medications. Examination by an orthopedic surgeon revealed no evidence of ligament or cartilage injury. An isokinetic evaluation

EVALUATION WORKSHEET

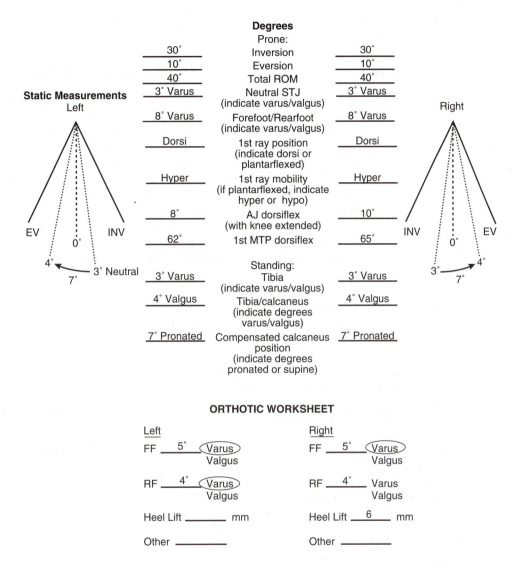

FIGURE 10–24. Evaluation form for Case 4: right medial knee pain, leg length discrepancy.

done previously indicated normal quadriceps and hamstring muscle strength. Figure 10–24 lists the findings of the biomechanical foot evaluation.

Gait analysis revealed no significant problems from heel strike to footflat, where pronation appeared to be normal; however, at push-off, the calcaneus remained in an everted position, indicating inability to resupinate. In addition to these findings, the patient was found to have a ⅜ of an inch shortening of the right lower extremity.

Based on these findings, Biothotic orthotic devices with 4° forefoot varus posts were constructed. Additionally, a 6-mm heel lift was added to the right orthotic. Over the next 2 weeks, the patient experienced gradual reduction in right-sided knee pain as she resumed her jogging. Over several weeks, the patient reported total absence of pain despite increasing her mileage to 25 miles per week.

5: Bilateral Knee Pain Associated with Running and Bicycling

A 29-year-old sales representative complained of bilateral knee pain that had persisted for several weeks and was associated with running. The patient was a triathlete who had recently increased his running mileage to about 35 miles per week, in addition to bicycling and swimming on a daily basis. He reported no history of knee pain. He stated that pain was greater on the left than on the right, but that both knees began to hurt after running 2 to 2.5 miles. The results of a thorough knee examination by an orthopedist were negative. Findings of the static evaluation are listed in Figure 10–25.

Gait analysis revealed signs of pronation throughout the entire stance phase. From heel strike to footflat, each calcaneus was at, or near, end-range pronation. Therefore, there was no normal pronation available from heel strike to footflat. Additionally, there was no resupination through push-off. The calcaneus remained everted, the naviculars were dropped downward and in toward the midline, and there was a sudden abduction of the foot at push-off. These findings indicated early, excessive pronation throughout the stance phase, probably secondary to forefoot varus and ankle joint equinus. Temporary orthotics were constructed. Forefoot varus posts of 6°, rearfoot varus posts of 4°, and heel lift of ¼ inch were added to each orthotic. The orthotics were designed to assist the STJ of each foot at heel strike by reducing some of the excessive pronation, thus allowing the STJ to pronate normally from heel strike to footflat. The forefoot posts were designed to assist with resupination at push-off by adding support to the first ray.

Over the next 3 weeks, the patient was able to gradually resume his normal running mileage. He reported total relief of right knee pain and "significant relief" of the left knee pain. At that time he was casted for rigid sports orthotics with the same prescription that was built into the temporary orthotics.

SUMMARY

Biomechanical orthotics may be useful in reducing the excessive forces of weight bearing for adults. These orthotics are not designed to change or correct foot abnormalities but to reduce pain and improve function of the foot during the stance phase of gait. The biomechanical orthotic has two components, a forefoot post and a rearfoot post. The purpose of the forefoot post is to support the forefoot deformity or bring the ground closer to the heads of the metatarsal bones. If the metatarsal heads are supported during maximum loading of the forefoot, abnormal forces can be reduced or eliminated.

The purpose of the rearfoot post is to position the rearfoot, or STJ, as close as possible to a neutral position. The function of the rearfoot post is most important at heel contact. If the rearfoot is prescribed correctly, it should prevent the STJ from starting

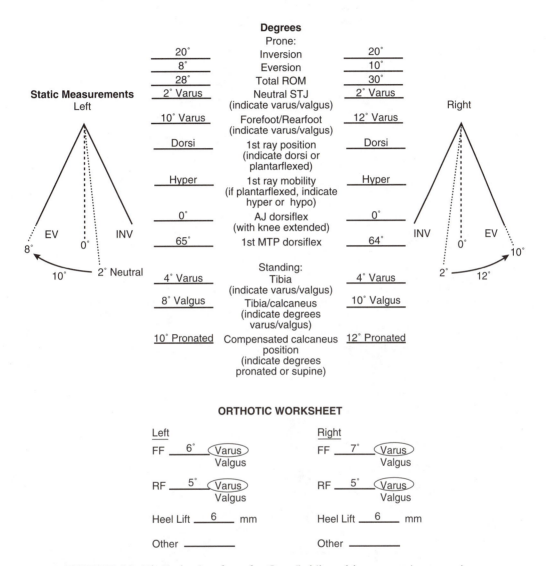

FIGURE 10–25. Evaluation form for Case 5: bilateral knee excessive pronation.

the stance phase in excessive pronation or excessive supination. At the same time, the rearfoot post must allow sufficient movement of the STJ.

A trial period of temporary posting is necessary to determine a more specific orthotic prescription. A more specific prescription means less adjustment time, greater patient satisfaction, more perceptible pain relief, and better patient compliance with the use of the foot orthotics. Table 10–1 summarizes the general characteristics of neutral cast orthotics.

Orthotics are prescribed for children to control excessive rearfoot movement in the stance phase of gait. Rigid materials are most commonly used to control move-

TABLE 10–1 Typical Progression of Orthotic Treatment

	Assessment	Treatment
Initial visit	History	Mold orthotic in subtalar joint neutral
	Static evaluation	Temporary posting
	Gait analysis	1–2 week trial
Second visit	Reevaluate	Adjust temporary posting
	Determine patient response and comfort	Grind, reglue as needed
Third visit	Reevaluate	Permanent posting
Follow-up visits	Reevaluate	Adjust or repost as needed
	Check for fit, comfort	Consider alternative orthotics
	Check for wear	(e.g., for dress shoes)
		Occasionally, cast for laboratory orthotics*
	Children: check for growth every 6–12 months	

*Criteria for casting: Toddlers and small children usually require rigidity (e.g., rohadur); excessive Biothotic wear and tear in <1 year; replacing previous casted orthotics.

ment. A medial flange and a lateral flange may be prescribed for severe hypermobile flatfoot deformities. Posting of the forefoot and rearfoot is discouraged in pediatric foot orthotics.

More research is needed in the area of foot orthotics. Valid and reliable methods are needed to help determine how orthotics alter foot function during the stance phase of gait.

REFERENCES

1. Blake, RL and Denton, JA: Functional foot orthoses for athletic injuries. J Am Podiatr Med Assoc 75:359, 1985.
2. Eggold, JF: Orthotics in the prevention of runners' overuse injuries. Physician Sports Med 9:125, 1981.
3. Rose, GK: Correction of the pronated foot. J Bone Joint Surg [Br] 40:674, 1958.
4. Weed, JG, Ratliff, FD, and Ross, SA: A biplanar grind for rearfoot posts on functional orthotics. J Am Podiatr Med Assoc 69:35, 1978.
5. McKenzie, DC, Clement, DB, and Taunton, JE: Running shoes, orthotics and injuries. Sports Med 2:334, 1985.
6. Smith, LS, Clark, TE, Hamill, CL et al: The effects of soft and semi-rigid orthoses upon rearfoot movement in running. Podiatr Sports Med 76:227, 1986.
7. Doxey, GE: Clinical use and fabrication of molded thermoplastic foot orthotic devices. Phys Ther 65:1679, 1985.
8. D'Ambrosia, RD: Orthotic devices in running injuries. Clin Sports Med 4:611, 1985.
9. Bates, BT, Osternig, LR, Mason, B et al: Foot orthotic devices to modify selected aspects of lower extremity mechanics. Am J Sports Med 7:338, 1979.
10. Subotnik, SI: The abuses of orthotics in sports medicine. Physician Sports Med 3:73, 1979.
11. Murphy, P: Orthoses: Not the sole solution for running ailments. Physician Sports Med 14:164, 1986.
12. Odom, RD and Gastwirth, B: Sand splint orthoses. J Am Podiatr Assoc 72:98, 1982.
13. Niehaus, PL: Sorbothotics: Soft tissue supplement orthotics. J Am Podiatr Assoc 15:46, 1985.
14. Helfand, AE: Basic considerations for shoes, shoe modifications and orthoses in foot care. Clin Podiatry 1:431, 1984.
15. Sperryn, PN and Reston, L: Podiatry and the sports physician—an evaluation of orthoses. Br J Sports Med 17:129, 1983.
16. Nigg, BM and Morlock, M: The influence of lateral heel flare of running shoes on pronation and impact forces. Med Sci Sports Exerc 19:297, 1987.
17. McCrea, JD: Pediatric Orthopaedics of the Lower Extremity. Futura Publishing, New York, 1985, p 317.
18. Subotnik, SI: Foot orthoses: An update. Physician Sports Med 11:103, 1983.

19. Hannaford, DR: Soft orthoses for athletes. J Am Podiatr Med Assoc 76:566, 1986.
20. Subotnik, SI: Foot orthotic control and the overuse syndrome. Arch Podiatr Med Foot Surg 2:207, 1975.
21. Carter, G: Foot orthoses: Simple prescriptions can mean dramatic pain relief. Aust Fam Physician 16:1104, 1987.
22. Scranton, PE, Pedegana, LR, and Whitesel, JP: Gait analysis: Alterations in support phase forces using supportive devices. Am J Sports Med 10:6, 1982.
23. Johanson, MA, Donatelli, RA, Wooden, MJ, et al: Effects of three different posting methods on controlling abnormal subtalar pronation. Phys Ther 74:149–159, 1994.
24. Brown, GP, Donatelli, RA, Catlin, PA, and Wooden, JM: The effect of foot orthoses on rearfoot mechanics. J Orthop Sports Phys Ther 21:258–267, 1995.
25. McCulloch, MU, Brunt, D, and Vander Linden, D: The effect of foot orthotics and gait velocity on lower limb kinematics and temporal events of stance. J Orthop Sports Phys Ther 17:2–10, 1993.
26. Eng, JJ and Pierrynowski, MR: The effect of soft foot orthotics on three-dimensional lower-limb kinematics during walking and running. Phys Ther 74:836–844, 1994.
27. Novick, A and Kelly DL: Position and movement changes of the foot with orthotics intervention during loading response of gait. J Orthop Sports Phys Ther 11:301–312, 1991.
28. Donatelli, RA, Hurlbert, C, Conaway, DJ, and St. Pierre, RK: Biomechanical foot orthotics: A retrospective study. J Orthop Sports Phys Ther 10:205, 1988.
29. Bordelon, LR: Hypermobile flatfoot in children. Clin Orthop 181:7, 1983.
30. Mereday, C, Dolan, CM, and Lusskin, R: Evaluation of the University of California Biomechanics Laboratory shoe insert in "flexible" pes planus. Clin Orthop 82:45, 1972.
31. Bleck, EE and Berzins, UJ: Conservative management of pes valgus with plantarflexed talus, flexible. Clin Orthop 122:85, 1977.
32. Nigg, BM, Eberle, G, Frei, D, et al: Gait Analysis and Sport Shoe Construction. Biomechanics VIA. University Park Press, Baltimore, 1978, p 303.
33. Cavanagh, PR: The Running Shoe Book. World Publications, Mountain View, CA, 1981, pp 83, 259.
34. Clarke, TE, Frederick, EC, and Hamill, D: The effects of shoe design parameters upon rearfoot movement in running. Med Sci Sports 15:376, 1983.
35. Bates, BT, James, SL, and Osternig, LR: Foot function during the support phase of running. Am J Sports Med 7:338, 1979.
36. Taunton, JE, Clement, DB, et al: A triplanar electrogoniometer investigation of running mechanics in runners with compensatory overpronation. Can J Appl Sports Sci 10:104, 1985.
37. Root, ML, Orien, WP, and Weed, JN: Clinical Biomechanics, vol II: Normal and Abnormal Function of the Foot. Clinical Biomechanics Corp., Los Angeles, 1977, pp 26–31.
38. Shaw, AH: The effect of a forefoot post on gait and function. J Am Podiatr Med Assoc 65:238, 1975.
39. Cowell, HR, Drennam, JC, Hensinger, RN, et al: Children's foot problems and corrections. Contemp Orthop 2:526, 1980.
40. Giannestras, NJ: Foot Disorders: Medical and Surgical Management, 2nd ed. Lea & Febiger, Philadelphia, 1973.
41. Helfet, AJ: A new way of treating flatfeet in children. Lancet 1:262, 1956.
42. Jahss, MH: Atlas of Orthotics: Biomechanical Principles and Applications. CV Mosby, St. Louis, 1975.
43. Jahss, MH (ed): Disorders of the Foot, vol I. WB Saunders, Philadelphia, 1982, p 1703.
44. Tachdjian, MO: Pediatric Orthopaedics. WB Saunders, Philadelphia, 1972.
45. Penneau, K: Pes planus: Radiographic changes with foot orthoses and shoes. Foot Ankle 2:299, 1982.
46. Kirby, KA: The medial heel skive technique: Improving pronation control in foot orthoses. J Am Podiatr Med Assoc 82:177–188, 1992.
47. Schoenhaus, HD: Hyperpronation control with a dynamic stabilizing innersole system. J Am Podiatr Med Assoc 82:149–153, 1992.
48. Aharonson, Z, Arcan, M, and Steinback, TV: Foot-ground pressure pattern of flexible flatfoot in children, with and without correction of calcaneovalgus. Clin Orthop 278:177–182, 1992.
49. Wenger, DR, Mauldin, D, Speck, G, and Lieber, RL: Corrective shoes and inserts as treatment for flexible flatfoot in infants and children. J Bone Joint Surg [Am] 71:800–810, 1989.
50. Gould, N, et al: Development of child's arch. Foot Ankle 9:241–245, 1989.

CHAPTER 11

Physical Therapy

Karen E. Davis, MPT, ATC
Jeff Cooper, MS, ATC
John C. Garbalosa, MMSc, PT

In this chapter, selected modalities and manual techniques of the physical therapy treatment for six theoretic case studies are presented to demonstrate the theory and application of the selected therapeutic techniques. The clinical decision-making model serves as the blueprint from which the selection of techniques is guided.[1]

The six case studies include a lateral ligamentous sprain, a bimalleolar fracture, calcaneal pain, and postsurgical status for hallux abductovalgus (HAV) correction, Achilles tendinitis, and Achilles tendon repair. Each case emphasizes a particular physical therapy technique or modality. The format consists of the presentation of evaluative findings, interpretation of these findings, a treatment plan, the patient response to the treatment plan, and some of the possible rationales for both the applied treatment and the observed changes.

The following material should not be taken as a definitive method for handling the problems presented but rather as a guideline for handling these therapeutic problems. Every effort has been made to support the clinical decisions with scientific and empiric evidence.

CASE STUDIES (TYPICAL PATIENT POPULATION)

CASE 1: LATERAL LIGAMENT SPRAIN

The central focus of this section is threefold: reduction of edema, restoration of movement, and prevention of reinjury of the ankle.

Initial Evaluation and Findings

The initial evaluation begins with the patient's history and includes a passive range of motion (ROM) test, manual muscle test (MMT), "figure-eight" girth measurement, palpation, visual inspection, pain assessment, and other specific tests (Table 11–1).

A 30-year-old recreational athlete sustained a plantar flexion, inversion, internal rotation injury to his right ankle while playing basketball. When the injury occurred, the athlete heard a popping noise. Subsequently, rapid edema about the right ankle ensued. A physician was consulted immediately after the injury by the athlete. The physician determined that there was no osseous involvement via roentgenogram. The diagnosis of the physician was moderate sprain of the lateral collateral ligaments of the right ankle.

Pain during movement of the right ankle, swelling of the right ankle, and decreased independence during ambulation were the patient's initial chief complaints. The patient did not have a history of trauma to the right ankle. Using a numeric pain scale of 0 to 10 (with 10 being excruciating pain and 0 being no pain), the athlete reported a pain level of 9. Figure 11–1 is the athlete's pain drawing. The drawing includes the plantar, anterior, and lateral aspects of the right ankle and foot as the symptomatic areas.

Visual inspection by the physical therapist of the athlete's lower extremities showed them to be remarkable for severe edema about the right ankle and forefoot. Ecchymosis was also present just distal to the lateral malleolus.

A severe restriction of active and passive ROM of the right ankle was present. Both passive and active movements reproduced the patient's pain. Passive ROM of the right ankle was 5° of dorsiflexion, 10° of plantar flexion, 5° of inversion, and 5° of eversion. The MMT of the lower leg musculature was within normal limits (WNL). Resisted eversion and plantar flexion reproduced the patient's pain symptoms, and he was unable to perform a standing toe raise with the affected limb.

Palpation of the right ankle and foot was markedly tender over the fibular attachment site of the anterior talofibular and calcaneofibular ligaments. An increase in the tissue temperature was evident over the lateral aspect of the right ankle joint.

TABLE 11–1 Case 1: Summary of Initial Evaluation and Weekly Progress

| | Passive Motion | | | | Girth | |
Week	Dorsiflexion	Plantar Flexion	Inversion	Eversion	Measurement (mm)	Pain Level*
Initial evaluation	5	10	5	5	66	9
1	5	20	5	5	61	7
2	10	25	10	10	58	0–1
3	10	25	10	10	55	0–1
4	15	47	23	10	55	0

*On a scale of 0 (no pain) to 10 (excruciating pain).

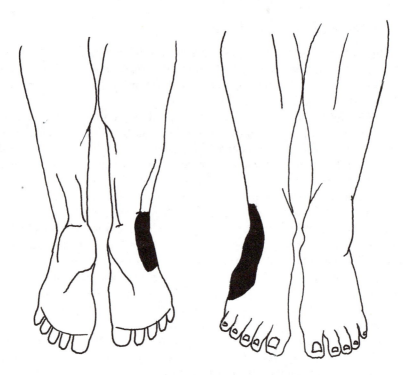

FIGURE 11–1. Pain drawing of patient in case 1.

Ligamentous stress testing of the right ankle joint did not demonstrate any increase in mobility when compared with the unaffected joint. Two ligamentous stress tests, the anterior drawer test (Fig. 11–2) and the calcaneal inversion test (Fig. 11–3), reproduced the pain complaints.[2] The figure-eight girth measurement about the malleoli, navicular tuberosity, and styloid process of the fifth metatarsal of the right ankle was 66 mm.

Interpretation

The evaluative findings confirmed that the lateral collateral ligaments of the right ankle—specifically the anterior talofibular and calcaneofibular ligaments—were involved. The tests of palpation, ligament stress, passive ROM, and MMT confirmed the involvement of those ligaments. Theoretically, these tests isolated the anterior talofibular and calcaneofibular ligaments.[2–4] The patient's history further supported the evaluative findings because the reported mechanism of injury is often associated with damage to the two involved ligaments.[2–5]

Treatment

The primary goals of treatment are to reduce edema and improve mobility while preventing further damage to the ankle. Given these goals, treatment initially consists of anti-inflammatory modalities. Anti-inflammatory treatments are indicated because of the presence of an active inflammatory and repair process, as evidenced by an increase in the tissue temperature and edema of the right

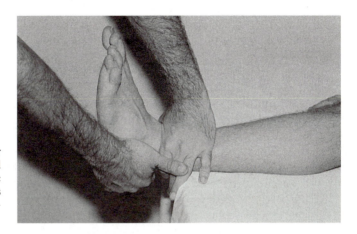

FIGURE 11–2. Anterior drawer test, case 1: Tibia and fibula are stabilized with one hand, while other hand grasps and forces the calcaneus anteriorly.

ankle.[2–4] Mobilizing the involved ankle joint prevents the deleterious effects of immobilization.[3,4,6]

Week 1

Treatment Plan. The first week of physical therapy consisted of treatments three times per week for cryotherapy in combination with electrotherapy, active joint mobilization exercises, and a home exercise program. During the first week, the patient was allowed to walk with axillary crutches bearing partial weight on the right ankle.

A typical treatment session during the first week began with placing the right lower extremity in an elevated position, packing the ankle and forefoot in ice, and applying high-voltage electrical stimulation (HVS) for 20 minutes. The HVS electrode pads were placed over each malleoli with the pulse rate set at 80 beats per second at an intensity of 150 volts and a negative polarity. After the cryotherapy treatment, the patient performed 45 repetitions of active plantar flexion—dorsiflexion exercises against manual resistance, as tolerated. Next, a 10-minute light effleurage massage was applied in a caudocephalad direction,

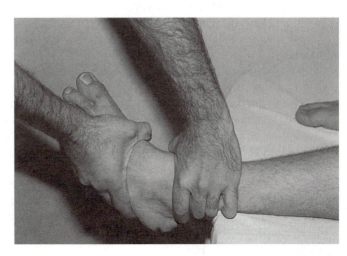

FIGURE 11–3. Inversion stress test, case 1: Tibia and fibula are stabilized with one hand, while other hand grasps and forces the calcaneus into inversion.

with the leg elevated. Treatment sessions ended with another 20-minute HVS and ice treatment. A compressive elastic stocking was applied to the foot and ankle at the end of the treatment session. The athlete was instructed to wear this at all times except during home exercise and icing sessions.

At home, the athlete iced the ankle and forefoot four times per day for 10 to 15 minutes, before and after performing his home exercises, and maintained the right lower extremity in an elevated position when not ambulating. The home exercise program consisted of active dorsiflexion and plantar flexion of the right ankle without resistance for 45 repetitions, two times per day, icing throughout the day. This was in addition to the hourly intermittent icing throughout the day. When ambulating, a heel-to-toe partial weight-bearing (PWB) gait pattern was used, and an air splint was worn. A compressive elastic sleeve was applied to be worn at all times except when exercising and icing. At night, the lower extremity was elevated by placing pillows beneath the foot on the mattress.

Treatment Results. At the end of the week, the passive ROM of the right ankle was 20° of plantar flexion with no changes in eversion, inversion, or dorsiflexion ROM. Ankle girth measurement was 61 mm, reduced by 5 mm. The patient's subjective pain level was 7. Palpation still revealed an increase in the tissue temperature about the lateral aspect of the right ankle.

Treatment Rationale. HVS and ice applied with the lower extremity elevated were chosen for the effects of HVS, cold, and elevation on blood flow. Cold is theorized to decrease vasodilator metabolism, encourage vasoconstriction, and increase blood viscosity.[2,7–10] Preliminary studies on the therapeutic effects of HVS are mixed.[11–14] There is some evidence in the literature that HVS alters hemodynamics.[11,12]

Reed,[12] in his animal experiment, concluded that HVS decreased the protein leakage from blood vessels via an as yet unknown mechanism. The decrease in protein leakage allows the lymphatics to remove excess fluid in the tissues and prevent further increase in fluid migration into the surrounding cells.

Michlovitz et al[11] noted a trend toward a reduction in edema and pain with the use of HVS in combination with ice; however, they were unable to detect a statistically significant difference between the effects of ice used alone and ice used in combination with HVS.

Elevation of a distal extremity reduces the gravitational forces that affect the cardiovascular system.[16] Massage is also reported to enhance venous and lymphatic drainage of the lower extremity.[17]

Active and passive exercise programs are performed to reverse the effects of immobilization on the connective tissues. Several authors have noted that prolonged immobilization of a joint leads to various undesirable biochemical and biomechanical changes in the surrounding connective tissues.[6,18–24] Mobilization of a joint through its ROM may prevent them.[6,22,25] A more complete discussion of the effects of mobilization is presented in the following section.

The home program adopts the same rationale as the clinical program, with one addition: protection of the right ankle. The ankle joint is protected with an air splint and PWB with axillary crutches. The compressive elastic sleeve provides some pressure to the ankle joint (preventing further increase in edema), whereas the air splint also offers some compression and prevents excessive inversion.[26,27] The air splint provides some compression to the ankle joint (preventing further increase in edema) and prevents the harmful effects of a loss of compression on hyaline cartilage. Hyaline cartilage is nutritionally dependent on alternating compression and decompression.[20,23] PWB also provides proprioceptive input to the ankle. Freeman and others[28-31] believe the loss of proprioception is one reason for the recurrence of ankle injuries.

Week 2

Treatment Plan. In the second week, the physical therapy program progressed, with the addition of proprioceptive exercises (Fig. 11–4) and the use of a bicycle ergometer. During the second week, the patient was seen three times for treatment. Tiltboard exercises were performed for 10 minutes during each treatment session. HVS and icing for 20 minutes before and after exercise were applied, as in week 1, as were manually resisted exercises to the dorsiflexors and plantar flexors. The patient was now allowed to fully weight bear (FWB) without using assistive devices. The air splint continued to be used whenever the athlete walked.

Gastrocsoleus stretches, toe curls, peroneal isometrics, and proprioceptive exercises were added to the patient's home exercise program. The gastrocsoleus stretching was performed two times per day for five repetitions, holding the gas-

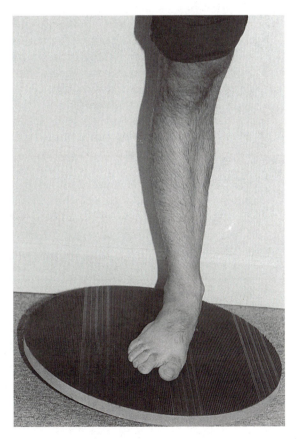

FIGURE 11–4. Proprioceptive exercises performed with case 1 standing on a tilt board. Case 1 is instructed to bring each edge of the board (one edge at a time) in contact with the floor in a circular fashion.

trocsoleus in a stretched position for 30 seconds for each repetition. Peroneal isometrics were performed two times per day for 30 repetitions, holding each repetition for 10 seconds. Toe curl exercises were performed with the patient in a sitting position with the toes resting on top of a towel lying on the floor. He curled the toes, bringing the opposite end of the towel closer to them. Toe curl exercises were performed for 30 repetitions, two times per day. The patient intermittently iced the right foot and ankle with the right lower extremity in an elevated position. Nighttime elevation of the lower extremity was also continued.

Treatment Results. By the end of week 2, the patient had minimal pain on active and passive ankle motion (pain level of 0 to 1). He continued to complain of some discomfort over the styloid process of the fifth metatarsal cuboid area. Edema was still present about the lateral aspect of the right ankle, as evidenced by the figure-eight girth measurement (58 mm). The passive ROM of the right ankle is 10° of dorsiflexion, 25° of plantar flexion, 10° of eversion, and 10° of inversion. The results of isokinetic tests of ankle dorsiflexion and plantar flexion performed at the end of the second week (as well as subsequent tests) are shown in Table 11–2. Ligament stress tests continued to show no excess of joint play. The anterior drawer test still provoked pain. No increase in tissue temperature was apparent with palpation when compared with the uninvolved extremity.

Treatment Rationale. The absence of complications in the second week of rehabilitation allowed the physical therapy program to progress accordingly. Proprioceptive exercises were initiated to rehabilitate the damaged mechanoreceptors in the joint capsule and accompanying ligaments.[27–29,31–33] Stimulation of the mechanoreceptor system of the injured joint may improve proprioception in the ankle. This improvement is accomplished by retraining the muscle-tendon mechanoreceptors or the undamaged joint mechanoreceptors, or both.[34] Several researchers have documented enhancement of proprioception of damaged joints through proprioceptive retraining.[29,33,34] These authors noted a decrease in position sense after inversion injury to an ankle. Following proprioceptive training using tiltboard, position sense improves.[29,33,34]

To maintain the athlete's cardiovascular endurance, a bicycle ergometer was used. Although cycling has not been shown to improve or maintain elite runners' conditioning, it does maintain cardiovascular endurance in moderately trained athletes.[35] It may also be effective in preventing muscle weakness in muscle groups adjacent to the injured lower extremity linkage system.[35,36] Dis-

TABLE 11–2 Case 1: Isokinetic Test Results (in foot-pounds)

Tests	Plantar Flexors*		Dorsiflexors*		Evertors†		Invertors†	
	Right	Left	Right	Left	Right	Left	Right	Left
1 (week 2)	20	56	0	20	—	—	—	—
2 (week 3)	—	—	—	—	10	21	10	22
3 (week 4)	49	54	19	21	—	—	—	—
4 (week 8)	51	54	19	21	18	20	21	22

*At 90° per second.
†At 60° per second.

use atrophy of the adjacent muscle groups as a result of immobilization of a joint has been reported.[36]

Isokinetic testing for weakness owing to disuse was performed. The results of the test (see Table 11–2) showed a strength deficit of the plantar flexors of 64% and of the dorsiflexors of 100%, as compared with the uninvolved side. The patient's isokinetic test results were also below the available norms. Scranton et al[37] and Davies[38] have demonstrated with isokinetic testing that the right ankle plantar flexors should exhibit between 30 and 72 foot-pounds of plantar flexion and 15 and 27 foot-pounds of dorsiflexion at 90° per second.

Ligament stress testing still revealed slight involvement of the anterior talofibular ligament secondary to the reproduction of pain on stressing the ligament. The inflammatory process most probably was no longer active, as suggested by the absence of palpated elevated skin temperatures. Gastrocsoleus stretching and peroneal isometric exercises at home were implemented to improve the flexibility of the gastrocsoleus complex and retard the potential disuse atrophy of the evertors of the right ankle.[2]

Week 3

Treatment Plan. Treatment sessions during week 3 continued to shift from passive to active forms of treatment. The patient was still seen three times per week. Treatments began and ended with the application of ice packs to the foot and ankle, without HVS, for 15 minutes. A warm-up period, consisting of cycling on a bicycle ergometer for 10 minutes, was followed by an isokinetic workout of 90 repetitions at 90° per second with the right ankle dorsiflexors and plantar flexors. The active portion of the treatment program ended with a 10-minute tiltboard workout.

An isokinetic test was done on the evertors and invertors of the right ankle at the end of the third week (Table 11–2). Based on the results of the test, an isokinetic strengthening program was initiated with the evertors and invertors of the right foot, consisting of 90 repetitions at 90° per second.

The home program during the third week was changed to a more functional exercise regimen. A "back to run" program was implemented, which consisted of gradual increase in running distance and agility skills. Progress in the program depends on the satisfaction of two criteria: absence of pain and absence of edema of the involved joint. The patient continued to ice the right foot and ankle before and after exercise and performed proprioceptive tiltboard exercises and gastrocsoleus stretching as before. Standing toe raises, for 45 repetitions six times per day, were added to the program. The use of the air splint for walking was gradually decreased.

The main focus of the treatment program is to simulate the patient's preinjury activities. His main deficits revolved around the loss of strength and reduction of cardiovascular endurance.

Treatment Results. By the end of the week, edema of the right ankle and forefoot could no longer be detected, either visually or by girth measurement. Girth of the right ankle was 55 mm. At this time, he experienced minimal pain only with inversion movements. The pain was located over the styloid process of the fifth metatarsal and cuboid bones. The anterior drawer test still reproduced complaints of pain.

Treatment Rationale. Ligamentous healing allowed the initiation of isokinetic testing and strengthening of the evertors and invertors of the ankle. The tensile strength of the ligaments at this point could be assumed to be sufficient to withstand the stress of eversion and inversion exercise.[39,40] Wong et al[41] demonstrated peak torque strength of between 14 and 24 foot-pounds for inversion and 14 and 22 foot-pounds for eversion at 60° per second.[41] Because of the normative data and the contralateral isokinetic test, an isokinetic strengthening program was instituted.

The back to run program was implemented to allow the musculoskeletal system to adapt to the new stresses placed on it, preventing further musculoskeletal injury. Also, the back to run program allowed the ankle to be stressed in a controlled manner, preventing premature return to full activity.[2,40,43] Further assurance of a safe return to full activity was afforded by the gradual discontinuation of the air splint.

Week 4

Treatment Plan. An isokinetic retest of the plantar flexors and dorsiflexors during week 4 revealed minimal deficits (49 foot-pounds and 19 foot-pounds, respectively, at 90° per second). In addition to using the bicycle ergometer for 10 minutes before exercise, the patient continued to strengthen the evertors and invertors of the right ankle using an isokinetic device for 120 repetitions at 90° per second. The foot and ankle were no longer iced. A modified cuboid whip manipulation (Fig. 11–5) was performed in an effort to decrease lateral plantar pain.[44] The athlete's home program now consisted of toe raises, eversion-inversion resis-

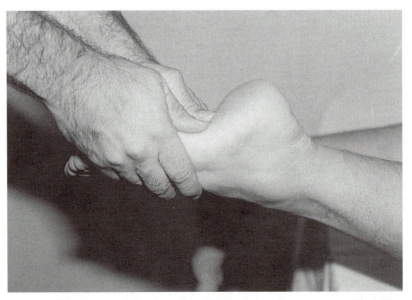

FIGURE 11–5. Modified cuboid whip manipulation. The therapist grasps the foot with both hands, placing both thumbs over the plantar aspect of the cuboid bone. From the starting position of knee flexion and ankle dorsiflexion, the therapist moves the lower leg into a position of knee extension and ankle plantar flexion and inversion while applying a superior force with the thumbs to the cuboid.

tive exercises using a large elastic band for 45 repetitions, tiltboard proprioceptive exercises, gastrocsoleus stretching, and agility skills. The agility skills consist of running figure-eight, back-pedaling, and zigzag patterns at varying speeds.

Treatment Results. Presently the patient has no complaint of pain. Minimal weakness was noted. The passive ROM of the right ankle was WNL (15° of dorsiflexion, 10° of eversion, 23° of inversion, and 47° of plantar flexion). Accordingly, active treatment was discontinued. A follow-up visit was planned in 4 weeks for a retest of the evertors and invertors.

Treatment Rationale. Although the patient still had some deficit in strength, he was discharged from active treatment because of economic constraints. A follow-up visit was planned to ascertain whether the observed strength deficits were problematic. Given the inability to reproduce the athlete's lateral cuboid pain through various tests of provocation of the ankle joint and the mechanism of injury, the cuboid bone was believed to be the source of the pain over the lateral cuboid area.[44]

Week 8

An isokinetic retest of the plantar flexors and dorsiflexors and evertors and invertors of the right ankle revealed clinically acceptable differences in strength (less than 10%; see Table 11–2). The patient's clinical evaluation was unremarkable, and he was discharged from active physical therapy.

CASE 2: BIMALLEOLAR FRACTURE

The use of mobilization techniques in the restoration of movement is the central theme of this section.

Initial Evaluation and Findings

A 26-year-old laborer sustained a bimalleolar fracture of the left ankle as a result of a fall from a ladder at home approximately 8 weeks earlier. On the date of injury, the laborer was admitted to the hospital by his physician. Open reduction with internal fixation of the fracture site was performed the same day. The postoperative hospital treatment course was uneventful. The patient reports being in a short-leg cast non–weight bearing (NWB) for 8 weeks. The cast was removed the day of his initial visit to the physical therapist.

The laborer's chief complaints were weakness, stiffness, and swelling of the left ankle. On a 0 to 10 numeric pain scale (with 10 being excruciating pain and 0 being no pain), the laborer reported a pain level of 5 that increased to 9 with movement of the left ankle. Table 11–3 is a summary of the evaluation and subsequent weekly reevaluation findings.

Marked atrophy of the left lower leg musculature was evident during visual inspection. The lower one third of the lower leg appeared to be slightly angulated in a varus direction. Slight edema of the left ankle was also visually noted.

During the initial evaluation, the strength of the lower extremity was not tested. The passive ROM of the left ankle was 0° of dorsiflexion, 5° of plantar flexion, 0° of eversion, and 0° of inversion. Pain was present when the extremes of all motions were reached.

TABLE 11–3 Case 2: Summary of Initial Evaluation and Weekly Progress

| Week | Passive Motion* | | | | Girth (mm) | Pain Level* |
	Dorsiflexion	Plantar Flexion	Inversion	Eversion		
Initial evaluation	0	5	0	0	60	5–9 with activity
1	5	20	5	5	59	2–7 with activity
2	9	33	10	10	57	1–8 with activity
4	12	41	18	10	57	1–8 with activity
28	5	10	5	5	58	4
29	12	25	11	10	56	0

*Measured on a scale of 0 (no pain) to 10 (excruciating pain).

Edema of the left ankle was confirmed during palpation of the ankle. Minimal tenderness was reproduced over the lateral malleolus during the palpatory examination. The mobility of the incision line was not restricted in any direction. The accessory joint play motions of anterior and posterior tibiofibular glide of the talus, superior and inferior glide of the metatarsals, and anterior and posterior glide of the tibia on the fibula at the inferior tibiofibular joint were limited (Figs. 11–6 to 11–8).[44,45] Joint play is a motion necessary for normal physiologic movement. Joint play is not under the voluntary control of the patient.[44] An example of joint play is the superior glide of the proximal phalanx of the first toe on the first metatarsal at the metatarsophalangeal joint.

Figure-eight girth measurements of the left and right ankles were 60 mm and 53 mm. Figure-eight girth measurements were performed as in Case 1.

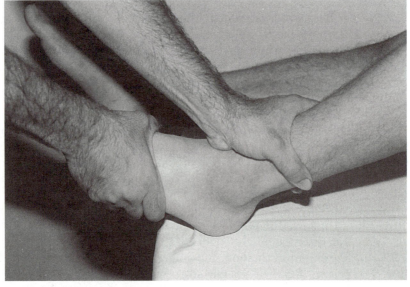

FIGURE 11–6. Tibiofibular posterior glide on talus. With one hand grasping the forefoot about the midtarsal joint, the examiner grasps and applies a posterior force on the tibia and fibula.

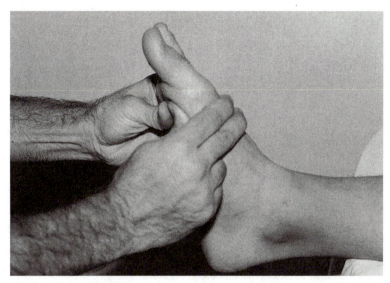

FIGURE 11–7. Superior intermetatarsal glide. The head and shaft of one metatarsal are grasped and stabilized with one hand. The other hand mobilizes the adjacent metatarsal, using the same hold as the stabilizing hand.

Interpretation

The history provided by the laborer had important implications for future treatments and explained some of the results seen during the initial evaluation. The use of long lever arms during mobilization techniques can be harmful. If too much force is generated by the use of long lever arms, the fracture ends could be displaced. Certain modalities, such as short-wave diathermy, are contraindicated for patients with internal fixation devices.[46]

The extended time of immobilization can be assumed to be the cause of the observed atrophy of the lower leg musculature.[21,24,47] The deficits noted in the passive ROM of the ankle joint can be partially attributed to the period of immobilization.[6,18,19,22,24,25] Another cause of the passive motion deficits of the ankle joint may be internal fixation devices.

Treatment

The primary goal of treatment is to improve the pain-free mobility of the ankle joint. Once an improvement in pain-free mobility is made, the secondary goals of increasing the strength of the lower leg musculature and increasing the patient's independence in gait can be addressed. The ultimate goal is to return the laborer to his previous functional status.

Week 1

Treatment Plan. Physical therapy treatment was given three times per week for the first week. The initial week of treatment consisted of warm whirlpool baths combined with active exercises in the whirlpool for 20 minutes; joint mobilization of the tibiofibular, talocrural, and intermetatarsal joints; and a home

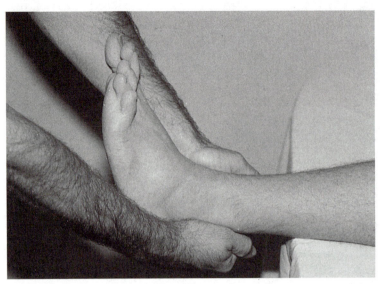

FIGURE 11–8. Posterior tibial glide on fibula. The examiner places the hypothenar eminence of the mobilizing hand over the medial malleolus and applies a posterior force. Simultaneously, the hypothenar eminence of the other hand is placed over the posterior surface of the lateral malleolus, and an anterior force is applied.

exercise program. The whirlpool exercise was drawing imaginary letters with the hallux.

Joint mobilization techniques for the inferior tibiofibular, talocrural, and intermetatarsal joints were simply a progression of the joint play test performed during the initial evaluation.[45–48] The main difference between the test and the treatment maneuvers was the addition of graded oscillations within the available joint play.[45–48] Inferior tibiofibular joint mobilization consisted of anterior and posterior glide of the tibia on the fibula (Fig. 11–8).[45] The talocrural joint mobilizations consisted of anterior and posterior glide of the tibia and fibula on the talus (Fig. 11–6) and long axis distraction of the talocrural joint (Fig. 11–9).[45] The intermetatarsal mobilizations consisted of superior and inferior glide of the metatarsals on each other (Fig. 11–7) and rolling of the forefoot (Fig. 11–10).[44,45] Mobilization treatments began with oscillatory forces of grade I and progressed immediately to grade IV forces.[48]

The home exercise program consisted of flexibility exercises, resistive exercises, cryotherapy, and protected gait. The flexibility exercise—gastrocsoleus stretching—is shown in Figure 11–11. To apply maximal stretch to the gastrocsoleus complex, the patient must keep the subtalar joint in a supinated position.[50,51] To ensure that this maximal stretch is attained, he was instructed to internally rotate his left lower extremity slightly and lean forward, bearing weight over the lateral aspect of the involved foot. The stretched position was held for 30 seconds for five repetitions, twice per day. Resistive exercises consist of eversion, plantar flexion, inversion, and dorsiflexion using an elastic material for resistance, performing the exercises for 45 repetitions for each motion, twice per day. The patient was encouraged to ice immediately after the completion of

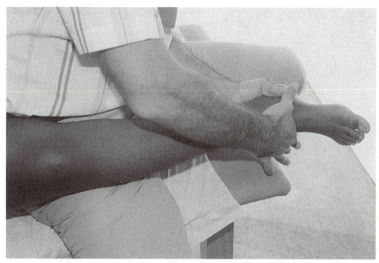

FIGURE 11–9. Long axis distraction of the talocrural joint. With the web space of one hand over the calcaneus and the web space of the other hand over the talar head, the examiner applies a force in a longitudinal direction to the lower leg.

flexibility and resistive exercises with the involved lower extremity elevated for 15 to 20 minutes. An air splint was applied to the ankle for walking.

Treatment Results. After the first week of treatment, passive ROM of the left ankle was 20° of plantar flexion, 5° of dorsiflexion, 5° of eversion, and 5° of inversion. The patient continued to have restrictions of the joint play of his talocrural joint. Intermetatarsal joint motion was WNL. A mild edema was still noticeable over the left lateral malleolus, as evidenced by the figure-eight girth measurement of 59 mm. The patient rated a decrease in his pain level from 5

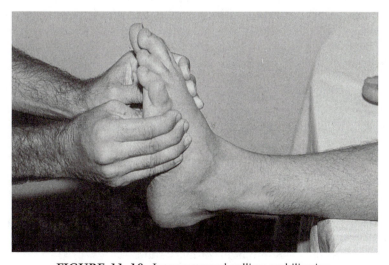

FIGURE 11–10. Intermetatarsal rolling mobilization.

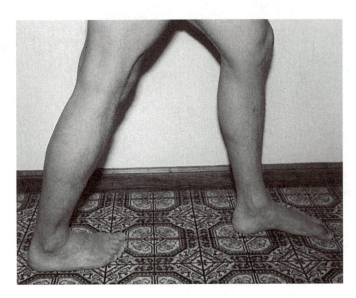

FIGURE 11–11. Gastrocsoleus stretching. Anterior leg should be flexed at the knee and hip with the posterior leg in hip and knee extension. The posterior leg should also be slightly internally rotated. The patient will then lean forward, keeping the heel of the posterior leg on the floor and the hip and knee in extension.

down to 2. The pain level increased from 2 to 7 during resistive activities with the foot (Table 11–3).

Treatment Rationale. Warm hydrotherapy was used because the effect of heat on connective tissues is to decrease their viscosity, which helps to reduce the stiffness in the ankle joint.[8,52] Elevated tissue temperatures in conjunction with stretching are thought to cause plastic deformation in connective tissues.[8,22,51,52] A secondary response to elevated tissue temperatures is an increase in oxygen uptake and blood flow to the heated tissues. Theoretically, these increases should make more nutrients available to the damaged tissues, thereby assisting in the healing process.[8,51]

During immobilization of a joint, several biochemical changes occur. These changes include a decrease in glycosaminoglycans (GAG) and water content and an increase in collagen cross-link formation.[6,18,19,22,25] The decreases in GAG and water lead to alterations in the viscous nature of connective tissue, causing an increase in the stiffness of the joint. The decreases also allow collagen cross-linking to occur, further diminishing the extensibility of the immobilized joint.[6,18,19,22,25]

Joint mobilization is purported to stimulate the production of GAG, thereby increasing the water content of connective tissue. The increase of both of these biochemical processes improves the mobility of the joint by decreasing the viscosity of involved tissues.[5,22] Other side effects of joint mobilization are the breaking of abnormal collagen cross-links and the stimulation of proper collagen fiber orientation.[6,22] All of these purported effects of joint mobilization ultimately lead to an increase in ROM.

Grade I mobilizations are believed to have effects on the nociceptive system of joints. These low-amplitude oscillatory mobilizations are believed to stimulate mechanoreceptors.[3,45] Stimulation of mechanoreceptors, primarily types I and II, has an inhibitory effect on the type IV nociceptors of the joint via certain spinal cord reflexes. Types I and IV mechanoreceptors are stimulated via grades I through IV mobilization forces.[3,45,53] Both the inhibition of pain and the reversal of the biochemical changes of immobilization improve joint mobility.

Ice after exercise was applied for two reasons: to prevent any adverse inflammatory response secondary to stretching and to maintain the plastic changes achieved during the stretch.[22,51] Maintenance of the observed clinical changes is accomplished at home by ROM exercises.

Week 2

Treatment Plan. Clinical sessions during the second week of physical therapy began with warm whirlpool treatments, as in the previous week. While in the whirlpool, the patient performed gastrocsoleus stretches along with his other ROM exercises. Once out of the whirlpool, he received joint mobilization techniques of long-axis talocrural distraction, anteroposterior talocrural glide, and inferior tibiofibular joint glides to the left ankle using grade I and IV forces. He was seen three times per week for physical treatment.

After the aforementioned mobilization therapy, resistive exercises against moderate manual resistance were applied by the physical therapist. The straight plane motions of eversion, inversion, plantar flexion, and dorsiflexion were resisted for 45 repetitions in each direction. The patient complained of discomfort over the area of the left lateral malleolus with the resisted eversion and plantar flexion motions.

On completion of the resistive phase of the treatment, the left ankle was placed in an active reflex treatment unit (ARTU, Universal Gym Equipment, Inc., Cedar Rapids, IA) for 20 minutes. The ARTU is a continuous passive motion, massage, and cooling device for the foot and ankle (Fig. 11–12). The extremes of all motions can be preset by the therapist to limit the degree of movement allowed by the ARTU. For the patient in Case 2, only the cooling and motion aspects of the machine were incorporated in treatment.

The home program was intensified by using a more resistive elastic material in the exercise program. The gait pattern progressed to FWB status with one axillary crutch. The laborer continued to use the air splint.

Treatment Results. At the end of week 2, the passive ROM was 10° of eversion, 10° of inversion, 9° of dorsiflexion, and 33° of plantar flexion. Slight edema was still noted about the lateral malleolus of the left ankle. The figure-eight girth measurement was 57 mm. Pain continued to occur with any type of resistive plantar flexion or eversion movement. Although the overall pain level was 1, the plantar flexion and eversion movements raised it to 7 or 8. The patient was now walking with FWB on the left lower extremity without any assistive devices except the air splint.

Treatment Rationale. The use of warm whirlpools continued secondary to the effects of heat on connective tissues, as previously mentioned. Static stretch was employed simultaneously with the whirlpool as a result of research indicating the benefits of prolonged low-load stretches in combination with heat.[21,22,51,52] Researchers have pointed out that low-load, long-duration stretches are more effective in attaining permanent plastic changes in connective tissues than high-load, short-duration stretches.[21,22,51,52] Joint mobilization techniques continued to be used for the same reasons previously mentioned.

Resistive exercises were now employed to regain the muscle strength of the lower extremity. Manually resisted exercises were initially employed because of

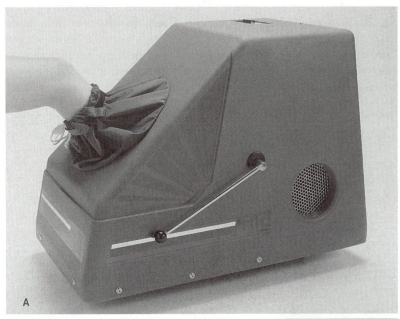

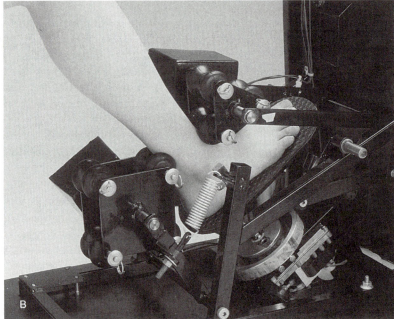

FIGURE 11–12. Active reflex treatment unit (ARTU).

weakness in the left lower leg. Given the foot-pounds needed to move the isokinetic device's extremity attachments, the therapist believed the laborer would
be unable to generate enough force to use the isokinetic device. Also the patient
experienced a great deal of discomfort when performing the manually resisted
eversion and plantar flexion exercises. Such discomfort is one contraindication
to the use of isokinetics.[39]

Employment of the ARTU was a result of the theorized effects on mobility and control of edema by the device. As has been noted previously, applying cold helps reduce or prevent the inflammatory response.[7–10] A second reason for the use of the ARTU was its theorized effect on the maintenance and improvement of passive mobility. Theoretically, joint mobility should improve through the use of a mobilization device such as the ARTU because of the positive effects of mobilization on connective tissue.[6,8,26,21,23,40] Although sound clinical research on the efficacy of the ARTU is lacking, it does promise to be an effective adjunct in the treatment of foot and ankle hypomobility and edema.

The gait pattern had progressed to FWB because of the progress in ROM. An air splint was still used to protect the ankle joint while the joint regained its strength, mobility, and position sense. The resistive portion of the home program was increased as a result of the improvement in lower leg strength.

Week 3

Treatment Plan. Warm whirlpool treatments in conjunction with static stretching and ROM exercises continued to be administered during week 3 of treatment, three times per week. As a result of the restoration of joint play motions, mobilization techniques were discontinued. A submaximal isokinetic exercise program was instituted along with a low-resistance bicycle ergometer workout. The submaximal isokinetic workout consisted of plantar flexion and dorsiflexion for 45 repetitions at 90° per second (Fig. 11–13). Eversion and inversion exercises continued against moderate manual resistance for 45 repetitions (Fig. 11–14). After the strengthening exercises, proprioceptive retraining exercises using a tiltboard were implemented for 10 minutes. All treatment sessions ended with a 20-minute session of the ARTU using only the cooling and passive motion features of the instrument.

The home program progressed with the addition of proprioceptive exercises and the use of a stronger elastic material during the strengthening phase.

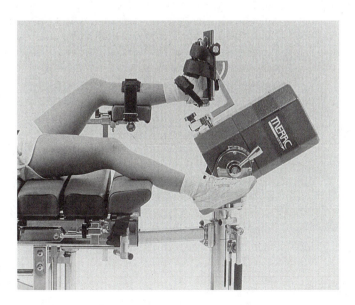

FIGURE 11–13. Inversion/eversion isokinetic workout.

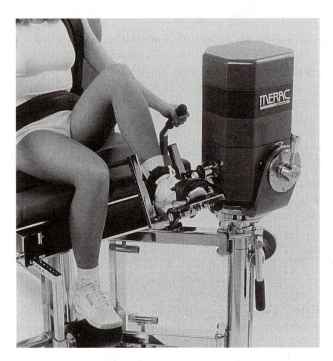

FIGURE 11–14. Plantarflexion/dorsiflexion isokinetic workout.

Another change in the home program was the addition of toe raises off the edge of a step for 45 repetitions. Aside from these adjustments, the home program remained unchanged.

Treatment Results. At the end of week 3, the laborer continued to complain of pain (level 8) over the lateral malleolus on forceful eversion and plantar flexion movements. Passive ROM was 10° of eversion, 16° of inversion, 12° of dorsiflexion, and 40° of plantar flexion. Minimal edema remained visible over the left lateral malleolus. It was barely detectable by figure-eight girth measurement (54 mm).

Given the patient's improvement, the main objectives of physical therapy were then to reduce the level of pain, improve left lower extremity strength, and maintain cardiovascular endurance.

Treatment Rationale. Submaximal isokinetic exercises were added to the clinical program in an attempt to increase the strength of the lower extremity. Maximal resistance was not administered owing to the increase in pain associated with manually resisted exercise, possibly as a result of the internal fixation devices. The posterolateral tendinous structures could have been pressed up against the fixation devices, causing an inflammatory response and the subsequent pain. Submaximal exercise is thought to cause less pressure against the fixation devices and therefore decreases the tendon irritation. Also the patient did not complain of discomfort while performing this type of exercise.

Given the improvement of joint play motion, mobilization treatments were discontinued. Proprioceptive exercises were implemented with the same rationale as in Case 1.

Week 4

Treatment Plan. The results of the isokinetic plantar flexion and dorsiflexion test performed at the beginning of week 4 (as well as subsequent tests) are shown in Table 11–4. As a result of the isokinetic test, an isokinetic exercise program was implemented, which consisted of plantar flexion and dorsiflexion for 90 repetitions at 90° per second. A bicycle ergometer was employed for 10 minutes before exercise. Whirlpool treatments were discontinued, and a static stretching program was implemented in place of the hydrotherapy. The proprioceptive and manually resisted eversion and inversion exercise regimen continued as before. A trial period of iontophoretic treatment with 1.0 mL of lidocaine (Xylocaine) (of local anesthetic) mixed with 0.5 mL of dexamethasone (of corticosteroid) was initiated. The drug electrode was placed just inferior to the lateral malleolus, and the dispersive pad was placed on the gastrocnemius muscle belly. A 2.7 mA current was used for 15 minutes during the iontophoretic treatment.[54] There was no change in the home program from the previous week. The patient continued to attend physical therapy three times per week.

Treatment Results. At the end of week 4, the patient had passive ROM of 12° of dorsiflexion, 41° of plantar flexion, 10° of eversion, and 18° of inversion. The isokinetic tests of his left plantar flexors and dorsiflexors revealed 15 foot-pound and 5 foot-pound of peak torque, respectively, at 90° per second (Table 11–4). Slight edema was still visible about the lateral malleolus of the left ankle. The patient continued to complain of pain (level 8) with resistive movements of the left ankle.

Treatment Rationale. The isokinetic dorsiflexion and plantar flexion program was based on the results of the test and the patient's ability to perform maximal efforts without experiencing symptoms. The tests revealed a deficit of over 10% compared with the contralateral extremity, indicating a need to strengthen the involved muscles.

Iontophoresis with a local anesthetic and corticosteroid was used for the drugs' anti-inflammatory and analgesic properties.[54,55] Several researchers using animal and human subjects have shown that ion transfer does occur across various membranes (e.g., skin).[56–60] Unfortunately, because of the inherent difficulties of such drug studies, the actual depth of penetration, concentration, and therapeutic levels achieved in humans have not as yet been determined.[52,55]

TABLE 11–4 Case 2: Isokinetic Test Results (in foot-pounds)

Tests	Plantar Flexors*		Dorsiflexors*		Evertors†		Invertors†	
	Right	*Left*	*Right*	*Left*	*Right*	*Left*	*Right*	*Left*
1 (week 4)	48	15	17	5	—	—	—	—
2 (week 28)	48	36	18	12	—	—	—	—
3 (week 30)	—	—	—	—	22	16	18	11
4 (week 31)	49	47	18	18	21	22	20	17
5 (week 33)	48	48	18	19	20	19	19	18

*At 90° per second.
†At 60° per second.

Some attempts have been made to determine the effectiveness of iontophoretic delivery of anti-inflammatory drugs for patients afflicted with various inflammatory conditions.[61,62] Harris[61] and Bertolucci[62] have indicated in their respective studies that iontophoretic treatment with anti-inflammatory medication effectively alleviates symptoms. Further definitive research on this modality is needed to determine its clinical effectiveness.

Week 5

Treatment Plan. The clinical portion of the treatment program consisted of iontophoresis as in week 4, isokinetic exercise workouts with the plantar flexors and dorsiflexors of the left foot, bicycle ergometer workouts, and proprioceptive exercises as before. ARTU and eversion-inversion exercises were discontinued. The home exercise program remained unchanged. The frequency of treatment remained as in week 4.

Treatment Results. By the end of the fifth week, ROM of the left ankle was WNL except for inversion and plantar flexion, which lacked 6° and 5° of motion, respectively, as compared with the contralateral extremity. Pain was still experienced on resisted eversion. Palpation over the posterolateral border of the ankle revealed point tenderness (pain level 8).

During week 5, the patient saw his physician for a follow-up visit. The physician believed that the fixation devices were irritating the posterolateral structures of the left ankle and decided that they should be removed. The patient was scheduled for surgery to remove the hardware in 3 months. At the physician's request, physical therapy treatments were discontinued, but the physician did instruct the laborer to continue his home exercise program.

Treatment Rationale. In the absence of any changes in the objective signs, the physical therapist believed the patient had received the maximum benefit from the ARTU and that modality was discontinued. Eversion and inversion exercises were discontinued because of the possibility that the posterolateral structures of the left ankle were being compressed against the fixation devices. This compression was believed to be the source of the patient's symptoms.

Week 28

Evaluative Findings. The patient returned for further treatment after the internal fixation devices were removed. After the hardware removal, the patient's leg was immobilized in an air cast for 4 weeks. At the end of the immobilization period, physical therapy treatment was reinitiated.

Active and passive ROM of the left ankle were again restricted: 5° of dorsiflexion, 10° of plantar flexion, 5° of inversion, and 5° of eversion. The joint play motion of anterior glide of the talus was slightly restricted. Slight edema was noted about the lateral and medial malleoli. A figure-eight girth measurement of the ankle revealed a 5-mm increase in girth when compared with the unaffected ankle. Palpation of the left ankle was unremarkable. The patient's chief complaints were stiffness, edema, and minimal (level 4) pain over the lateral malleolus.

Treatment Plan. Office treatments consisted of the ARTU for 20 minutes before and after exercise, ultrasound followed by joint mobilization and static stretching, bicycle ergometer, submaximal isokinetic exercise with the plantar flexors and dorsiflexors, and manually resisted eversion and inversion. The mobilization treatment consisted of anterior and posterior tibiofibular glide on the talus using grade I and IV oscillatory forces. The home program remained unchanged from week 5. The patient was seen three times per week for treatment.

Treatment Results. By the end of the week, the patient had passive ROM of 25° of plantar flexion, 12° of dorsiflexion, 10° of eversion, and 11° of inversion. No restriction was noted in any joint play motion. An isokinetic test performed at the end of the week revealed a 25% deficit of the plantar flexors and a 34% deficit of the dorsiflexors, when compared with the unaffected side (Table 11–4). Pain was no longer noted with eversion or inversion movements of the left ankle. Figure-eight girth measurement of the left ankle was 56 mm, a 3-mm decrease from the beginning of the week.

Treatment Rationale. The ARTU was reimplemented for the device's effect on the reduction of edema. Isokinetic exercise was implemented because of the strength deficits noted.

The main goals of therapy were an increase in strength (to within 10% of the uninvolved lower extremity's strength), the absence of edema of the involved ankle, and the restoration of pain-free ROM.

Week 30

Treatment Plan. An isokinetic test was performed to ascertain the strength of the evertors and invertors of the left ankle (Table 11–4). Based on the results of that test, an isokinetic exercise program was implemented (Fig. 11–13). The isokinetic program consisted of 45 repetitions at 90° per second. The ARTU continued to be used after exercise and the bicycle ergometer before exercise. The home program remained unchanged except for the addition of a walking program. The patient was to walk daily, increasing the distance by a quarter mile every other day until he was ambulating a maximum of 2 miles.

Treatment Results. The isokinetic test of the evertors and invertors of the left ankle revealed deficits of 39% and 27%. Figure-eight girth measurement of the left ankle revealed no increase in girth as compared with the uninvolved ankle (54 mm). ROM of the left ankle was 40° of plantar flexion, and all other movements were WNL. The patient had no complaints of pain in the left ankle but reported some pain over the medial aspect of the left knee.

Treatment Rationale. Because of the significant differences in strength between the involved and uninvolved extremities, an isokinetic exercise program for the evertors and invertors was initiated. Plantar flexion and dorsiflexion workouts continued because of strength deficits in these muscles.

Week 31

Treatment Plan and Results. An isokinetic retest of the lower leg musculature revealed only a 15% deficit of the evertors of the left ankle (see Table 11–4). Plantar flexion ROM continued to exhibit a loss of 6° as compared with the unaffected side. The patient continued to complain of left medial knee pain that was exacerbated by increased activity (e.g., cycling, walking). The pain remained localized to the medial aspect of the left knee. A biomechanical foot evaluation (see Chapter 6) was performed (Fig. 11–15). As a result of the foot evaluation, temporary foot orthotics were fabricated, to be used for 2 weeks, at which time

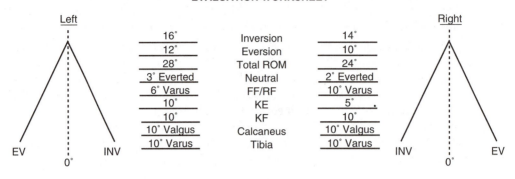

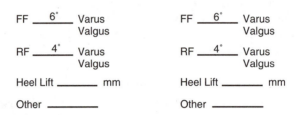

FIGURE 11–15. Biomechanical foot evaluation for case 2. KE = dorsiflexion with knee extended; KF = dorsiflexion with knee flexed.

the physical therapist was to evaluate their effectiveness. During week 31, the laborer was seen three times.

Based on the foot evaluation, the foot was posted medially 8 mm in the left forefoot, 4 mm in the left rearfoot, 6 mm in the right forefoot, and 4 mm in the right rearfoot (Fig. 11–15). Active treatment for strengthening and stretching was discontinued. The patient was followed only to evaluate the effectiveness of the orthotics and to determine whether his current strength deficits were causing any difficulties.

Treatment Rationale. Given the patient's previous activity level and his home exercise program, the therapist believed that the current strength deficits were not significant enough to warrant further active treatment. The therapist believed the home program would restore the patient's strength.

Biomechanical foot orthotics were fabricated to reduce the abnormal mechanics of the lower extremity. The angulation of the lower one third of the tibia and fibula, in combination with the forefoot varus deformity, might make it difficult for the subtalar joint to compensate for the deformities.[63,64] Several studies have indicated that angular deformities of the lower leg greater than 9° can cause alterations in the mechanics of the lower kinetic chain that could produce symptoms.[63,64] To assist the subtalar joint in its compensatory role, the forefoot and rearfoot were posted medially. Theoretically, medial posting decreases the amount of pronation that would otherwise occur to compensate for the forefoot varus.[63–68] If no angular deformity of the lower leg is present, the subtalar joint should have enough compensatory ability to allow the lower kinetic chain to function normally.[69]

Week 33

Permanent orthotics were fabricated using the same posting as in the temporary orthotics. At this time, the patient had no complaints of pain. The excessive pronation of the subtalar joint was effectively controlled by the biomechanical orthotics. An isokinetic retest revealed a 5% deficit of the evertors only (Table 11–4). Based on the results obtained from the isokinetic test and the biomechanical foot evaluation, the patient was discharged from physical therapy.

CASE 3: CALCANEAL PAIN

The use of modalities to ameliorate pain and inflammation are the focus of this case.

Initial Evaluation and Findings

A 36-year-old woman began experiencing pain along the medial plantar aspect of her right heel approximately 4 weeks earlier. Figure 11–16 is the pain drawing completed by this patient. The onset of pain was insidious. The patient stated that she experienced no pain while walking but that if she sat for a prolonged period the pain would return on standing. The pain would awaken her in the middle of the night. The pain is worse in the morning than at night. At times, it radiates into the digits of the right foot. The patient rated her pain level at 8 on a numeric scale of 0 to 10 (10 being excruciating pain and 0 being no pain).

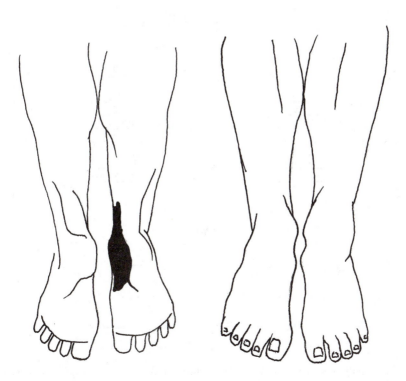

FIGURE 11–16. Pain drawing of patient in case 3.

On visual inspection, the lower extremities were unremarkable. Decreased dorsiflexion of the right foot as compared with the left was noted during passive ROM testing. Dorsiflexion of the right foot was 5°. Results of the hyperpronation test and Tinel's sign were negative. The remainder of the evaluation was unremarkable. The hyperpronation test was performed by taking the calcaneus of the involved foot and maximally everting it. This position was maintained for 30 to 60 seconds.[70]

Palpation of the right foot revealed marked point tenderness over the plantar aspect of the anteromedial border of the right calcaneus. The patient stated that palpation over this area reproduced her symptoms. Dorsiflexing the toes and palpating the medial aspect of the calcaneus increased the severity of the symptoms.

A biomechanical foot evaluation was performed. The results are presented in Figure 11–17. Forefoot varus of 10° in the right foot and 6° in the left foot was noted. Subtalar joint motion was 24° in the right foot and 28° in the left. The left subtalar joint had 12° of eversion and 16° of inversion, whereas the right joint had 10° of eversion and 14° of inversion. Standing still, the patient demonstrated 10° of calcaneal valgus bilaterally and 10° of tibial varus bilaterally. During the gait analysis, she exhibited excessive pronation at heel strike of the right foot, and the feet remained in pronation throughout the stance phase of gait.

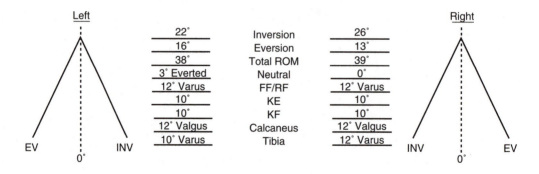

EVALUATION WORKSHEET

Left			
	22°	Inversion	26°
	16°	Eversion	13°
	38°	Total ROM	39°
	3° Everted	Neutral	0°
	12° Varus	FF/RF	12° Varus
	10°	KE	10°
	10°	KF	10°
	12° Valgus	Calcaneus	12° Valgus
	10° Varus	Tibia	12° Varus

EV   0°   INV   INV   0°   EV

ORTHOTIC WORKSHEET

FF ___7°___ Varus   FF ___7°___ Varus
           Valgus   Valgus

RF ___3°___ Varus   RF ___3°___ Varus
           Valgus   Valgus

Heel Lift _____ mm   Heel Lift _____ mm

Other _____   Other _____

FIGURE 11–17. Biomechanical foot evaluation for case 3. KE = dorsiflexion with knee extended; KF = dorsiflexion with knee flexed.

Interpretation

An analysis of the evaluation findings revealed several perpetuating, predisposing, and precipitating factors. One such factor was tightness of the Achilles tendon–gastrocsoleus complex, which might cause an increase in pronation of the rearfoot.[49,50,70–72] Excessive pronation of the subtalar joint added further tensile stress, overloading the plantar fascia and possibly leading to an inflammatory condition at its insertion on the calcaneus.[70–74] The degree of forefoot varus in the right foot can be another source of strain to the plantar fascia for the same reason as a tight gastrocsoleus complex, excessive pronation.[66,67] Given the absence of signs of tarsal tunnel involvement (negative Tinel's sign and hyperpronation test) and given the results of palpation, the plantar fascia was assumed to be the source of pathology.[70,72,73]

If left untreated, the inflammatory condition caused by the stress on the plantar fascia could have led to compression of the posterior tibial nerve as it divides in the tarsal tunnel into the medial and lateral plantar nerves.[70,71] Some authors believe that excessive pronation of the subtalar joint overstretches the tibial nerve and that such overstretching itself leads to fibrotic changes within the tunnel. The increase in fibrotic changes or nerve compression ultimately causes the patient's symptoms.[70,71]

Treatment

The major goal of treatment was to reduce the patient's level of pain. The therapist attempted to accomplish this by controlling the abnormal mechanics of the foot, decreasing the inflammatory condition at the calcaneus, and improving the flexibility of the gastrocsoleus.

Week 1

Treatment Plan and Results. Treatment began with iontophoresis with lidocaine and dexamethasone administered as in Case 2, with the drug electrode over the medial plantar aspect of the calcaneus followed by ice massage over the same area. Temporary orthotics were fabricated on the initial visit. The orthotics were posted medially 6 mm in the forefoot area and 4 mm medially in the rearfoot area bilaterally (Fig. 11–17). Ultrasound treatment in combination with a static stretch is administered to the gastrocsoleus area for 10 minutes.[75] The ultrasound treatment is followed by the application of cold with the patient in the same position as in the ultrasound treatment for 20 minutes. The patient was seen for three visits during the first week of treatment. She was instructed in a home exercise program of gastrocsoleus stretching and frequent ice massage to the heel during the day. At the end of week 1, she reported a 50% reduction in her symptoms and a pain level of 4. The medial plantar aspect of her heel was less tender to palpation.

Treatment Rationale. Iontophoresis with a local anesthetic and corticosteroid was implemented in an attempt to decrease the inflammatory process in the heel.[54,56,61,62,72] Ice was used following the iontophoretic treatment to help reduce blood flow to the area, possibly reducing the amount of medication removed from the local area by the circulatory system.[7–9,72,73] Temporary orthotics were employed to decrease the excessive pronation in the subtalar joint, thereby reducing the tensile forces on the plantar aponeurosis. It was hoped that reducing the tensile forces would eradicate the precipitating factor of excessive pronation.[70,72,73,76]

Ultrasound treatments in conjunction with a stasis stretch were used to facilitate the increase in flexibility of the gastrocsoleus complex.[51,52,75] Wessling et al[75] noted improvement in the dorsiflexion of healthy women when this method of stretching was used. The average increase in dorsiflexion was on the order of 4.7° to 7.7° after 1 week of treatment. Cold was applied after stretching, to maintain the plastic deformation of the gastrocsoleus complex.[22,51,52]

To maintain and increase the flexibility of the gastrocsoleus complex, the patient was instructed to continue with the stretching program at home. Ice was also applied at home to reduce inflammation.

Week 2

Iontophoretic treatment and gastrocsoleus stretching, as previously noted, were continued three times per week. At the end of week 2, the patient reported an 85% improvement in her symptoms. Her pain level was 2. The passive ROM of dorsiflexion was 10°. The patient reported that the temporary orthotics were valuable in ameliorating her symptoms.

Week 3

Treatment Plan and Results. Semirigid permanent orthotics were fabricated using the Orthofeet system (Orthofeet Inc., Hillsdale, NJ). They were posted medially in the forefoot and rearfoot. The forefoot and rearfoot are bilaterally posted 6 mm and 4 mm, respectively. On reevaluation of the right foot, a pain level of 0 was reported. Point tenderness was no longer present. Dorsiflexion of the right foot was 10° with the knee extended and flexed. Active physical therapy was discontinued as a result of the improvement.

Treatment Rationale. The choice of a permanent orthotic device was made because of the reduction in symptoms and the temporary orthotic's ability to control the abnormal mechanics in the lower kinetic chain. The patient was scheduled for a follow-up visit in 3 weeks.

Week 6

At the follow-up visit, the patient had no complaint of symptoms. ROM measurements of the right ankle revealed 10° of dorsiflexion bilaterally. The patient was instructed to continue using the permanent orthotics and performing gastrocsoleus stretching. She was discharged from active physical therapy at that time.

CASE 4: HALLUX ABDUCTOVALGUS

The following section emphasizes the treatment of the metatarsophalangeal (MTP) joint after surgery.

Initial Evaluation and Findings

During the initial interview, the patient, a 45-year-old woman, stated that she underwent surgery approximately 4 weeks earlier for correction of an HAV deformity in her right first MTP joint. No internal fixation device was in place in the first metatarsal, and no other significant history was reported. The chief complaints were pain (level 7–8), stiffness, and edema in the right first MTP joint.

Visual inspection of the right foot revealed a moderate degree of edema about the first MTP joint and forefoot. The incision lines over the dorsal and medial aspects of the joint were intact. The patient wore a cast shoe.

Passive and active ROM testing revealed decreased arthrokinematic and osteokinematic mobility of the intermetatarsal and first MTP joints of the right foot. Pain was felt at the extremes of flexion and extension of the first MTP joint. The ROM of the first MTP was 20° of extension and flexion to neutral (0°).

Palpation of the forefoot and MTP area of the right foot revealed marked tenderness over the joint line of the first MTP. An increase in the tissue temperature was also noted over the first MTP joint. Girth measurement at the level of the metatarsal heads of the right forefoot was 27 mm, as compared with the left forefoot, which had 23 mm.

Interpretation

An analysis of the evaluation findings revealed the need to reduce the edema of the forefoot and improve the mobility of the first MTP joint. For normal gait to occur, at least 60° of motion is necessary in the first MTP joint.[77,78]

Treatment

The major goals of therapy, therefore, were to increase the mobility of the first MTP to at least 60° of extension, reduce the edema of the forefoot, and prevent recurrence of the HAV deformity.

Week 1

Treatment Plan. The first week of physical therapy consisted of the ARTU for 20 minutes, using the massage rollers and the cooling features of the machine. This treatment was followed by a 10-minute effleurage massage to the forefoot area with the lower extremity elevated and intermetatarsal joint play mobilization. The forefoot treatment was followed by the facilitation of passive pain-free ROM of extension and flexion for the first MTP. Figure 11–18 illustrates long-axis distraction mobilization administered to the first MTP joint using grade I oscillatory forces after the facilitation of passive pain-free ROM.[45] The treatment program ended with another 20-minute ARTU session. The patient was seen three times during the first week.

She was instructed in a home exercise program consisting of self-mobilization of MTP flexion and extension within the pain-free range. She was also instructed to keep the lower extremity elevated and to apply ice packs to the right forefoot for 10 to 15 minutes intermittently throughout the day.

Treatment Results. At the end of week 1, the patient had 35° of first MTP extension. The girth of the forefoot was 25 mm, and the subjective pain level had decreased to 6.

Treatment Rationale. Cold and massage were applied in an effort to reduce the amount of edema in the forefoot and first MTP.[2,7,9,17,79] The mobilization pro-

EVALUATION WORKSHEET

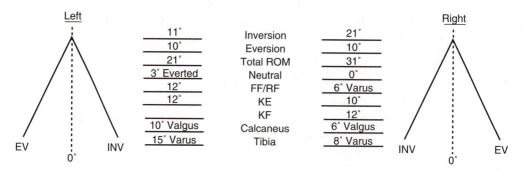

Left		Inversion	21°	Right
	11°	Inversion	21°	
	10°	Eversion	10°	
	21°	Total ROM	31°	
	3° Everted	Neutral	0°	
	12°	FF/RF	6° Varus	
	12°	KE	10°	
		KF	12°	
	10° Valgus	Calcaneus	6° Valgus	
	15° Varus	Tibia	8° Varus	

EV   INV   INV   EV
        0°   0°

ORTHOTIC WORKSHEET

Left   Right

FF __8°__ Varus   FF __6°__ Varus
          Valgus   Valgus

RF __4°__ Varus   RF __4°__ Varus
          Valgus   Valgus

Heel Lift _____ mm   Heel Lift _____ mm

Other _____   Other _____

FIGURE 11–18. Biomechanical foot evaluation for case 4. KE = dorsiflexion with knee extended; KF = dorsiflexion with knee flexed.

gram was an effort to provide nutrition to the joint, break adhesions, and realign collagen fibers along appropriate lines of stress.[20–23,79]

Week 2

Treatment Plan. Clinic sessions continued to emphasize the use of cryotherapy before and after exercise using the ARTU and joint mobilization. Mobilization treatments progressed to include grade IV long-axis distraction and superior glide of the proximal phalanx of the hallux on the first metatarsal using grade I and grade IV forces (Fig. 11–19).[44] The home exercise program progressed to walking in tennis shoes, gastrocsoleus stretching, and standing MTP stretch. Standing MTP stretch is accomplished while standing by simply raising the heel of the involved foot while keeping the hallux on the floor. The remainder of the home exercise program remained unchanged. The patient was seen three times per week.

Treatment Results. After the second week of treatment, the patient had 40° of first MTP extension. The girth measurement of the right forefoot was 25 mm, a 2-mm difference from the unaffected foot.

The treatment progressed by the addition of more aggressive stretches as a result of the degree of osseous healing. At that time, the therapist believed the patient could safely tolerate the standing stretch and superior glide mobilization treatment.

Week 3

Figure 11–18 shows the results of the biomechanical foot evaluation performed by the therapist, from which a forefoot varus deformity of 12° was noted

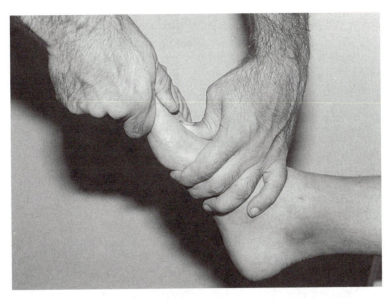

FIGURE 11–19. Long axis distraction of first MTP joint. The shaft of the first metatarsal is grasped by one hand and stabilized. The other hand will apply a longitudinal directed force to distract the MTP joint.

bilaterally. In the gait evaluation, the therapist found that the patient pronated excessively late in the gait cycle, at toe-off. Temporary orthotics were prescribed. The orthotics were posted medially in the forefoot (7 mm) and rearfoot (3 mm; Fig. 11–18). The patient was fitted with a pair of semirigid permanent orthotics that were posted identically to the temporary orthotics (Fig. 11–19). Because the initial goals were achieved and there were no symptoms, the patient was discharged from further physical therapy treatments.

After 4 weeks of treatment, the patient exhibited 60° of extension of the first MTP joint. No difference was detected in the girth measurement of the forefoot area, and the subjective pain rating was 0. Clinic treatments in weeks 3 and 4 remained unchanged, as did the home exercise program. The patient was seen two times per week.

CASE 5: ACHILLES TENDINITIS

The identification of both training errors and biomechanical contributors to Achilles tendinitis are discussed in this section. The rehabilitation of the Achilles tendon–gastrocsoleus complex is the primary focus.

Initial Evaluation and Findings

An 18-year-old high school cross-country runner presented with complaints of chronic right Achilles tendon pain. She reported an insidious gradual onset of symptoms that were first noticed with uphill running. Her symptoms were now present with all running and climbing stairs. The athlete reported that she had taken 2 months off from running and had recently doubled her mileage in an

attempt to remain a competitive member of the team. As a fourth year return-
ing cross-country team member, she did not have a significant history of similar
or related injuries.

During the initial evaluation, she removed a pair of worn running shoes
and reported she had not purchased a new pair of running shoes yet this season. On visual inspection, her posture appeared normal. No significant tibial or
calcaneal deviations were noted.

Passive ROM measurements were 4° of dorsiflexion for the right ankle and
7° for the left, both measured with the knee extended. Bilateral hamstring tightness was noted, and a modified Thomas test revealed bilateral hip flexor and
quadriceps flexibility deficits. Lower extremity strength was WNL with gross
manual muscle tests except for the gastrocsoleus on the right. The athlete was
unable to perform a single leg raise on the right, limited by pain. During a dou-
ble-leg toe raise, she reported an increase in symptoms primarily during the
lowering or eccentric phase.

Palpation revealed tenderness, localized swelling, and a mild thickening of
the Achilles tendon approximately 4 cm proximal to the Achilles tendon insertion into the calcaneus. A moderate decrease in stance time and push-off on the
right was observed during gait analysis. A biomechanical foot evaluation was
not performed at this time.

Interpretation

An analysis of the subjective history and evaluative findings indicated that
training errors and gastrocsoleus insufficiency were the two primary contributors to this injury. Training errors are a commonly known contributor to overuse
injuries, specifically Achilles tendinitis.[43,80] Clement et al[80] demonstrated training errors as a primary cause of injury to the Achilles tendon in more than 75%
of cases studied. An increase in pain with running up hill and climbing stairs
demonstrated the athlete's limited dorsiflexion. Both of these activities require
adequate flexibility. Limits in dorsiflexion ROM place extra eccentric forces on
the Achilles tendon.[80]

Given the amount of training errors, a negative history of similar or related
injuries, and apparently normal postural alignment, a biomechanical foot assessment was not performed. It is important to note, however, that functional overpronation is one of the leading etiologic factors in running-induced injuries,
specifically Achilles tendinitis.[43,80–82] An appropriate evaluation and orthotic
treatment are necessary in some cases. Excessive overpronation produces a
whipping action or bowstringing of the Achilles tendon contributing to
microtears.[80] It has been shown that there is a vascular watershed region of the
tendon approximately 2 to 6 cm proximal to its osseous insertion. These findings
are compared with Rathburn and McNab's findings[84] in the rotator cuff. Vascular blanching or wringing out vessels in the tendon with excessive overpronation may contribute to degenerative changes.

Treatment

The goals of treatment were first to decrease the local inflammation and
increase the flexibility of the lower extremity, specifically the Achilles tendon
gastrocsoleus complex, and second to correct training errors.

Week 1

Treatment Plan. Physical therapy was given three times per week during the first week. This initial week of treatment consisted of phonophoresis, gastrocsoleus stretching, anterior tibialis strengthening, cycling on a bicycle ergometer, ice massage, and a home program.

Ultrasound with a 10% hydrocortisone cream with a 50% duty cycle, at 0.5 W/cm^2, 3 MHz × 5 minutes was applied to the injured site of the tendon. Dorsiflexion resistive exercises with a large elastic band were performed for three sets of 30 repetitions; hamstring and iliopsoas/quadriceps stretches were performed; and an interval training program was done on the bicycle ergometer for 20 minutes. Five minutes of gastrocsoleus stretching with the knee bent and with the knee straight preceded a 10-minute ice massage. The ice massage was performed with a static stretch of the gastrocsoleus. Gastrocsoleus and lower extremity stretching, dorsiflexion resistive exercises, cycling, and ice were incorporated into the athlete's daily home program. The athlete was not permitted to run or perform any physical activities other than those in physical therapy or her home program.

Heel lifts 12 mm were given to the athlete to wear in both shoes during the symptomatic phases of treatment. The athlete was instructed to purchase a new pair of running shoes with a firm, well-fitted heel counter and a moderately flared heel.

Treatment Results. Passive dorsiflexion ROM was 8° for the right ankle and 10° for the left ankle by the end of the first week. Achilles tenderness to palpation and swelling was minimal. General lower extremity flexibility was improving.

Treatment Rationale. Phonophoresis with 10% hydrocortisone was used in an attempt to decrease the inflammatory process and facilitate healing. A 50% duty cycle at an intensity of less than 1.0 W/cm^2 was used for the delivery of the medication and the nonthermal effects of the ultrasound.[85] According to Dyson,[85] these nonthermal effects include the stimulation of tissue regeneration, soft tissue and bone repair, changes in cell metabolism, and the promotion of pain relief. A 3-MHz frequency was used because the target tissue is superficial, lying 1 to 2 cm beneath the skin's surface. There is a greater attenuation and absorption of energy and superficial structures with a higher ultrasound frequency.[91]

Dorsiflexors were strengthened to balance the powerful plantar flexors. Imbalances between the pretibial muscles and the gastrocsoleus have been associated with running injuries.[86] Lower extremity stretching of the hamstrings and iliopsoas/quadriceps was instituted to improve the overall lower kinetic function. Alterations in muscle function, including poor flexibility, can predispose or precipitate musculoskeletal injuries.[87,88]

Interval training on the bicycle ergometer served to maintain the athlete's cardiovascular status and lower extremity strength.[35,36] Gastrocsoleus stretching with both the knee straight and flexed served to stretch the gastrocnemius and soleus portions of the Achilles tendon. Stretching all muscle groups after cycling served to maintain the plastic deformation of those tissues gained during treatment.[22,51,52] Placing the Achilles tendon on static stretch during icing served to maintain the plastic deformation while reducing any inflammation provoked during treatment. The athlete was asked to perform the home program to maintain and increase slowly gains made during the treatment session. It is reasonable to request a high school student to perform a home program once daily and expect compliance.

Heel lifts of 12 to 15 cm relieved tension on the Achilles tendon during the symptomatic phase.[80] Lifts were placed in both shoes to prevent a secondary leg length discrepancy. A firm, well-fitted heel counter and moderately flared heel provide adequate rearfoot stability. It is the author's belief that with consistent continued wear, running shoes should be replaced every 4 to 6 months. Excessive shoe wear has been implicated as a factor in overuse injuries.[89]

Week 2

Physical therapy was continued three times per week during the second week. Phonophoresis treatments continued with the ultrasound parameters changed to a continuous duty cycle, and the tendon was placed on static stretch for these treatments. Resistive plantar flexion exercises were added using the large elastic band. Cycling followed by low-intensity noninterval Stairmaster workouts for 5, 10, and 15 minutes completed each physical therapy visit. The resistive plantar flexion exercises were added to the home program.

Treatment Results. At the end of week 2, the athlete reported a significant overall decrease in her symptoms. She exhibited pain-free ambulation up hills and climbing stairs. Passive dorsiflexion equaled 12° bilaterally.

Treatment Rationale. The thermal effects of ultrasound were desired at this stage of rehabilitation. These thermal effects include an increase in tissue extensibility, blood flow, and nerve conduction velocity as well as decreases in pain and spasm.[90] Ultrasound in combination with a prolonged static stretch was implemented for reasons stated in Case 3.

Muscle atrophy of the gastrocsoleus is inevitable following an Achilles tendon injury,[81] and resistive plantar flexion exercises begin to retrain the gastrocsoleus complex in a controlled manner. Cardiovascular fitness was maintained with cycling and challenged with the Stairmaster. It is the author's opinion that the Stairmaster serves as an interim between the non–weight-bearing activity of cycling and the loads sustained during running. With full contact of both feet on the pedals of the Stairmaster, weight bearing is achieved with a reduced amount of force on the tendon compared with running.

Stretching and ice completed all treatments. The resistive plantar flexion exercises were added to the athlete's home program.

Week 3

Treatment Plan. Physical therapy was given three times per week for the third week. A warm whirlpool was used during the initial 10 minutes of treatment before a 10-minute warm-up period on the bicycle ergometer. Next, all stretching exercises preceded toe raises. The athlete performed double and single leg toe raises. Three sets of 20 repetitions were performed using 0, 10, and 20 pounds increasing on each consecutive day of treatment. Three sets of 10 repetitions of eccentrics were performed by the athlete raising up with two legs and lowering herself with the involved side. Eccentrics were performed with 0, 5, and 10 pounds increasing on each consecutive day of treatment. Stairmaster workouts were increased to interval training of moderate intensity for 20, 25, and 30 minutes on each consecutive day of treatment. All lower extremity stretches and icing of the Achilles tendon completed each treatment session. Concentric toe raises were added to the home program.

Treatment Results. The athlete experienced delayed onset muscle soreness 12 hours after the first eccentric training session. The Achilles tendon was not painful to palpation or at the end range of passive dorsiflexion.

Treatment Rationale. Warm hydrotherapy was used for the heating effects on connective tissue reported in Case 2. Strengthening of the Achilles tendon gastrocsoleus complex was progressed. In restoring a body part to preinjury status, Arnheim and Prentice[92] denote muscle strength as one of the most important factors. The maximal load of an eccentric contraction is placed on the Achilles tendon during the landing phase of running following foot strike[80]; therefore, eccentrics were added to the program.

Delayed onset muscle soreness was experienced possibly from muscle damage and swelling of the connective tissue after eccentric exercise.[93] Eccentrics were performed only three times that week during therapy and not added to the home program to allow adequate time for recovery.

Week 4

Treatment Plan. Physical therapy continued three times per week. Sessions were similar to those during week 3 except the Stairmaster was replaced with light jogging on the treadmill, 0% incline for 10, 20, and 30 minutes increasing each consecutive day of treatment. The speed of the treadmill was 1 mile per hour less than her last season's average mile time. New running shoes were worn. The home program remained unchanged.

Treatment Results. The athlete was pain free before, during, and after each treatment session.

Treatment Rationale. Progressive increases of running distance at submaximal levels were used to increase gradually the stress on the Achilles tendon without reinjuring the tissue.

Week 5

Treatment Plan. Physical therapy continued three times per week. An isokinetic test was performed on the plantar flexors and dorsiflexor of the ankle. The right plantar flexors presented with a 10% deficit when compared with the left. Hydrotherapy was discontinued. Five minutes of cycling preceded stretching exercises. Treadmill running, 0% incline, was performed for 15, 25, and 35 minutes progressing on each consecutive day of treatment. The running speed was increased to tolerance. The athlete was instructed to begin running on flat even surfaces and to increase her mileage slowly. Her return to running included the following guidelines: Run every other day for 2 weeks; run a maximum of 5 days per week for the following month; stop running if pain is experienced while running; replace lost time with stationary cycling; and decrease the distance and speed on the next run. For pain after running, the athlete decreased the workout by 50% and increased at a rate of 10% per week, and each workout was preceded by a warm-up and stretch period and followed by a cooldown, stretch, and ice.

Treatment Results. By the end of week 5, the athlete had returned to her average running speed and distance without aggravation of her symptoms. The athlete was ready to return to training with her team and was discharged from physical therapy.

Treatment Rationale. Sufficient dorsiflexion ROM and soft tissue healing was achieved, and cycling served as a practical and appropriate method of warming up. Isokinetic testing of the ankle demonstrated sufficient strength for the plantar flexion strengthening to be continued with the home program. The running guidelines should facilitate a return to competitive level without the risk of reinjury.[94]

CASE 6: ACHILLES TENDON REPAIR

Rehabilitation of a surgically repaired Achilles tendon is examined in this section. Predisposing and precipitating factors are identified and discussed.

Initial Evaluation and Findings

A 45-year-old computer programmer ruptured his left Achilles tendon while playing racquetball 7 weeks ago. The patient reported he had played racquetball one to two times per month for the past year and had been experiencing some occasional left heel and calf pain but attributed it to his poor physical condition. On injury, he heard a loud pop and experienced a pain similar to that of being struck with his partner's racquet on the back of the heel. The intensity of the pain decreased; however, he was unable to walk without assistance. He underwent an open repair for a type II rupture and end-to-end anastomosis within 1 week of the initial injury. Following surgery, he was casted above the knee for 2 weeks followed by a below-the-knee cast for 2 weeks. A gradual increase in dorsiflexion was used during the casting. The patient then wore a compressive elastic bandage and a lower leg walking boot, which maintained the ankle joint in a neutral position. At this point, the patient was PWB, progressing to FWB by the sixth postoperative week. The patient performed active ankle dorsiflexion out of the walking boot daily, and a splint was worn at night.

The initial evaluation revealed a 2-cm increase in the figure-eight girth measurements of the left ankle when compared with the right. A 5-cm scar appeared on the posteromedial aspect of the lower leg. Distal pulses and sensation were intact. Gross MMTs demonstrated decreases in left lower extremity strength, although only marked atrophy of the gastrocsoleus complex was noted.

Interpretation

The history given was typical for many cases of Achilles tendon ruptures. It is well noted that many of these injuries occur in middle-aged individuals participating in recreational sports requiring sudden acceleration or jumping.[95,96] These individuals are usually not in adequate physical condition and often have sedentary occupations. Research supports chronic degeneration as a precipitating factor in Achilles tendon ruptures.[95-98] This patient's reports of chronic tendonitis-like symptoms support the literature.

Type II injuries are classified as greater than a 50% rupture, up to a 3-cm defect, and are successfully anastomosed followed by a series of castings.[97,98] It is recommended that a series of cast changes take place following surgical repair to dorsiflex the foot progressively to stretch the muscle tendon unit and slow the progression of atrophy.[95]

The mild edema is common after an open repair, and the extended period of immobilization and non–weight bearing contributed to the strength decreases.[21,24,47]

Treatment

The primary goal of treatment is to regain gradually strength and tension to the Achilles tendon.

Week 1

Treatment Plan. The first week of therapy consisted of three treatment sessions per week, including warm whirlpools, pulsed ultrasound, active ROM ankle exercises, passive dorsiflexion, isometrics for plantar flexion, progressive resistive exercises for the remainder of the left lower extremity, and cryotherapy.

The patient performed active ROM exercises while in the warm whirlpool for 20 minutes at the start of each treatment session. Pulsed duty-cycle ultrasound treatments were given as in Case 5. The therapist carefully applied a manual low-load prolonged stretch to the Achilles tendon–gastrocsoleus complex for 5 to 10 minutes, progressing each treatment session. Isometrics were performed in a neutral position. Progressive resistive exercises were used to strengthen the remainder of the left lower extremity. With the foot and ankle elevated, 20 minutes of ice with a compression wrap terminated each treatment session. The patient wore his compressive elastic bandage at all times outside of therapy.

A home program consisting of passive dorsiflexion stretching with a towel for a 30-second hold repeating 10 times, active ankle ROM exercises, isometrics, and icing for 15 minutes in a slightly dorsiflexed position or at least neutral was implemented.

Treatment Results. At the end of the first week, passive dorsiflexion equaled 5° with the knee straight and 7° with the knee bent. Figure-eight girth measurements were 1 cm apart.

Treatment Rationale. Warm hydrotherapy, active ROM exercises, and manual controlled passive ROM exercises were implemented for reasons mentioned in Case 2. The pulsed ultrasound was used for its nonthermal effects on tendon healing discussed in Case 5. Disuse atrophy and secondary weakness of the adjacent muscle groups were addressed by the isometrics and progressive resistive exercises. Elevation, compression, and ice have all been mentioned in previous cases for their effectiveness in edema and pain reduction as well as maintenance of deformation in plastic tissue. The home program is intended to maintain progress gained in therapy sessions.

Weeks 2 and 3

Treatment Plan. Physical therapy sessions continued three times per week, and treatments were similar to those during week 1. Ultrasound treatments were given with a continuous mode. Standing heel cord stretching was added with the knee straight and the knee bent; however, the patient always maintained 50% or more of his body weight on the uninvolved extremity. Mild resistive ankle exercises were introduced using a large elastic band for plantar flexion, dorsiflexion, inversion, and eversion of the ankle. The patient wore his walking boot and placed the pedal under the midfoot during stationary biking. The standing heel cord stretches were added to the home program.

Treatment Results. Increases in dorsiflexion equaled 10° and 12° with the knee extended and flexed, respectively. Figure-eight girth measurements were equal bilaterally.

Treatment Rationale. The thermal effects of ultrasound discussed in previous cases were now desired. By 8 and 9 weeks postoperatively, sufficient tendon healing had taken place to apply the increased stress of weight-bearing stretches, light resistive exercise, and non–weight-bearing exercise. Cycling promoted cardiovascular fitness and strengthening of the lower extremity.[35,36]

Weeks 4, 5, and 6

Treatment Plan. The walking boot was removed at the beginning of week 4. Ultrasound treatments were discontinued. All resistive exercises were increased to tolerance, and stationary biking was performed without the walking boot. Stairmaster workouts at mild intensities were added during week 5, and eccentric strength training of the gastrocsoleus complex began during week 6 following parameters given in Case 5.

Treatment Results. Increases in dorsiflexion equaled 16° and 20° with the knee extended and flexed, respectively. Isokinetic testing of the lower quarter demonstrated symmetry of all muscle groups except the plantar flexors. The left plantar flexors had a 30% deficit when compared with the right.

Treatment Rationale. Progression to ambulation without the walking boot was appropriate and reasonable for the length of time since surgery. Stairmaster workouts and eccentrics were appropriate for reasons discussed in Case 5.

Weeks 7, 8, 9, and 10

Treatment Plan. A biomechanical foot assessment was performed and temporary orthotics fabricated. Strengthening and stretching progressed and a "back to run" program was initiated during week 10. Physical therapy sessions were reduced to two times per week.

Isokinetic strengthening of the plantar flexors and dorsiflexors was initiated. The back to run program resembled that in Case 1. A biomechanical foot assessment revealed a 10° forefoot varus deformity bilaterally and overpronation of the left foot throughout the stance phase.

Temporary orthotics were fabricated with medial posting of the forefoot and rearfoot with a 12-mm heel lift.

Treatment Results. The isokinetic deficit was reduced to 18% for the left plantar flexors. The patient was asymptomatic during his back to run program.

Treatment Rationale. Isokinetic strengthening facilitated a reduction in the plantar flexor strength deficit. The orthoses warranted by the static and dynamic biomechanical foot assessment limited his overpronation. Functional overpronation is one of the three most prevalent etiologic factors in Achilles tendinitis according to Clement.[80]

Week 11

The patient was seen once and casted for permanent orthotics. On reassessment, dorsiflexion ROM was 20° and isokinetic strength deficits were less than 15% for the left plantar flexors. The patient was discharged from therapy and periodically followed for orthotic fabrication.

SPECIAL CASES (INJURIES IN PROFESSIONAL SPORTS)

The following cases are presented to compare the similarities and differences in treating the professional athletes and the typical patient population. Rationales for the various treatments are not given in detail in this section; however, references from the previous six cases may be applied.

CASE 1: INSERTIONAL ACHILLES TENDINITIS

A 31-year-old professional baseball player complained of acute left heel pain and dysfunction after running bases.

History

The injury occurred during the eighth inning of game 70 in a 162-game schedule. The game was the third in a three-game series. The previous sequence of field surfaces included 10 games on artificial surfaces, 3 on natural surfaces, and a return to an artificial surface for the present series.

This athlete wore a cleated shoe that caused similar problems with other players secondary to its deep heel rake and lack of adequate heel flair. The lift on the shoe was 24 mm.

Interpretation

Contributing factors of this injury included a prolonged playing schedule, playing surface changes, and an offending shoe design. The effects of fatigue and deconditioning contribute to the high injury periods often experienced in professional baseball. These periods occur in mid-June, when approximately 65 to 80 games have been played, and then again in mid-August, when approximately 120 to 135 games have been played.

Initial Evaluation and Significant Findings

On evaluation, there was edema present in the area of the distal Achilles tendon and the site of insertion to the calcaneus. ROM for plantar flexion and dorsiflexion was equal; however, the involved side was painful with forced dorsiflexion. The athlete demonstrated acute pain directly over his calcaneus. The remaining ankle examination was unremarkable. The athlete related his heel being sore for a number of games but tolerated the situation and performed without dysfunction. This athlete had been treated for a similar injury to his right heel during spring training two seasons prior.

Immediate care was to place the injured area in ice and to elevate the ankle. After the initial treatment, the injury was prepared for travel by placing the ankle in a compressive wrap and adequate ice to prevent further edema owing to air travel. Arrangements were made to be evaluated by an orthopedist the following day.

On the physician's evaluation, the athlete was placed on an oral anti-inflammatory medication, and it was suggested that a magnetic resonance imaging (MRI) should be performed. The MRI scan was scheduled for the athlete's return home in 4 days.

Treatment

The treatment plan was to control the pain, reduce the inflammation, reduce the edema, develop increased ROM in dorsiflexion, increase strength, and, importantly, alter the causative factors within the physical therapist's control. Treatment continued with the introduction of electrical stimulation (ES), contrast baths limited to body temperature, passive motion, aggressive hamstring stretching, and mild heel cord stretching.

ES was introduced with an H-Wave (Electronic Waveform Lab., Inc.). A pattern of interference using two channels with pad placement, insuring coverage of the painful bone site, and developing the interference at the critical zone of the Achilles was employed. The frequency was set to 1 and the intensity between 7 and 9 for the first 20 minutes. This was followed by 10 minutes of a frequency of 10 with the intensity set to tolerance that was increased to tolerance at 1-minute intervals for the next 2 minutes.

ES treatment was followed by a contrast bath beginning with a body temperature whirlpool for 5 minutes followed by immersion in ice for a period of 1 minute. The sequence continued reducing the whirlpool time by a minute a cycle (i.e., 5/1–4/1–3/1–2/1–1/1).

Passive motion was then initiated for the ankle using a basic ROM series involving (1) dorsiflexion with knee flexion, (2) dorsiflexion with knee extension, (3) eversion, (4) planter flexion with knee extension, (5) plantar flexion with knee flexion, and (6) inversion. This pattern of motion was repeated in repetitions of 10 for a period of not less than 20 minutes per treatment. This was followed by hamstring stretching.

The athlete was compressed, elevated, and placed in ice at the conclusion of the treatment. This protocol was followed for the first 3 days of treatment, whereupon the temperatures of the contrast bath slowly increased and the ROM exercises slowly developed into a resistive process.

MRI was performed on the fifth day postinjury and revealed the following: chronic Achilles tendinitis with an interstitial tear of the lateral aspect of the distal Achilles tendon, Achilles edema, and edema of the marrow at the calcaneus at the insertion of the Achilles tendon. The athlete was also examined by the team orthopedist and was counseled as to his return to play.

Treatment was accelerated to include a tiltboard and controlled treadmill jogging.

Summary

It is beyond the physical therapist's ability to control the playing surface or the frequency of change from one surface to the other. The athletic shoe has to be a major component in this circumstance. A shoe had to be found with a reduced heel rake, and a heel lift was added to the rearfoot. The player's shoes were fitted with a lift between the spike plate and the sock liner that consisted of a combination of ½ inch of Temperstick foam and ⅛ inch of adhesive foam. The authors have found this combination to be satisfactory when compressed by the player's body weight. The athlete returned to play on the fifth night and continued being treated for the next 5 weeks.

CASE 2: LATERAL LIGAMENT SPRAIN

A 23-year-old professional baseball player injured his left ankle while base running.

History and Initial Evaluation

The injury occurred during game 70 of a 162-game schedule. As the athlete rounded first base following a base hit, he planted his left foot squarely on the top of the base and rolled his ankle into plantar flexion and inversion. He was immediately removed from the field for an evaluation.

The athlete was examined by a physician and diagnosed with a sprain of the lateral ankle ligaments with a +1 anterior drawer sign. Radiographs were deferred until the next morning to allow more time for edema reduction and therefore a more accurate assessment.

Immediate Care

The athlete's ankle was placed in a compression wrap with ice and elevated for 20 minutes following the physician's examination. The ankle was then placed in a compression boot for 40 minutes. This ice and compression 60-minute cycle was repeated again before the athlete was transported from the stadium. A new compression wrap and protective brace were applied before leaving for the hotel. Three more cycles of ice followed by compression were administered at the team's hotel.

Treatment and Return to Play

Initial radiographs were negative for fractures, and treatment began the next day. The treatment plan was to continue to control the edema, control the pain, maintain the active ROM, and restore strength to the affected ankle.

The first day of treatment included changing the compression wrap and replacing it with new material. Before the application of this wrap, electrodes were placed both medially and laterally on the ankle distal to the malleolus. The leads were freed through the compression material so they could be accessed. ES cables were connected to the electrodes and taped for safety. The entire limb was placed in a compression boot and elevated. The cables connected to the ES (Intelect VMS, Chattanooga Corp.). ES was introduced at 200 pulses per seconds at a level of sensation for the first 20 minutes of the 40-minute compression cycle.

After the compression cycle, the ankle was passively moved in the manner previously described for three sets of 10 repetitions. The ankle was then placed in ice and again evaluated. This protocol was repeated four times during the first day.

The second day of treatment included the previous modalities with the addition of heel and toe walking. Resistance was added to the planes of motion in the third set of the manual exercises that were tolerable.

The third day of treatment, the athlete was able to run in place, and an incline board was introduced. The athlete was required to run in place to a count of 50 in all four directions on the incline board. Resistance was added to two sets of the manual exercise.

On the fourth day, a contrast bath and ultrasound were added. The tiltboard was added for both range and strength. The athlete was now confident enough to begin working at his playing skills.

On the seventh day, the athlete and physical therapist returned to the home stadium. The player was evaluated by the team orthopedist and counseled that he could return to play when the athlete felt confident he could perform at the skill level that was necessary to compete.

Treatments were reduced to twice a day and now included the use of continuous passive movement equipment for both plantar flexion/dorsiflexion and inversion/eversion. Trampoline running was added to the incline board.

Base running was added at day 8. The ankle was protected with standard athletic tape in a basket weave manner. A double heel lock with double figure-eight was done in elastic tape. A brace (Active Ankle, Medical Biomet, Inc.) was used in conjunction with the tape. The athlete returned to play the following day. Treatments were continued for the following 6 weeks.

SUMMARY

Similarities and differences exist in the treatment of professional athletes and the average patient population. Injuries to the foot and ankle are often caused by overuse or improper training. Pain and edema reduction; restoration of motion, strength, balance, and function; and provision of proper support to promote healing are all necessary in treating any type of patient. Although functional goals and outcomes vary between the professional athlete and the average patient population, the rationale for effective treatment remains the same.

Several pathologic entities have been identified in this chapter. Some possible corresponding treatments for these pathologic entities have been highlighted in a clinical scenario. The scientific basis for each of the employed treatments was developed.

The reader is urged to remember that there are many ways to approach the various clinical problems discussed here. This chapter is not intended to be a definitive statement on the best (or only) way to treat the identified problems but rather as a guide with which to approach the foot using physical therapy modalities. Until such time as scientific research is available affirming the best way to treat a particular problem, clinicians must explore all feasible treatment approaches.

REFERENCES

1. Wolf, SL (ed): Clinical Decision Making in Physical Therapy. FA Davis, Philadelphia, 1985.
2. Roy, S and Irwin, R: Sports Medicine: Prevention, Evaluation, Management, and Rehabilitation. Prentice-Hall, Englewood Cliffs, NJ, 1983.
3. Kessler, RM and Hertling, D: The ankle and hindfoot. In Kessler, RM and Hertling, D: Management of Common Musculoskeletal Disorders: Physical Therapy Principles and Methods. Harper & Row, Philadelphia, 1983, p 448.
4. O'Donoghue, DH: Injuries of the ankle. In O'Donoghue, DH: Treatment of Injuries to Athletes. WB Saunders, Philadelphia, 1976, p 698.
5. Ruch, JA, Downey, MS, and Malay, DS: Ankle fractures. In McGlamry, ED (ed): Comprehensive Textbook of Foot Surgery, vol 2. Williams & Wilkins, Baltimore, 1987.
6. Donatelli, R and Owens-Burkart, H: Effects of immobilization in the extensibility of periarticular connective tissue. J Orthop Sports Phys Ther 3:67, 1981.
7. Kowal, MA: Review of physiological effects of cryotherapy J Orthop Sports Phys Ther 5:66, 1983.
8. Lehman, JF, Warren, CG, and Scham, SM: Therapeutic heat and cold. Clin Orthop 99:207, 1974.
9. Michlovitz, SL: Cryotherapy: The use of cold as a therapeutic agent. In Michlovitz SL (ed): Thermal Agents in Rehabilitation. FA Davis, Philadelphia, 1986.
10. Starkey, J: Treatment of ankle sprains by simultaneous use of intermittent compression and ice packs. Am J Sports Med 4:142, 1976.
11. Michlovitz, S, Smith, W, and Watkins M: Ice and high-voltage pulsed stimulation in treatment of acute lateral ankle sprains. J Orthop Sports Phys Ther 9:301, 1988.
12. Reed, BV: Effect of high-voltage pulsed electrical stimulation on microvascular permeability to plasma proteins: A possible mechanism in minimizing edema. Phys Ther 68:491, 1988.
13. Bettany, JA, Fish, OR, and Mandel, FC: Influence of high voltage pulsed direct current on edema formation following impact injury. Phys Ther 70:219, 1990.
14. Griffin, JW, Newsome, LS, Sralka, S, and Wright, PE: Reduction of chronic post traumatic hand edema: A comparison of high voltage pulsed current, intermittent pneumatic compression, and placebo treatments. Phys Ther 70:279, 1990.
15. Cosgrove, KA, Alon, G, Bell, SF, et al: The electrical effect of two commonly used clinical stimulators on traumatic edema in rats. Phys Ther 72:227, 1992.
16. Sims, D: Effects of positioning on ankle edema. J Orthop Sports Phys Ther 8:30, 1986.
17. Beard, G and Wood, EC: Effects of massage. In Beard, G and Wood, EC: Massage: Principles and Techniques. WB Saunders, Philadelphia, 1965, p 46.
18. Akeson, WH, Amiel, D, and Woo, S: Immobility effects of synovial joints: The pathomechanics of joint contracture. Biorheology 17:95, 1980.
19. Enneking, W and Horowitz, M: The intra-articular effects of immobilization on the human knee. J Bone Joint Surg 54A:973, 1972.
20. McDonough, AL: Effects of immobilization and exercise on articular cartilage: A review of literature. J Orthop Sports Phys Ther 3:2, 1981.
21. Perry, J: Scientific basis of rehabilitation. Instr Course Lect 34:385, 1985.
22. Sapega, AA, Quedenfeld, TC, Moyer, RA, et al: Biophysical factors in range of motion exercise. Phys Sports Med 9:57, 1981.
23. Salter, RB, Simmonds, DF, Malcolm, BW, et al: The biological effect of continuous passive motion on the healing of full-thickness defects in articular cartilage. J Bone Joint Surg 62A:1232, 1980.
24. Tabary, JC, Tabary, C, Tardieu, C, et al: Physiological and structural changes in the cat's soleus muscle due to immobilization at different lengths by plaster casts. J Physiol 224:231, 1972.
25. Woo, S, Matthews, JV, Akeson, WH, et al: Connective tissue response to immobility: Correlative study of biomechanical and biochemical measurements of normal and immobilized rabbit knees. Arthritis Rheum 18:257, 1975.
26. Glick, JM, Gordon, RB, and Nishimoto, D: The prevention and treatment of ankle injuries. Am J Sports Med 4:136, 1976.
27. Tropp, H, Askling, C, and Gillquist, J: Prevention of ankle sprains. Am J Sports Med 13:259, 1985.
28. Freeman, MAR: Instability of the foot after injuries to the lateral ligament of the ankle. J Bone Joint Surg 47B:669, 1965.
29. Freeman, MAR: Treatment of ruptures of the lateral ligaments of the ankle. J Bone Joint Surg 47B:661, 1965.
30. Kay, DB: The sprained ankle. Current therapy. Foot Ankle 6:22, 1985.

31. Milch, LD: Rehabilitation exercises following inversion ankle sprains. J Am Podiatr Med Assoc 76:577, 1986.
32. Gross, MT: Effects of recurrent lateral ankle sprains on active and passive judgements of joint position. Phys Ther 67:1505, 1987.
33. Freeman, MAR, Dean, MRF, and Hanham, IWF: The etiology and prevention of functional instability of the foot. J Bone Joint Surg 47B:678, 1965.
34. DeCarlo, MS and Talbot, RW: Evaluation of ankle joint proprioception following injection of the anterior talofibular ligament. J Orthop Sports Phys Ther 8:70, 1986.
35. Moroz, DE and Houston, ME: The effects of replacing endurance running training with cycling in female runners. Can J Sports Sci 12:131, 1987.
36. Nicholas, JA and Hershman, EB (eds): The Lower Extremity and Spine in Sports Medicine. CV Mosby, St. Louis, 1986.
37. Scranton, PE, Whitesel, JP, and Farewell, V: Cybex evaluation of the relationship between anterior and posterior compartment lower leg muscles. Foot Ankle 6:85, 1985.
38. Davies, GJ: Subtalar joint, ankle joint, and shin pain testing and rehabilitation. In Davis GJ (ed): A Compendium of Isokinetics in Clinical Usage and Clinical Notes. S&S Publishers, LaCrosse, WI, 1984, p 123.
39. Arem, AJ and Madden, JW: Effects of stress on healing wounds: I. Intermittent non-cyclical tension. J Surg Res 20:93, 1976.
40. Levenson, SM, Geever, EF, Crowley, IV, et al: The healing of rat skin wounds. Ann Surg 161:293, 1965.
41. Wong, DLK, Glasheen-Wray, M, and Andrew, LF: Isokinetic evaluation of the ankle invertors and evertors. J Orthop Sports Phys Ther 5:246, 1984.
42. Brody, DM: Part III: Rehabilitation of the injured runner. Instr Course Lect 33:268, 1984.
43. James, SL, Bates, BT, and Ostering, LR: Injuries to runners. Am J Sports Med 6:40, 1978.
44. Mennell, JM: Joint Pain: Diagnosis and Treatment Using Manipulative Techniques, ed 1. Little, Brown, Boston, 1964.
45. Wooden, MJ: Mobilization of the lower extremity. In Donatelli, R and Wooden, MJ (eds): Orthopedic Physical Therapy. Churchill Livingstone, New York, 1989.
46. Kloth, L: Shortwave and microwave diathermy. In Michlovitz, SL (ed): Thermal Agents in Rehabilitation. FA Davis, Philadelphia, 1986, p 177.
47. Cooper, RR: Alterations during immobilization and regeneration of skeletal muscle in cats. J Bone Joint Surg 54A:919, 1972.
48. Maitland, GD: Peripheral Manipulation, ed 2. Butterworths, Boston, 1977.
49. Michael, RH and Holder, LE: The soleus syndrome: A cause of medial tibial stress (shin splints). Am J Sports Med 13:87, 1985.
50. Tiberio, D: Evaluation of functional ankle dorsiflexion using subtalar neutral position. A clinical report. Phys Ther 67:995, 1987.
51. Michlovitz, SL: Biophysical principles of heating and superficial heat agents. In Michlovitz, SL (ed): Thermal Agents in Rehabilitation. FA Davis, Philadelphia, 1986, p 99.
52. Warren, GC, Lehman, JF, and Koblanski, JN: Heat and stretch procedures: An evaluation using rat tail tendon. Arch Phys Med Rehab 57:122, 1976.
53. Wyke, B: The neurology of joints. Ann R Coll Surg Engl 41:25, 1967.
54. Kahn, J: Ionotophoresis. In Principles and Practice of Electrotherapy. Churchill Livingstone, New York, 1987, p 153.
55. Boone, DC: Applications of Ionotophoresis. In Wolf S (ed): Clinics in Physical Therapy: Electrotherapy. Churchill Livingstone, New York, 1986, p 99.
56. Gangarosa, LP, Park, NH, Fong, BC, et al: Conductivity of drugs used for iontophoresis. J Pharm Sci 67:1439, 1978.
57. Glass, JM, Stephen, RL, and Jacobson, SC: The quantity and distribution of radiolabeled dexamethasone delivered to tissue by iontophoresis. Int J Dermatol 19:519, 1980.
58. Puttemans, FJM, et al: Iontophoresis: Mechanism of action studied by potentiometry and x-ray flurorescence. Arch Phys Med Rehab 63:176, 1982.
59. Tregeat, RT: The permeability of mammalian skin to ions. J Invest Dermatol 46:16, 1966.
60. Zankel, HT, Cress, RH, and Kamin, H: Iontophoresis studies with a radioactive tracer. Arch Phys Med Rehab 40:192, 1959.
61. Harris, PR: Iontophoresis: Clinical research in musculoskeletal inflammatory conditions. J Orthop Sports Phys Ther 4:109, 1982.
62. Bertolucci, LE: Introduction of antiinflammatory drugs by iontophoresis. A double blind study. J Orthop Sports Phys Ther 4:103, 1982.
63. Olerod, C: The pronation capacity of the foot: Its consequences for axial deformity after tibial shaft fractures. Arch Orthop Trauma Surg 104:303, 1985.
64. Ting, AJ, et al: The role of subtalar motion and ankle contact pressure changes from.angular deformities of the tibia. Foot Ankle 7:290, 1987.
65. Donatelli, R: Normal biomechanics of the foot and ankle. J Orthop Sports Phys Ther 7:91, 1985.
66. McPoil, TG and Knecht, HG: Biomechanics of the foot in walking: A functional approach. J Orthop Sports Phys Ther 7:69, 1985.

67. Root, ML, Orien, WP, and Weed, JH: Normal and Abnormal Function of the Foot: Clinical Biomechanics, vol 2. Clinical Biomechanics Corporation, Los Angeles, 1977.
68. Subotnick, SI: Biomechanics of the subtalar and midtarsal joints. J Am Podiatr Med Assoc 65:756, 1975.
69. Garbaloser, JC, et al: The frontal plane relationship of the forefoot to the rearfoot in an asymptomatic population. J Orthop Sports Phys Ther 20:200–206, 1994.
70. Bordelon, RL: Subcalcaneal pain: A method of evaluation and plan for treatment. Clin Orthop 177:49, 1983.
71. Kushner, S and Reid, DC: Medial tarsal tunnel syndrome: A review. J Orthop Sports Phys Ther 6:39, 1984.
72. Kwong, PK, et al: Plantar fasciitis: Mechanics and pathomechanics of treatment. Clin Sports Med 7:119, 1988.
73. McBryde, AM: Plantar fasciitis. Instruc Course Lect 278, 1984.
74. Sarrafian, S: Functional characteristics of the foot and plantar aponeurosis under tibiotalar loading. Foot Ankle 8:4, 1987.
75. Wessling, KC, DeVane, DA, and Hylton, CR: Effects of static stretch versus static stretch and ultrasound combined on triceps surae muscle extensibility in healthy women. Phys Ther 67:675, 1987.
76. Shikoff, MD, Figura, MA, and Postar, SE: A retrospective study of 195 patients with heel pain. J Am Podiatr Med Assoc 76:71, 1986.
77. Biossonault, W and Donatelli, R: The influence of hallux extension on the foot during ambulation. J Orthop Sports Phys Ther 5:240, 1984.
78. Bojsen-Moller, F and Lamoreux, L: Significance of free dorsiflexion of the toes in walking. Acta Orthop Scand 50:471, 1979.
79. Clanton, TO, Butler, JE, and Eggert, A: Injuries to the metatarsophalangeal joints in athletes. Foot Ankle 7:162, 1986.
80. Clement, DB, Taunton, JE, and Smart, GW: Achilles tendinitis and peritendinitis: Etiology and treatment. Am J Sports Med 12:179–184, 1984.
81. Galloway, MT, Joki, P, and Dayton, OW: Achilles tendon overuse injuries. Clin Sports Med 11:771–782, 1992.
82. Buchbinder, MK, Napora, NJ, and Briggs, EW: The relationship of abnormal pronation to chondromalacia of the patella in distance runners. J Am Podiatr Assoc 69:159–162, 1979.
83. Lagerern, C and Lindholm, A: Vascular distribution of the Achilles tendon—an angiographic and microangiographic study. Acta Chir Scand 116:491–495, 1958/59.
84. Rathburn, JR and McNab, I: The microvascular pattern of the rotator cuff. J Bone Joint Surg 52B:540–553, 1970.
85. Dyson, M: Therapeutic applications of ultrasound. In Nyberg, WL, Ziskin MC (eds): Biological Effects of Ultrasound (Clinics in Diagnostic Ultrasound). New York, Churchill Livington, 1985.
86. Michlovitz, SL (ed): Thermal Agents in Rehabilitation. Philadelphia, FA Davis, 1986.
87. Subtonick, SI: The shin splints syndrome of the lower extremity. Podiatr Sports Med 66:43, 1976.
88. James, SL and Brubaker, CE: Biomechanics of running. Orthop Clin North Am 4:605, 1973.
89. Elliot, B and Achland, T: Biomechanical effects of fatigue of 10,000 meter running techniques. Res Quart Exer Sports 52:160, 1981.
90. Clancy, WG: Runner's injuries. Am J Sports Med 8:137, 1980.
91. Gannm, N: Ultrasound concepts. Clin Management 11:64–69, 1991.
92. Arnheim, DD and Prentice, WE: Principles of Athletic Training, ed 8. Mosby-Year Book, St. Louis, 1993.
93. Armstrong, RB, Ogilvie, RW, and Schwane, JA: Eccentric exercised-induced injury to rat skeletal muscle. Proceedings of the American Physiology Society, 1983.
94. Brody, DM: Techniques in the evaluation and treatment of the injured runner. Orthop Clin North Am 13:541–588, 1982.
95. FitzGibbons, R, Hefferon, J, and Hill, J: Percutaneous Achilles tendon repair. Am J Sports Med 21:724–747, 1993.
96. Landvater, S and Renstrom, P: Complete Achilles tendon ruptures. Clin Sports Med 11:741–756, 1992.
97. Kuwada, G: Critical analysis of tendo Achilles repair using Achilles tendon rupture classification system and repair. J Foot Ankle Surg 32:611–614, 1993.
98. Kvist, M, Jozsa, L, and Jarvinen, M: Vascular changes in the ruptured Achilles tendon and paratendon. Int Orthop 16:377–382, 1992.
99. Reinherz, RP, Granoff, S, and Westerfield, M: Pathologic afflictions of the Achilles tendon. J Foot Surg 30:117–121, 1991.

CHAPTER 12

The Application of Kinetic Chain Rehabilitation in the Lower Extremities

Bruce Greenfield, MMSc, PT, OCS
J. Gregory Bennett, MS, PT

Rehabilitation is essential to restore normal function after musculoskeletal injury or surgery. The application of skilled rehabilitation has evolved over the last 10 years into a sophisticated array of exercise and motor learning strategies that has resulted in a large body of scientific principles of exercise application and progression. These principles have been applied to treating orthopedic injuries and postsurgical cases with varying degrees of success and have empowered rehabilitation specialists to be adept clinical decision makers and to be well versed in current trends of rehabilitation. One of the most intriguing principles in rehabilitation is the use of kinetic (kinematic) chain concepts in exercise prescription.[1–8]

The hip, knee, and ankle joints compose the lower extremity kinetic chain. Movement of all three of these joints in unison represents a kinetic chain movement and can be used for lower extremity exercise in addition to traditional exercises, such as seated quadriceps muscle extensions that isolate one link in the kinetic chain.[2] Kinetic chain training differs from traditional training in several areas, and the rehabilitation specialist should consider the characteristics of each exercise mode in formulating a rehabilitation program (Table 12–1).

The purposes of this chapter are to review the characteristics of kinetic chain training, review the application of kinetic chain training in rehabilitation, develop an understanding of the interdependency and interrelationship of lower kinetic chain movement to the foot and ankle, and incorporate the information into case studies.

TABLE 12–1 Open Kinematic Chain and Closed Kinematic Chain Exercises: Differential Features

Exercise Mode	Characteristics	Advantages	Disadvantages
Open Kinematic Chain	Single muscle group	Isolated recruitment	Limited function
	Single axis and plane	Simple movement pattern	Limited function
	Emphasize concentric contraction	Isolated recruitment	Limited function
	Non–weight bearing	Minimal joint compression	Less proprioception and joint stability with increased joint shear forces
Closed Kinematic Chain	Multiple muscle groups	Functional recruitment	Difficult to isolate
	Multiple axes and planes	Functional movement patterns	More complex
	Balance of concentric and eccentric contractions	Functional contractions	Loss of control of target joint
	Weight-bearing exercise	Increased proprioception and joint stability	Compressive forces on articular surfaces

From Greenfield, BH and Tovin, BJ: The application of open and closed kinematic chain exercises in rehabilitation of the lower extremity. J Back Musculoskel Rehabil 2:38–51, 1992, with permission.

TERMINOLOGY

Kinetic chain terminology was derived originally for linkage analysis in mechanical engineering, set forth by Reuleaux.[9] In the link concept, rigid overlapping segments are connected in series by pin joints. The system is considered closed if both ends are connected to an immovable framework, thus preventing translation of either the proximal or distal joint center. The result is a system in which movement at one joint produces movement at all other joints in a predictable manner and is called a closed kinetic chain (CKC). Steindler[10] proposed that, in the human body, each limb could be thought of as a chain consisting of rigid overlapping segments connected by a series of joints. He observed that when the foot or hand meets considerable resistance, muscle recruitment and joint motion differ from that seen when the foot or hand can move without restriction. Steindler believed the difference was significant enough to warrant distinguishing the two conditions with separate terms. Specifically an open kinetic chain (OKC) exists when the peripheral joint of the extremity can move freely, such as when waving the hand or moving the foot forward in the swing phase of gait. A CKC exists whenever the foot or hand meets resistance, such as in the chin up or rising from a squat. From a strictly mechanical perspective, one can argue that neither exercise is CKC because either the proximal or distal segment moves in each situation. Conversely, one could argue that both exercises are CKC exercises because the peripheral limb meets resistance in each situation.[2] Indeed, Steindler pointed out that a true CKC exists only during isometric exercise because, by definition, neither proximal nor distal segment can move in a closed system. Therefore, OKC exercises may be more aptly described as traditional exercise training, and CKC training can simply be referred to as kinetic chain exercises. For the purpose of being consistent with the literature, however, this chapter continues to use the nomenclature of OKC and CKC exercises.

THEORETIC BASIS FOR CLOSED KINETIC CHAIN EXERCISES

To accomplish a treatment goal, the rehabilitation specialist should consider all the factors associated with the patient's case: the nature of the musculoskeletal injury, the type of surgery, healing and biomechanical constraints, the patient profile and personality, and the exercise mode. When choosing a mode of kinetic exercise, the characteristics associated with either an OKC or CKC exercise must be considered. The following section reviews biomechanical, neuromuscular, and other factors associated with kinetic exercises. The reader should refer to Chapters 1 and 2 for an in-depth analysis of ankle and foot anatomy and biomechanics to facilitate understanding of this section.

Kinematics

Kinematics is the term used to describe a body in motion regardless of the forces that produce the motion.[11] When a body moves, it does so in accordance with its kinematics, which in the human body takes place through arthrokinematics (movement of the joint surfaces) and osteokinematics (movement of the long bones).[12] Human kinematics occurs as a result of synchronous movement of body parts, that is, human performance of all functional tasks results from linked segments of skeletal levers rotating about their anatomic joint axes. Such fundamental motion is influenced by muscle, gravitational, ground reaction, inertial, and joint reaction forces.[13] The differences in biomechanical forces and other physical and motor parameters between CKC and OKC movements in the lower extremity can be illustrated during functional activities.

SQUAT

The squat is a popular CKC exercise for rehabilitation.[2,3,14] The squat produces simultaneous movement in the ankle, knee, and hip joints. As shown in Figure 12–1A, knee flexion is accompanied by hip flexion and ankle dorsiflexion. Conversely, knee extension is accompanied by hip extension and ankle plantar flexion. The simultaneous movement of the three joints in the lower extremity results in an integrated and predictable movement pattern. In contrast to an OKC, in which osteokinematic movement can be isolated to one joint in the kinetic chain (Fig. 12–1B), the integrated movement in CKC exercises requires functional stability and mobility in the lower extremities. Joint motion that occurs only in one plane is designated as 1° of freedom of motion; in two planes, 2° of freedom of motion; and in three planes, 3° of freedom.[15] The lower extremity and trunk together possess 25° or more of freedom. Weakness or dysfunction in one joint in the kinetic chain may result in an altered or aberrant pattern of movement. Because of the multiple joint requirements to produce a CKC movement, a squat becomes a useful screening evaluation for potential areas

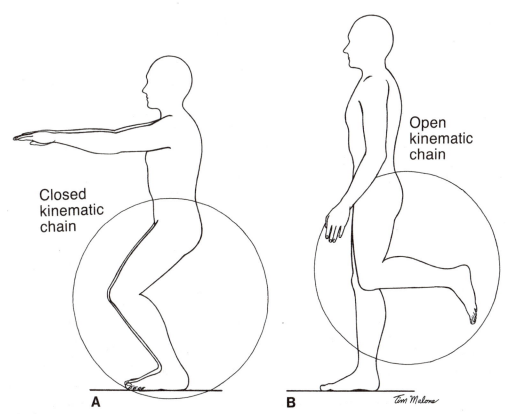

FIGURE 12–1. Closed and open kinematic chains. (*A*) In the closed kinematic chain, knee flexion is accompanied by hip flexion and ankle dorsiflexion. (*B*) Knee motion in an open kinematic chain may occur with or without motion at the hip and ankle. Knee flexion is accompanied by hip flexion but no motion has occurred at the ankle. (From Norkin and Levangie,[11] p 69, with permission.)

of dysfunction as well as a functional assessment for motor performance of the lower extremities. Conversely the ability to isolate movement in a single joint in an OKC is advantageous for early rehabilitation after major orthopedic injury and prolonged immobilization or in the infirm or elderly patient, in whom there is a loss of total leg strength, range of motion (ROM), and proprioception.

WALKING

Walking is a pure kinetic chain activity that requires integrated and synchronous movement of the joints in the lower extremities. For example, during gait, as many as 14 segments (bones) of the trunk and lower extremity can be involved.[13] Movement of the foot and ankle during stance influences and accommodates the position and movement of the bones and joints in the lower extremities. A review of the gait mechanics would be extensive, and the reader should refer to excellent texts[11,16,17] and Chapter 4 in this text for a complete analysis. A review of the effect of subtalar joint motion on the lower leg during stance, however, provides an excellent example of the kinetic chain concept. Tibial rotation occurs during the stance phase of walking. Walking results in a series of transverse rotations in the bones of the lower extremites. Inman found the tibia to rotate an average of 19°.[16] Because the foot is fixed to the ground, the subtalar joint becomes a torque converter for the transverse rotation of the tibia (see Fig. 1–11).[18] At heel strike, the tibia is rotating internally, and the talus adducts and plantar flexes; the result is calcaneal eversion. This movement is CKC pronation. From midstance to toe-off, the tibia is rotating externally, and the talus simultaneously abducts and dorsiflexes; the result is calcaneal inversion. This movement results in CKC supination. OKC pronation in the foot and ankle results from dorsiflexion, eversion, and abduction at the ankle, subtalar, and midtarsal joints, whereas OKC supination results from plantar flexion, inversion, and adduction in the same joints. These movements can be produced relatively independent from segmental rotation in the tibia or femur.

Kinetics

Examination of forces and their effects on the body is the study of kinetics.[11] The external forces acting on the body are inertia, gravity, and the ground reaction force. Inertia is that element of a body that resists a change in state (a speeding up or slowing down). Gravity force is the point at which a single force of magnitude (weight of the body) is applied to the body. Ground reaction force is defined as the force that acts on the body as a result of the interaction with the ground.[19] The internal forces are created primarily by the muscles. The summation of these forces produces a joint reaction force. Joint reaction forces are equal and opposite forces that exist between adjacent bones of a joint. The actual joint reaction force changes throughout the ROM, as the angle of the joint changes relative to the ground, combined with the magnitude and direction of muscle action. Joint reaction forces can result in compressive, shear, and tensile forces.[19]

KNEE JOINT

Studies performed primarily at the knee joint[5,20–22] indicate that shearing is the primary joint reactive force during OKC exercises, whereas compressive joint reactive forces dominate during CKC exercises. Grood et al[5] used cadaveric specimens to ascertain that maximal anterior tibial translation occurred at 30° of OKC knee extension. Butler et al[22] found the amount of anterior tibial translation and the forces on the anterior cruciate ligament (ACL) were greatest from 30° to full OKC knee extension. Both Arms et al[20] and Renstrom et al[21] found that posterior tibial translation occurred between 90° and 60° of OKC knee extension, followed by anterior tibial translation from 60° to full knee extension.

A study by Yack et al[7] compared the amount of anterior tibial displacement that occurred in ACL-deficient knees during two types of exercises: OKC resisted exercises and a parallel squat, a CKC exercise. Subjects had significantly greater anterior tibial translation from 64° to 10° in the OKC knee extension exercise compared with the parallel squat, which produced primarily tibiofemoral compressive forces. Lutz et al[14] compared tibiofemoral shear and compression forces using a load cell and a free force diagram in five healthy subjects during OKC knee extension and a squat exercise. The authors found that during OKC extension, maximum posterior shear force (resisting force for anterior tibial translation) of 285 occurred at 30° of knee flexion, and maximum anterior shear forces (resisting force for posterior tibial translation) of 1780 N occurred at 90° of knee flexion. The CKC exercise produced significantly less posterior shear force at all angles of knee flexion when compared with the OKC exercise. In addition, the CKC exercise produced significantly less anterior shear force at all angles except 30° when compared with the OKC exercise. Analysis of tibiofemoral compressive forces revealed that the CKC exercise produced significantly greater compressive forces at the same angles that the OKC exercises produce shear forces. The authors deduced that the compressive forces produced in the CKC exercise resulted from the axial orientation of the applied ground reaction force and muscular cocontraction.

PATELLOFEMORAL JOINT

The patellofemoral joint undergoes compressive forces during CKC activities.[23,24] Reilly and Martens[23] reported that retropatellar compressive forces ranged from 0.5 times body weight during normal walking to 3.3 times body weight climbing stairs. Deep knee bends produced patellofemoral compressive forces 7.8 times body weight. This information has important clinical implications in CKC training. Although compressive forces produced during a squat stabilize the various joints in the lower extremities, the same compressive forces may be deleterious and painful in patients with patellofemoral dysfunction or pathology of the retropatellar surface. During the application of kinetic chain exercises, the rehabilitation specialist should consider the type of forces produced in each joint in the kinetic chain. A weak link (pathologic or dysfunctional joint) in the kinetic chain necessitates modification of the kinetic training mode. In patients with patellofemoral dysfunction, the squat should be limited to quarter range, and the patient is instructed to keep the lower legs vertical to the weight-bearing surface and the knees behind the toes (Fig. 12–2).[25]

HIP AND ANKLE JOINTS

Few data are available that compare joint reaction forces of the ankle and hip between the CKC and OKC. Cavanagh[26] reported that the ground reaction force through the foot and ankle in the midstance of running is 250% to 400% body weight. Stauffer et al[27] reported that with the larger articular surface of the talus in the ankle mortise, the ankle is able to withstand compression forces during gait of as much as 450% of body weight with little incidence of hyaline cartilage damage. Sammarco et al[28] and McCullough and Burge[29] have demonstrated that rotatory stability of the ankle is increased by the application of axial loads during weight bearing.

Results of a study of hip forces by Rydell[30] found that OKC hip flexion with a subject supine increased compressive forces on the hip 1.0 to 1.5 times body weight. Activities such as squatting, sitting, and even sitting in low chairs produced a small force at the hip joint.[31] Only during the stance phase of walking are compressive forces on the weight-bearing hip large, ranging from 3.5 to 5.5 times body weight.[32,33]

FORCE DIAGRAM

Forces are vectors that have a point of application, magnitude, and direction.[11] Force vectors acting on a human body can be illustrated using a force diagram. A force diagram includes all the forces and torques acting on a body.[2]

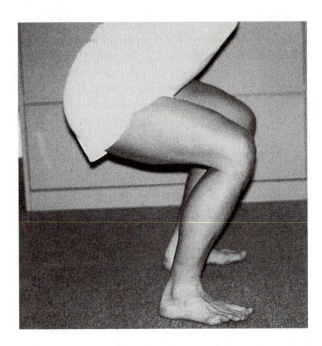

FIGURE 12–2. Squat mechanics— knee/tibial position. The knees should not pass over the toes in a sagittal plane. With the knees in this position, the alignment of the tibial bones relative to the supporting surface is nearly vertical, which results in minimal strain to the patellofemoral joint. (From Greenfield,[25] p 125, with permission.)

Figure 12–3 is a force diagram of the seated knee extension exercise (OKC). The system has been simplified such that only three forces are acting on the tibia: the applied force (A), the quadriceps muscle force (M), and the joint reaction force (R). If the tibia is in equilibrium, the line of application of all three forces must pass through a common point (d). Therefore, if the direction and point of application of M and A are known, the direction of R can be determined. Vector R can then be resolved into its components e—f (compression) and e—g (shear). In Figure 12–3, the shear force of the femur is directed posteriorly, inducing an anterior tibial translation.

MUSCLE COCONTRACTION

CKC exercises induce muscle cocontraction.[2,14] Although authors have shown that cocontraction of the hamstrings does occur during OKC knee extension,[21,34] Draganich et al[35] demonstrated that the contraction is only 10% to 20% of maximal isometric contraction. Figure 12–4 schematically demonstrates muscular cocontraction during a squat.[2] Consider a force A applied to the distal tibia. Because the hip and knee are unconstrained, the force created a flexion moment at both joints. A moment is calculated as product of a force and the perpendicular distance between the line of force to the axis of rotation of the joint.[19] The hamstrings contract to stabilize the hip, and the quadriceps contract to stabilize the knee. Activity in the biarticular hamstring muscle, induced for hip stability, helps neutralize the tendency of the quadriceps to cause anterior tibial translation. A similar phenomenom occurs at the ankle joint as the force A is applied to the bottom of the foot. Tension in the gastrocnemius muscle (biarticular muscle that crosses both the ankle and knee joints), which would be induced to stabilize the ankle joint flexion moment, has an indirect effect on reducing anterior knee translation. Analysis of muscle electromyographic (EMG) activity during a squat by Lutz et al[14] indicated that cocontraction of the hamstrings and quadri-

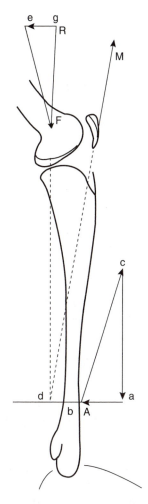

FIGURE 12–3. Force diagram for sitting knee joint extension. A = applied force; R = joint reaction force; f = knee instant center of rotation; a, b, c, = triangle formed by force vectors in equilibrium: used to determine length of unknown vector, R; d = common point of intersection of three-force system in equilibrium: e—g = shear component of R; e—f = normal component of R.

ceps occurred through the range but was maximum between 30° and 60° of knee flexion. A key element in the squat exercise is to maintain hip flexion with lumbar spine lordosis to produce the hip flexion moment necessary to activate the hamstrings (Fig. 12–5).[25]

In another study, Morrison[36] investigated knee muscle power output and dissipation. He found that maximum power output about the knee joint was produced by the knee flexor muscles at heel strike and loading response while walking down a ramp. Also during this period, maximum power dissipation occurred through the knee extensors. This action, according to Morrison, is an excellent example of muscle concontraction during a functional activity.

The effect of cocontraction on joint stability was examined by Markolf et al.[37] The authors studied the effects of maximum isometric contraction of the knee joint muscles on the overall stiffness of the tibiofemoral joint. Joint stiffness can be defined as the change in the force per unit change in displacement of the joint. Subjects' knees were tested for anteroposterior and varus-valgus displacement. The authors found that on average the stiffness of the tibiofemoral joint was increased by a factor of 2.2 to 4.2 when the subjects made a maximal isometric contraction of the hamstring and

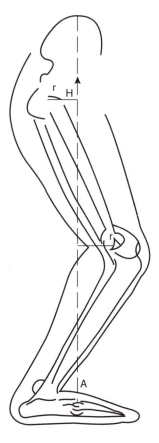

FIGURE 12–4. Diagramatic representation of the induction of muscular cocontraction due to flexion moments caused by applied force. A = applied force; rH = hip moment arm; rK = knee moment arm.

quadriceps muscle, compared with when the muscles were relaxed. In humans, the muscles around the joints in the lower extremities are activated simultaneously in a wide range of motor activities.[38] Concontraction of these muscles presses the articulating surfaces of joints together and contributes to increased, but in many cases equal, distribution of compressive forces.

CONCURRENT SHIFT

CKC training has been reported to reproduce what Palmitier et al[2] call the concurrent shift of biarticular muscles that occurs during the simultaneous hip, knee, and ankle action of locomotion. Palmitier et al explain the concurrent shift. Simultaneous hip and knee extension occurs when rising from a squat. The rectus femoris and the hamstring muscles are both active. As the hip extends, the rectus femoris muscle lengthens while the hamstrings shorten, but as the knee extends, the rectus femoris shortens as the hamstrings lengthen. The result at the muscular level might be called a pseudoisometric contraction, owing to simultaneous concentric and eccentric contractions at opposite ends of each muscle.[10] This so-called concurrent shift and the resultant pseudoisometric contraction cannot be reproduced with isolation exercises.

The concurrent shift has added significance in muscle training based on research of evidence of task-specific functional groups of motor units within a single muscle in cats.[39-43] Muscle compartmentalization has been reported to be present in biarticu-

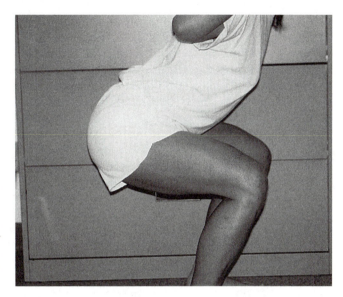

FIGURE 12–5. Squat mechanics—pelvic position. The pelvis is positioned in an anterior tilt to maintain the lumbar lordosis. Flexion at the hip and knee joints results in cocontraction of the hamstrings and quadriceps muscle. (From Greenfield,[25] p 125, with permission.)

lar muscles, with each compartment being predominantly composed of one specific muscle fiber type. One may deduce that activation of separate muscle compartments occurs functionally during a concurrent shift of biarticular muscles.

MUSCLE CONTRACTION

Table 12–2 lists and describes the characteristics of muscle contraction types and modes. The literature indicates that eccentric muscle action is essential during lower kinetic chain function,[16,44,45] and a review of foot and ankle muscle action in Chapters 1 and 4 illustrates the eccentric muscle action of the various muscles during gait. Although OKC chain training can incorporate eccentric training, only CKC training

TABLE 12–2 Modes of Open Kinematic Chain Exercise

Mode	Characteristics	Angular Velocity	Resistance
Isometrics	Muscle contracts without osteokinematic joint movement	Fixed at 0° per second	Accommodating but not quantified: dependent on amount of force applied
Isotonics			
Concentrics	Dynamic contraction with muscle shortening	Accommodates to effort	Preset and quantified
Eccentrics	Dynamic contraction with muscle lengthening	Accommodates to effort	Preset and quantified
Isokinetics	Dynamic contraction	Preset and quantified in degrees per second	Accommodating to effort and quantified in Newton-meters or foot-pounds

From Greenfeld, BH and Tovin, BJ: The application of open and closed kinematic chain exercise in rehabilitation of the lower extremity. J Back Musculoskel Rehabil 2:38–51, 1992, with permission.

incorporates eccentric muscle action under functional conditions. These conditions include a temporal pattern of muscle recruitment, time rate of tension development of muscle contraction, optimum muscle tension requirements, and dynamic muscle flexibility. An in-depth analysis of muscle action is beyond the scope of this chapter, and the reader is referred to works by Mann and Inman,[44] Inman,[16] and Perry.[45] The following theoretic model presented by Norkin and Levangie[11] partially explains muscle action during walking.

EMG is often used in conjunction with force plates, cinematography, and electrogoniometry to pinpoint the exact moment when a particular muscle is acting during gait. Static analysis used to determine the effects of the force of gravity on the body during erect static posture is used to analyze gravitational forces during walking. When the gravity line is located at a distance from the joint axis, a gravitational moment is created around a joint, which disturbs the equilibrium of the joint. To prevent motion at the joint, specific muscles act to oppose the moment, thereby maintaining equilibrium. During walking, joint movement is necessary. According to Norkin and Levangie, gravitational moments are desirable if they tend to produce motion in a desired direction and undesirable if they produce motion in an undesired direction. Norkin and Levangie offer the following examples: If flexion of the knee is necessary during a certain phase of gait and there is a flexion moment acting at the knee, the flexion moment is desirable. Muscular activity may be required to control knee flexion. If control is necessary, an eccentric muscle contraction of the knee extensors is required to control the flexion (Fig. 12–6A). If, conversely, there is a flexion moment at the knee and knee extension is the desired motion, a concentric contraction of the knee extensors is necessary to oppose the flexion moment and to produce knee extension (Fig. 12–6B).

Consider how this concept of muscle action applies to gait. The type of muscle activity that occurs during gait depends on the nature of the moment acting around

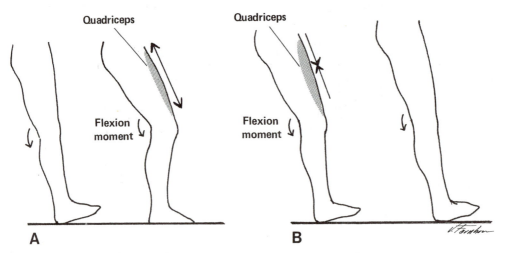

FIGURE 12–6. (A) There is a flexion moment at the knee and knee flexion is the desired motion; therefore, an eccentric contraction of the quadriceps muscle is necessary to control the amount of knee flexion. (B) There is a flexion moment acting around the knee and extension is the desired motion; therefore, the quadriceps muscle must work concentrically to counteract the flexion moment and to produce knee extension. (From Norkin and Levangie,[11] p 468, with permission.)

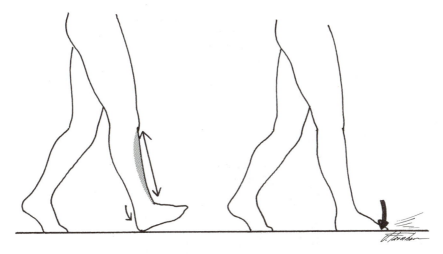

FIGURE 12–7. In the period of gait from heel strike to foot flat there is a plantarflexion moment acting around the ankle. Plantarflexion is the desired motion that is necessary to position the foot on the supporting surface. The dorsiflexors act eccentrically to control plantarflexion and to prevent the foot from slapping to the ground in an uncontrolled motion. (From Norkin and Levangie,[11] p 468, with permission.)

the joints during stance and the direction of the desired motion. In the period of gait from heel strike to midstance, there is a plantar flexion moment acting around the ankle because the line of gravity falls posterior to the axis of the ankle joint. Plantar flexion is a desired motion that is necessary to put the foot on the floor so that it is in a position to receive the body weight. The foot slaps the floor in an uncontrolled fashion, however, unless muscle activity (eccentric activity of the ankle dorsiflexors) and the precise time (temporal variable) are used to control the plantar flexion (Fig. 12–7). A different situation exists at the knee joint during the same interval of stance. In this period, the knee is extending as it moves from about 15° of flexion during heel strike to 5° of flexion in midstance. There is a flexion moment at the knee, and flexion is the undesired motion. A concentric contraction of the extensors with precise timing at midstance is necessary to counteract the flexion moment and to produce knee joint extension.

Proprioception

Anatomic studies[46,47] indicate the presence of articular innervation and sensory receptors in the capsule and ligaments in the synovial joints. Table 12–3 classifies and describes the four major sensory or mechanoreceptors in synovial joints. Studies have also indicated that muscle mechanoreceptors (muscle spindles) possess more of a role as proprioceptive and kinesthetic sense organs than was previously believed.[48,49]

Joint mechanoreceptors and muscle spindles apprise the central nervous system of joint position sense, movement, changes of movement of a joint, and, in some cases, changes in intraligamentous tension. Proprioception describes awareness of posture, movement, changes in equilibrium, and mechanical inertia that generate pressures and strains at the joints.[50] Proprioceptive input, such as that provided by

TABLE 12–3 Positional Sense Receptors

Type	Characteristics	Function
Ruffini endings	Spray-type nerve endings receiving strong stimulation with sudden joint movement. After slight adaptation initially, a steady signal is transmitted	Static joint position sense and initial rate of movement
Golgi tendon receptor (organ)	Less numerous than Ruffini endings, found primarily in tendons and ligaments. These organs are stretch sensitive with similar response properties to Ruffini endings	Reflexive alteration of muscle tone to "brake" excessive movement
Pacinian corpuscles	Detect the rate of rotation of the joint with extremely rapid adaptation	Provides sensory feedback regarding the rate of acceleration/deceleration
Free nerve ending	Found primarily in the skin put also in other tissues, free nerve endings detect and are sensitive to changes in touch and pressure	Sensitive to application of noxious stimuli

the afferent neural system in synovial joints and muscle spindles, primarily functions in an adaptive role. This afferent neural input enables motor strategy changes based on information provided by changes in body position.[51]

Several studies have illustrated the deleterious effects of joint injury resulting in the loss of proprioception and kinesthetic awareness.[52-55] A study by Wyke[55] showed marked postural changes in a boy with apparent alteration of afferent impulses from the ankle capsule following injury to the lateral aspect of the capsule. The postural deficit persisted despite an otherwise complete recovery, with restoration of normal strength and ROM and with no residual pain. The boy complained of the ankle "giving-way." Barrack et al[52] found perceptual deficits manifested in altered joint position sense in patients with ACL-deficient knees compared with their uninvolved knees.

Freeman[56] advocates the use of coordination exercises on a balance board for patients with chronic ankle "instability" in the absence of demonstrable structural instability. France et al[57] examined lower extremity balance enhancement in normal individuals after training on a balancing device and found improved pretest to posttest balance and stability skills.

PROTECTIVE MUSCLE REFLEX

A number of studies have shown that ligament stretches do not exert much influence on the skeletomotor system, at least at moderate loads.[49,58-61] The effects on the gamma muscle spindle system, however, seem to be frequent and potent and to be elicited at low mechanical stimulation intensities. The standard stimulation of the cruciate ligaments, for example, used in the investigations by Johansson et al[49] and Sojka et al[61] consisting of a tonically applied low (5–40 N) traction force, indicates that most of the observed effects on the spindle afferent responses were caused by slowly adapting receptors with low thresholds to stimulation (type I). The articular mechanoreceptors at low loads of stress are therefore involved in the normal reflex coordination of muscle tone in posture and movement, and these receptors operate polysynaptically via the gamma motor neuron loop and are elicited during weight-bearing (CKC) training. The result is that this reflex regulates muscle tone and stiffness around a joint for movement and stability. Solomonow et al[34] elicited reflex contraction of the hamstring muscles when sagittal translation in ACL-deficient knees was provoked. The results indicate a protective reflex mechanism of muscles that can be elicited during CKC training to protect ligaments and stabilize a joint. The protective reflexes are putatively facilitated by stressing type III mechanoreceptors (high threshold, slowly adapting; see Table 12–3), which excite the agonist (hamstring) and inhibit the antagonist muscle (quadriceps) of the involved ligament (ACL). Solomonow et al, however, reported that large loads (around 130 N) had to be applied to the ACL to evoke a reflex change in the EMG signals from the hamstrings and quadriceps muscle.

MYOTATIC STRETCH REFLEX

Studies have shown that an eccentric muscle contraction immediately preceding a concentric muscle contraction significantly increases the force generated concentrically.[62–65] The mechanism is called a stretch shortening contraction and occurs during plyometric training (a quick powerful movement involving prestretching or countermovement).[64] The force generated during the stretch-shortening cycle is due to two mechanisms: (1) prestretching the elastic or noncontractile portion of the muscle, which results in stored energy that is then quickly released, and (2) elicitation of the myotatic stretch reflex.

The myotatic stretch reflex is a proprioceptive reflex. Proprioceptors, including muscle spindles and Golgi tendon organs (GTOs), are located within the muscle and provide afferent information about the degree of muscular distortion. Muscle spindles are small complex organs located within the muscle fibers and have both afferent and efferent innervation.[67] When the muscle spindle is activated via stretching, a sensory afferent response is evolved and transmitted to the spinal cord, which, in turn, sends impulses back to the skeletal muscle causing a motor response. Shortening of the muscle relieves the stretch on the muscle spindles contained within the muscle, thereby removing the stimulus from the stretch reflex. The myotatic reflex is the only monosynaptic reflex in the body, with a loop time of approximately 30 to 50 ms.[67]

The GTOs are located within muscle tendons near the point of attachment to the muscle. Activation of GTOs inhibits the muscle. Owing to the GTO series alignment with the contractile muscle fibers, activation of these proprioceptors occurs with stretch. When deformation or tension is produced, sensory impulses are transmitted to the spinal cord and cerebellum. The arrival of these impulses at the spinal cord causes inhibition of the alpha motor neurons of the contracting muscle and synergists, thereby limiting force development. The complex interplay of both muscle and joint proprioceptors to elicit position sense and to modulate muscle force for coordinated and safe movement is best facilitated during functional or CKC training.[66]

Motor Learning

Motor learning is a primary goal of rehabilitation and entails the acquisition or reacquisition of skilled or coordinated movement.[68,69] Coordination is defined as the process by which movement components are sequenced and organized temporally and their relative magnitudes determined to produce a functional movement pattern or synergy.[68] A musculoskeletal system has the potential to move in multiple directions and use multiple muscles to produce a desired motion. Different neural pathways within the central nervous system influenced by vestibular, ocular, or joint proprioceptive input may produce the same coordinated movement. Studies by Keshner[69,70] demonstrated that different muscle recruitment patterns were induced with experimental manipulation of the environment that produced the same desired motion. To function with appropriate movement behaviors in a changing environment, the central nervous system must be able to identify and perceive sensory input under different conditions. Keshner suggests that therapeutic intervention provide different environmental circumstances that require multiple adaptive responses. She warns that overlearning a specific task can inhibit adaptation of motor responses; that is, one should not make the patient so comfortable with a single response pattern that he or she attempts to use that response even when it interferes with the generation of a more appropriate response. By progressively altering specific movement tasks and environments during CKC training, altering overall afferent neural system input to the central nervous system, and facilitating appropriate muscle recruitment and movement patterns, clinicians can improve the flexibility and variety of motor responses.

Summary

The previous section delineates the influence of OKC and CKC movements on the biomechanical and neuromuscular responses of the lower extremities. The clinician should understand the characteristics, and therefore the advantages and disadvantages, of closed and open kinetic training during rehabilitation. OKC training in general imposes less stress on the joint and isolates muscle activity without the influence of muscle forces imposed on the entire lower extremity during weight bearing. In most cases, OKC exercises are used early in rehabilitation. CKC training results in a functional training effect by producing cocontraction around a joint, compressive forces, recruitment of multiple joints and muscle groups, concurrent eccentric and concentric muscle action, proprioceptive input, and learning for motor skill reacquisition.

APPLICATION OF KINETIC CHAIN TRAINING

The application of kinetic chain training in rehabilitation is to progress the patient to CKC training. By advancing from OKC to CKC training, rehabilitation follows a functional progression. This concept has been defined by Keggerreis[71] as an ordered sequence of activities enabling the acquisition or reacquisition of skills required for safe, effective performance for function and athletics.

SAID Principle

The functional progression incorporates the principle of exercise specificity and is based on the SAID (specific adaptations to imposed demands) principle.[72] According to this principle, the body adapts to activities based on the type of imposed stresses and is specific to the type of training performed. Functional exercises must, therefore, simulate the specific activity that the individual is required to perform.

Exercise Progression

CKC training has been reported as the only way to reproduce the biomechanical, neuromuscular, and learning responses for function in lower extremities.[73] As with any rehabilitation program, however, timely progression of exercise is critical to the outcome. Judicious implementation and monitoring of exercise advancement is crucial to the period of rehabilitation. The phases and time period of soft tissue healing must be considered in the presence of ligamentous disruption or following surgical intervention, as these phases dictate guidelines for exercise progression. In addition, the clinician should continuously monitor the patient's signs and symptoms in response to the exercise. Table 12–4 is an example of a time-based exercise program that considers the phases of soft tissue healing and uses a functional exercise progression. These are general guidelines and should be modified based on each individual case. The initial treatment intervention is designed to ameliorate the acute phase of injury, with specific attention directed at eliminating swelling, pain, loss of motion, and weakness. At the same time, the clinician designs the rehabilitation program to accommodate the phases of healing. As physical parameters improve and

TABLE 12–4 Time and Criteria-Based Exercise Progression

Phase	Characteristics	Goals	Treatment
Phase I	Inflammatory stage of healing Maximum protection Lasts 1–10 days	Reduce pain Decrease edema/effusion Increase ROM	Ice Compression, elevation Passive ROM
Phase II	Fibroplasia stage of healing Protected mobilization Lasts 10 days to 6 weeks	Increase ROM Prevent muscle atrophy by initiating strengthening	Whirlpool, partial ROM (mobilization and stretching), assisted ROM Multiple angle isometrics, light weight isotonics
Phase III	Maturation stage of healing Minimal protection Lasts 6–12 weeks	Improve muscle performance Improve flexibility Improve proprioception	Full range isotonics, multiple speed isokinetics; closed kinetic chain Balance exercises
Phase IV	Late maturation Return to function Lasts 12–16 weeks	Restore normal muscle performance Restore normal flexibility Return to function	Advanced closed kinetic chain exercises

ROM-Range of motion.
From Greenfield, BH and Tovin, BJ: The application of open and closed kinematic chain exercises in rehabilitation of the lower extremity. J Back Musculoskel Rehabil 2:38–51, 1992, with permission.

healing progresses, exercises are implemented in a hierarchical manner from less to more stressful and complicated movement patterns and within the progression of functional training. Ultimately the patient is training in movement patterns that elicit the motor responses in an integrated fashion to replicate normal function.

Summary

Exercise selection and progression depend on the nature of the injury and the needs of the patient. The first objective is to choose an exercise that meets the goals of treatment in a safe, effective manner. The second objective is to ensure that the exercises chosen are progressed in a manner that allows a patient to return to a preinjury level of function. Although each individual's preinjury level of function is different, each rehabilitation program should incorporate CKC exercises.

CASE STUDY

The following case study demonstrates clinical decision making for exercise progression during OKC and CKC training.

CASE: INVERSION ANKLE SPRAIN

Subjective Findings

A 20-year-old female Division I basketball player twisted her ankle during a basketball game. The patient reported rebounding the ball and landing on a teammate's foot; her right ankle subsequently "turned in." She reported that she felt a loud snap on the outside of her ankle, fell to the ground, and experienced almost immediate swelling. She was carried off the court by her athletic trainer, and her ankle was wrapped in an ace wrap and placed in ice water for 30 minutes. There was no obvious external deformities; she was taken to a nearby hospital emergency room; radiographs were negative for fracture. She was placed in an ankle immobilizer, instructed to keep her limb elevated for the night above her heart, and was seen the next morning by the school team physician.

Subsequent medical examination revealed:

1. 2+ edema dorsolateral ankle and foot
2. Ecchymosis
3. Talar tilt test with peroneal nerve block indicated 22° opening measured from the tibial plafond on x-ray

Diagnosis

Diagnosis was Lauge-Hansen supination-adduction (SA) injury with probable complete tear of the anterior talofibular ligament (ATFL) and calcaneal-fibular ligament (CFL).[74] The result was 3+ instability in her lateral ankle. SA injuries occur when the supinated foot is forced medially, tensing the fibular collateral ligaments of the ankle. Tear of this ligament complex or avulsion fracture of the

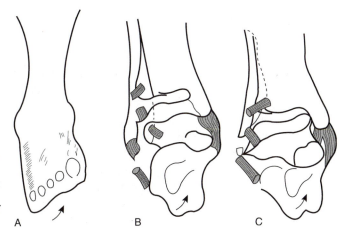

FIGURE 12–8. Lauge-Hansen classification: supination-adduction injuries. (*A*) Supinated foot tending to go into tibial flexion. (*B* and *C*) Stage one: rupture of the lateral ligament.

fibula constitutes the first stage of SA. In the second stage, the tibal malleolus suffers compression fracture (Fig. 12–8).

Because of the severe instability and the fact that the patient was an athlete with high functional demands on the lower extremities, the surgeon decided to perform a lateral ankle stabilization procedure, known as a split peroneal brevis lateral ankle stabilization (SPLAS).[75] The basic approach to surgery was to cut a strip of the distal end of the attached peroneal brevis tendon and reroute the tendon strip through the fibular bone and attach the tendon to the talus. The reattached tendon strip replaces the torn ATFL. The patient was initially casted in a plaster cast below the knee for 3 weeks to allow initial healing (early fibroplasia); the cast was subsequently removed, and the patient was placed in an air boot, partial weight bearing with crutches. The air boot contains small air cells that provide a compressive force to the foot and ankle to reduce edema. The patient was referred to physical therapy.

Initial Physical Findings

1. 2+ edema dorsolateral ankle and foot and posterior ankle
2. Indurated surgical scar along the lateral ankle
3. Minimal active and passive talocrural ankle motion
4. Restricted subtalar joint motion and midtarsal joint mobility
5. Atrophy of the gastrocnemius-soleus muscle group
6. Tight Achilles tendon
7. Atrophy of the vastus medialis oblique (VMO) and vastus lateralis (VL) muscle in the involved lower extremity
8. 3/5 muscle strength of all the major muscle groups in the ankle-foot complex
9. Passive straight leg raise (SLR) right = 50° (limited by hamstring muscle tightness) and left = 90°
10. Antalgic and unsteady gait without assistive devices—the patient was unable to balance during bilateral standing without significant "swaying" of the entire body for more than 10 seconds; the "swaying" occurred in a matter of seconds with eyes closed.

Assessment

The primary physical findings to treat in priority order included: (1) Reduce and eliminate edema; (2) promote functional scar during healing by facilitating normal realignment of collagen fibers in the scar; (3) restore both active and passive talocrural joint motion and restore mobility to both the subtalar and the midtarsal joints; (4) reestablish muscle balance by stretching tight muscles and strengthening weak muscles; (5) facilitate joint mechanoreceptor input and muscle sensory input to the central nervous system.

The contributing factors were as follows:

Early Fibroplasia and Nonfunctional Scar. Full healing of the reconstruction occurs in approximately 6 to 8 weeks postsurgery with the maturation period extending 6 months to a year.[76] Therefore, exercise progression is implemented with caution for the next few weeks and then progressed as physical parameters improve and the healing graft matures and gains tensile strength.

Division I College Basketball Player. The high functional demands that this patient requires from her lower extremities results in an intensive functional training program. Therefore, once the initial physical problems of swelling, loss of motion, pain, and weakness are addressed, and as soft tissue healing permits, exercises are implemented to prepare the patient for aggressive CKC training. The time table for treatment, therefore, is rather long, perhaps extending for 4 to 6 months postsurgery. A program design of this length is sometimes difficult to justify to insurance companies in view of the cost of treatment; the clinician must act as a strong advocate for the patient to all concerned parties so that proper treatment time is allocated.

Treatment

Initial Treatment

Initial treatment for the first 3 to 6 weeks after surgery was designed to improve the physical deficits delineated in the assessment. Because this chapter emphasizes kinetic chain training, a detailed analysis of initial treatment is not reviewed, and the reader is referred to Chapter 11. There are some important kinetic chain treatment strategies, however, to underscore early in the care of this patient. As pain and swelling subsided, the patient was quickly progressed to low-level CKC exercises. Early bilateral weight shifts with the eyes open and closed (Fig. 12–9) were effective to begin to stress the ankle joint capsule and facilitate mechanoreceptor input. The patient was also instructed to roll onto the balls of her feet to perform a modified heel raise exercise (Fig. 12–10). The clinician should continually monitor the ankle and foot for increased pain and swelling. During this period, OKC rehabilitation was directed at preparing the patient for aggressive CKC training; flexibility, eccentric muscle strength, and normal arthrokinematics are all essential to progress CKC training safely and effectively.

Week 6 to 12

Motion of the joints in the foot and ankle were approaching normal; edema was less than 1+, muscle strength was 3+ to 4/5 with manual testing, and there was proper recruitment of the VMO and VL muscles during quadriceps muscle

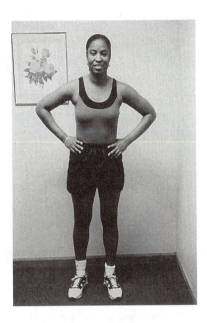

FIGURE 12–9. Early bilateral weight shifts.

contraction.[77] The patient was able to stand without any discernible imbalance (swaying) for over 30 seconds. She was full weight bearing with an air cast and without assistive devices.

Goals of treatment were to maximize motion and strength in her ankle and entire lower extremity, continue to improve proprioceptive input, and improve functional motor skills and movement patterns. The patient performed isokinetic training in all movement patterns and at various speeds. Surgical tubing exercises were used to facilitate eccentric strength control. The patient used balance

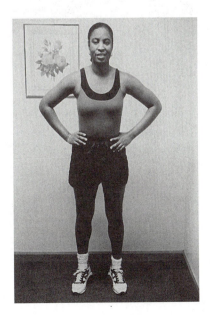

FIGURE 12–10. The patient was instructed to perform parial heel raises by rolling unto the balls of her feet. The position can be held for a 2-second count.

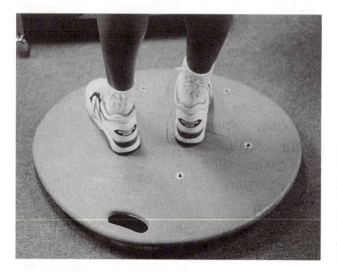

FIGURE 12–11. The patient is using a balance device to facilitate ankle joint proprioception. She was instructed to keep the board balanced on a hemispherical pivot and not allow the edges of the board to touch the floor. She was encouraged not to look at her feet.

devices to facilitate proprioceptive input (Fig. 12–11). Resisted heel raises (Fig. 12–12) and leg presses (Fig. 12–13) were used to facilitate total lower extremity strengthening. The patient was progressed to quarter squats to facilitate cocontraction and concurrent eccentric and concentric muscle action (Fig. 12–14). The Stairmaster is an excellent CKC training device to facilitate total lower strengthening and cardiovascular conditioning. The patient was instructed to retrowalk on the Stairmaster and to restrain from holding onto the handles to increase difficulty and improve proprioception and balance. (Fig. 12–15). All exercises were performed without the air cast to maximize motor control.

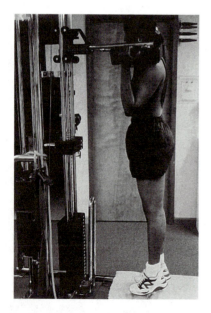

FIGURE 12–12. Resisted heel raises.

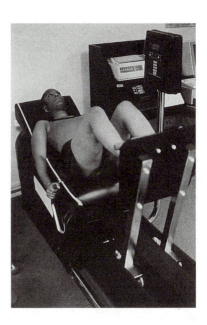

FIGURE 12–13. Leg presses in a supine position.

Week 12 to 16

At 12 to 16 weeks, CKC training was progressed. The patient was instructed in single leg heel raises, the sliding board, and jogging on a minitramp (Figs. 12–16 to 12–18). Plyometric training was emphasized to facilitate and maximize the stretch-shortening cycle, enhance neuromuscular control, and improve speed and power. Preplyometric testing was performed and divided into two categories: static stability and dynamic movement testing. The three basic static tests are one-legged standing, single-leg quarter squats, and single-leg half squats. An

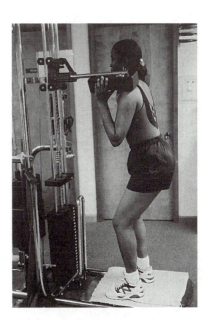

FIGURE 12–14. Standing one-quarter squats. Note that the lower leg should remain perpendicular to the floor and the knees are positioned behind the toes.

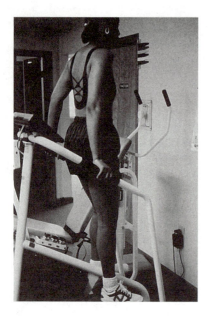

FIGURE 12–15. Retro walking on the Stairmaster.

individual should be able to perform one-legged standing for 30 seconds with eyes opened and closed before the initiation of a plyometric program. The purpose of the static stability testing is to determine the patient's ability to stabilize the torso and control the body. Dynamic movement testing assesses the individual's ability to produce explosive coordinated movement, and the test is designed to mimic a motor requirement of the patient. For example, a basketball player should be able to perform a series of standing jumps before implementing a full plyometric program.

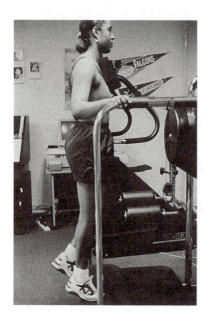

FIGURE 12–16. Single-leg heel raises. The exercise should be performed on a raised platform to allow a pre-stretch to the gastrocnemius-soleus muscles.

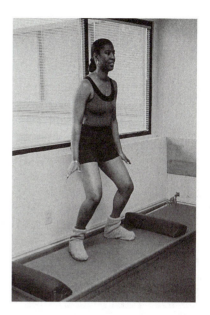

FIGURE 12–17. Sliding board exercise is excellent for proprioception, agility, and cardiovascular endurance. The patient is instructed in time bout training; she starts with three 30-second time bouts and progresses to three 2-minute time bouts.

Few protocols exist for plyometric training and progression,[78] so the clinician should design a program that replicates the motor needs of the patient. Guidelines include: Plyometric training should be specific to the goals established for the athlete (for example, if the goal is to improve vertical jump, jumping would be the best method of training); quality of work is more important than quantity; exercise intensity should be a maximal level; the greater the amplitude or intensity, the greater the recovery time; and plyometric training may have its greatest benefit at the conclusion of the normal workout. This

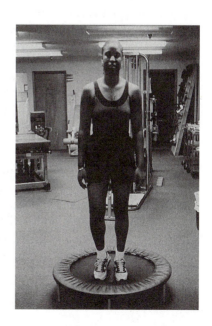

FIGURE 12–18. Jogging on a minitramp.

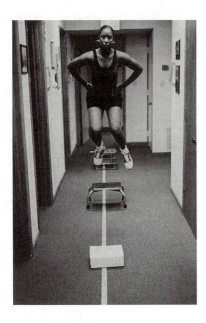

FIGURE 12–19. Bounding exercise.

approach best replicates exercise under a partial to total fatigue environment; when the proper technique can no longer be demonstrated, maximum volume has been achieved; initially, exercises of low motor complexity and stress should be introduced progressing to high-intensity training; high-intensity plyometrics should be limited to twice weekly to avoid injury or overuse.

Because this patient was an athlete, high ballistic movements, such as in-place jumping, hops, and jumps, and cutting, were emphasized. Initially the patient performed side-to-side or lateral jumping over a 6-inch height. Time bouts are useful in plyometrics; she was instructed to perform a 30-second time bout and progressed to three 30-second time bouts. A metronome can be used to maintain pace, beginning with a slow speed of one jump every 2 to 3 seconds to a jump each second. Once the patient was performing three sets of 30-second time bout training at a quick pace, the height was increased but limited to approximately 1 foot. Bounding involves jumping over a preset height across a distance and facilitates muscle power and speed (Fig. 12–19). As the patient improved her speed and movement, she was progressed to cutting exercises, including figure-eights and cariocas. During these exercises, it was important initially that her ankle was taped and she wore her air cast.

Week 16 to 24

Functional training continued; the complexity and demands increased, and sports-specific drills using a basketball were incorporated into her program. The clinician continued to monitor for any significant recurrence of swelling, pain, or loss of motion. Mild swelling was expected during this phase, and the patient was instructed to ice for approximately 20 minutes after training.

Discharge Parameters

Discharge parameters should always include a compilation of several physical and functional tests, including isokinetic tests (less than 10% side-to-side difference in all muscle groups), full and painless ROM, and functional testing. The series of hop tests developed by Noyes et al[19] seem to have a relatively high correlation with function. These tests include single leg hop for distance, single leg hop along 6 m for time, and triple leg hop for distance. Bilateral comparisons with the uninvolved lower extremity should be within 85% of all tests.

Summary of Case

This case represented a typical case of an athletic patient that demonstrated a program design incorporating CKC training. The patient was progressed initially based on soft tissue healing time constraints and correction of common physical findings of edema, loss of motion, pain, and loss of strength. Functional training was the major focus in the middle and later stages of rehabilitation and was progressed in a manner that slowly stressed and challenged the neuromuscular system to allow for the proper timing of motor skill reacquisition in a safe, effective manner.

CONCLUSION

This chapter reviewed the terminology, basic concepts, and principles of kinetic training. The principles of biomechanical forces, muscle forces and contraction modes, proprioception, learning, and exercise specificity all must be considered in the manner in which they interact during OKC and CKC training. Analysis of these variables under the two kinetic chain training modes clearly indicates the functional demand and skill that occurs in CKC training. CKC training produces a large array of motor responses in an integrated manner that simply cannot be replicated during OKC training. The implication is that all rehabilitation programs must be designed to incorporate functional or CKC training.

REFERENCES

1. Shelbourne, KD and Nitz, P: Accelerated rehabilitation after anterior cruciate ligament reconstruction. Am J Sports Med 18:292, 1980.
2. Palmitier RA, et al: Kinetic chain exercise in knee rehabilitation. Sports Med 11:402, 1991.
3. Henning, CE, Lynch, MA, and Glick, JR: An in vivo strain gauge study of elongation of the anterior cruciate ligament. Am J Sports Med 13:22, 1985.
4. Seto, JL, et al: Rehabilitation of the knee after anterior cruciate ligament reconstruction. J Orthop Sports Phys Ther 11:8, 1989.
5. Grood, ES, et al: Biomechanics of knee extension exercise. J Bone Joint Surg 66A:725, 1984.
6. Yasuda, K, et al: Muscle weakness after anterior cruciate reconstruction using patellar and quadriceps tendons. Bull Hosp Joint Dis Orthop Inst 51:175, 1991.
7. Yack, JH, Collins, CE, and Whieldon, TJ: Comparison of closed and open kinetic chain exercise in the anterior cruciate ligament–deficient knee. Am J Sports Med 21:49, 1993.
8. Fanton, GS: Rehabilitation of the knee after anterior cruciate ligament surgery. Phys Med Rehabil 4:639, 1987.
9. Gowitzke, BA and Millner, S: Scientific Basis of Human Movement. Williams & Wilkins, Baltimore, 1988, pp 1–3.
10. Steindler, A: Kinesiology of the Human Body Under Normal and Pathological Conditions. Charles C. Thomas, Springfield, IL, 1973, p 63.
11. Norkin, CC and Levangie, PK: Joint Structure and Function: A Comprehensive Analysis. FA Davis, Philadelphia, 1989.

12. Warwick, R and Williams, PL: Gray's Anatomy. 35th British edition. Churchill Livingstone, New York, 1973, p 406.
13. Deusinger, RH: Biomechanics of clinical practice. Phys Ther 64:1860, 1984.
14. Lutz, GE, Palmitier, RA, and Chao, EYS: Comparison of tibiofemoral joint forces during open-kinetic-chain and closed-kinetic-chain exercises. J Bone Joint Surg 75A:732, 1993.
15. Brunstrom, S: Clinical Kinesiology. FA Davis, Philadelphia, 1962, pp 1–48.
16. Inman, VT: The Joints of the Ankle. Williams & Wilkins, Baltimore, 1976.
17. Root, ML, Orien, WP, and Weed, JN: Clinical Biomechanics. Vol 11: Normal and Abnormal Function of the Foot. Clinical Biomechanics, Los Angeles, 1977.
18. Inman, VT and Mann, R: Biomechanics of the foot and ankle. In Inman, VT (ed): DuVries' Surgery of the Foot, ed 3. CV Mosby, St. Louis, 1973.
19. Rodgers, MM and Cavanagh PR: Glossary of biomechanical terms, concepts, and units. Phys Ther 64:1886, 1984.
20. Arms, SW, et al: The biomechanics of anterior cruciate rehabilitation and reconstruction. Am J Sports Med 12:8, 1984.
21. Renstrom, P, et al: Strain within the anterior cruciate ligament during hamstring and quadriceps activity. Am J Sports Med 14:83, 1986.
22. Butler, DL, et al: On interpretation of our anterior cruciate data. Clin Orthop 196:26, 1985.
23. Reilly, DT and Martens, M: Experimental analysis of the quadriceps muscles force and patello-femoral joint reaction forces for various activities. Acta Orthop Scand 43:126, 1972.
24. Hungerford, DS and Barry, M: Biomechanics of the patellofemoral joint. Clin Orthop 144:9, 1975.
25. Albert, MS: Principles of exercise progression. In Greenfield, BH (ed): Rehabilitation of the Knee—A Problem-Solving Approach. FA Davis, Philadelphia, 1993, p 125.
26. Cavanagh, PR: The biomechanics of lower extremity action in distance running. Foot Ankle 7:197, 1987.
27. Stauffer, RN, Chao, EYS, and Brewster RC: Force and motion analysis of normal, diseased and prosthetic ankle joints. Clin Orthop 127:189, 1977.
28. Sammarco, GJ, Burstein, AH, and Frankel, VA: Biomechanics of the ankle: A kinematic study. Orthop Clin 4:75, 1973.
29. McCullough, CJ and Burge, PD: Rotatory stability of the load-bearing ankle. J Bone Joint Surg 62B:460, 1980.
30. Rydell, N: Biomechanics of the hip joint. Clin Orthop 92:6, 1973.
31. Deusinger, RH: Development of Baseline Mechanical Parameters for Selected Functional Activities. Doctoral Dissertation. Iowa City, IA, The University of Iowa, 1981.
32. Paul, JP: The biomechanics of the hip joint and its clinical relevance. Proceedings of the Royal Society of Medicine 59:943, 1966.
33. Paul, JP: Loading on the head of the human femur. J Anat 105:943, 1966.
34. Solomonow, M, et al: The synergistic action of the anterior cruciate ligament and thigh muscles in maintaining joint stability. Am J Sports Med 15:207, 1987.
35. Draganich, LF, Jaeger, RJ, and Knalji, AR: Coactivation of the hamstrings and quadriceps during extension of the knee. J Bone Joint Surg 71A:1075, 1989.
36. Morrison, JB: The mechanics of muscle function in locomotion. J Biomech 3:431, 1970.
37. Markolf, KL, Graff-Radford, A, and Amstatz, HC: In vivo knee stability: A quantitative assessment using an instrumental clinical testing apparatus. J Bone Joint Surg 60A:664, 1978.
38. Baratta, R, et al: Muscular coactivation: The role of antagonistic musculature in maintaining knee stability. Am J Sports Med 16:113, 1988.
39. English, AW, Wolf, SL, and Segal, R: Compartmentalization of muscles and their motor nuclei: The partitioning hypothesis. Phys Ther 73:857–867, 1993.
40. Wolf, SL, Segal, RL, and English, AW: Task-oriented EMG activity recorded from partitions in human lateral gastrocnemius muscle. J Electromyogr Kinesiol 3:87–94, 1993.
41. English, A: An electromyographic analysis of compartments in cat lateral gastrocnemius muscle during unrestrained locomotion. J Neurophysiol 52:114, 1984.
42. English, A and Ledbetter, W: A histochemical analysis of identified compartments of cat lateral gastrocnemius muscle. Anat Rec 204:123, 1982.
43. English, A and Weeks, O: Compartmentalization of single motor units in cat lateral gastrocnemius. Exp Brain Res 56:361, 1984.
44. Mann, RA and Inman, VT: Phasic activity of intrinsic muscles of the foot. J Bone Joint Surg 46A:469, 1964.
45. Perry, J: Kinesiology of lower extremity bracing. Clin Orthop 102:18, 1974.
46. Gardiner, E: The innervation of the knee joint. Anat Rec 101:109, 1948.
47. Wyke, BD: Articular neurology: A review. J Physiother 58:94, 1972.
48. Hutton, RS and Atwater, SW: Acute and chronic adaptations of muscle proprioceptors in response to increased use. Sports Med 14:406, 1992.
49. Johansson, H, Sjolander, P, and Soijka P: Activity in receptor afferents form the anterior cruciate ligament evokes reflex effects on fusimotor neurones. Neurosci Res 8:54, 1990.
50. Sherrington, CS: The Integrative Action of the Nervous System. Cambridge Press, London, 1948.

51. Gentile, A: Skill acquisition: Action, movement, and neuromotor processes. In Carr, JH, Shepherd, RB, and Gordon, L (eds): Movement Science: Foundations for Physical Therapy in Rehabilitation. Aspen Publishers, Rockville, MD, 1987, pp 93–154.
52. Barrack, RL, Skinner, HB, and Buckley, SL: Proprioception in the anterior cruciate deficient knee. Am J Sports Med 17:1, 1987.
53. Freeman, MAR and Wyke, BD: Articular contributions to limb muscle reflexes. An electromyographic study of normal and abnormal influences of ankle-joint mechanoreceptors upon reflex activity on gastrocnemius muscle in cat. J Physiol 171:20, 1964.
54. Friden, T, Zatterstrom, R, and Zindstrand, A: Disability in anterior cruciate ligament insufficiency. An analysis of 19 untreated patients. Acta Orthop Scand 61:131, 1990.
55. Wyke, B: The neurology of joints. Ann R Coll Surg Engl 41:25, 1967.
56. Freeman, MAR: Treatment of ruptures of the lateral ligament of the ankle. J Bone Joint Surg 47B:661, 1985.
57. France, EP, et al: Preliminary clinical evaluation of the Breg K. A. T. Effects of training in normals. Isokin Exerc Sci 2:133, 1992.
58. Andersson, C and Stener, B: Experimental evaluation of the hypothesis of ligamentomuscular protective reflexes: II: A study in cats using the mediocollateral ligament of the knee joint. Acta Physiol Scand 48:(suppl) 166:27, 1959.
59. Grabiner, MD, et al: Electromyographic study of the anterior cruciate ligament–hamstrings synergy during isometric knee extension. J Orthop Res 7:152, 1989.
60. Pope, DF, Cole, KJ, and Brand, RA: The ACL does not contribute to monosynaptic reflexes in the cat. 35th ORS Annual Meeting, Las Vegas, 1989.
61. Sojka, P, et al: Fusimotor neurones can be reflexly influenced by activity in receptor afferents from the posterior cruciate ligament. Brain Res 483:173, 1989.
62. Asmussen, E and Bonde-Peterson, F: Storage of elastic energy in skeletal muscles in man. Acta Physiol Scand 91:335, 1974.
63. Bosco, C and Komi, PV: Potentiation of the mechanical behavior of the human skeletal muscle through prestretching. Acta Physiol Scand 106:467, 1979.
64. Cavanga, G, Saibene, F, and Magaria, R: Effect of negative work on the amount of positive work performed by an isolated muscle. J Appl Physiol 20:157, 1965.
65. Bobbert, MF: Drop jumping as a training method for jumping ability. Sports Med 9:7, 1990.
66. Voight, ML and Draovitch, P: Plyometrics. In Albert, M (ed): Eccentric Muscle Training in Sports and Orthopedics. Churchill Livingstone, New York, 1991, pp 45–73.
67. Guyton, AC: Organ Physiology. Structure and Function of the Nervous System, ed 2. WB Saunders, Philadelphia, 1976.
68. Scholz, JP: Dynamic pattern theory—some implications for therapeutics. Phys Ther 70:827, 1990.
69. Keshner, EA: Controlling stability of a complex movement system. Phys Ther 70:844, 1990.
70. Keshner, EA, Woolacott, MH, and Debu, B: Neck and trunk responses during postural perturbations in humans. Exp Brain Rex 71:455, 1988.
71. Keggerreis, S: The construction and implementation of a functional progression as a component of athletic rehabilitation. J Orthop Sports Phys Ther 4:14, 1983.
72. Wallis, EL and Logan, GA: Figure Improvement and Body Conditioning Through Exercise. Prentice Hall, NJ, Engelwood Cliffs, 1964.
73. Nyland, J, et al: Review of the afferent neural system of the knee and its contribution to motor learning. J Orthop Sports Phys Ther 19:2, 1994.
74. Kelikian, H and Kelikian, AS: Disorders of the Ankle. WB Saunders, Philadelphia, 1985, p 68.
75. Johnson, KA: Surgery of the Foot and Ankle. Raven Press, New York, 1989.
76. Frank, C, et al: Medial collateral ligament healing. Am J Sports Med 11:380, 1983.
77. Voight, ML, and Weider, DL: Comparative reflex response times of vastus obliquus and vastus lateralis in normal subjects and subjects with extensor mechanism dysfunction: An electromygraphic study. Am J Sports Med 19:131, 1991.
78. Chu, D: Plyometric Exercise. NSCA Journal 6:56, 1984.
79. Noyes, FR, Barber, SD, and Mangine, RE: Abnormal lower limb symmetry determined by function hop tests after anterior cruciate ligament rupture. Am J Sports Med 15:513, 1991.

CHAPTER **13**

Surgical Intervention

Paul V. Spiegl, MD
Karen S. Seale, MD

In this chapter, some of the surgical options for management of several pathologic conditions of the lower extremity are discussed. These include pes cavus, pes
planus, hallux valgus, hallux rigidus, deformities of the lesser toes, ankle instability,
advanced arthritis of the foot and ankle, and extrinsic abnormalities of the lower
extremity. This chapter does not attempt to give specific details of every condition or
to cover all possible solutions to any given problem. Rather it is intended to help the
nonsurgeon who desires a better understanding of the indications, contraindications,
and mechanics of orthopedic surgery of the foot and ankle.

The first priority of surgery is to relieve pain. Other goals include maintaining
stability, preserving strength, and improving mobility. Frequently, these goals are at
odds, and compromises must be made.

An understanding of normal biomechanics of the foot and ankle and a thorough
examination of the patient to determine the pathomechanics are essential to determine
the most appropriate surgical procedure in a given situation. The ultimate clinical
selection of an operation, however, is also made with regard to the patient's age,
lifestyle, expectations, and other underlying health problems. A discussion of these
clinical factors and the decision-making process involved is beyond the scope of this
chapter.

PES CAVUS

The cavus foot deformity represents a spectrum of difficulties ranging from mild
elevation of the medial arch to a severe elevation with numerous associated deformities, which may include hindfoot varus, calcaneal dorsiflexion, tight plantar fascia,
forefoot adductus, a plantar flexed first ray, and claw toes. There are many causes of

cavus, including congenital, neuromuscular, and soft tissue contracture. The severity of the pes cavus deformity and patient symptoms underlying disorders dictate the treatment required.

In the cavus foot, stiffness in the subtalar joint diminishes the impact-absorbing capability of the foot and its ability to accommodate weight-bearing stresses. In the more mildly symptomatic patient, pressure-absorbing orthotic devices and shoe modifications are sufficient. With greater degrees of deformity, accommodation becomes less practical. As surgical intervention is planned, the cause of the pes cavus must first be determined. Each component of the cavus deformity must be assessed so that the major components can be corrected. Chapter 2 reviews the mechanics of abnormal supination and the components of pes cavus deformity.

CASE STUDY

A 24-year-old white woman with Charcot-Marie-Tooth disease presented with complaints of repeated ankle sprains that had become so severe that she was unable to negotiate level terrain safely (Fig. 13–1). Treatment with appropriate devices and shoe modifications had been unsuccessful. Biomechanical evaluation revealed three major components: heel varus, pes cavus, and great

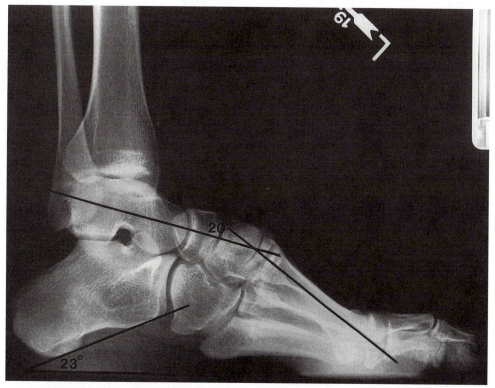

FIGURE 13–1. Preoperative radiograph of patient with heel varus and pes cavus.

toe clawing. Surgical options to improve the biomechanics and restore more normal function are discussed for each component.

The patient demonstrated two factors contributing to abnormal rearfoot function: limited subtalar motion with excursion from neutral to varus and an increase in the angle of inclination of the calcaneus (or dorsiflexion of the heel), which further accentuated the high arch.

Clinical evaluation of the midfoot revealed a tight plantar fascia, which was palpable along the longitudinal arch on passive dorsiflexion of the metatarsophalangeal (MTP) joints, and a rigidly plantar flexed first ray. The hindfoot varus locked the transverse tarsal joints. This increased the mechanical advantage of the peroneus longus as it passed around the calcaneocuboid joint to insert on the first metatarsal, accentuating plantar flexion of the first ray.

Evaluation of the forefoot revealed hyperextension deformities of all the MTP joints, particularly the first; mild dorsal MTP joint contractures and plantar prominence of the metatarsal heads; and flexion deformities of the interphalangeal joints.

In this particular case, attention was first directed to correction of the hindfoot varus deformity. A lateral closing wedge osteotomy of the calcaneus was performed. The tuberosity fragment into which the Achilles tendon inserts was translated laterally, thus providing a valgus shift in the biomechanical axis of the hindfoot. The tuberosity fragment was also shifted proximally to decrease the angle of inclination of the calcaneus. The osteotomy was rigidly fixed with two screws, which did not cross the subtalar joint, allowing normal function of the subtalar joint (Fig. 13–2). In addition, the plantar fascia was released from its origin on the calcaneus to prevent tethering and to allow repositioning of the calcaneal tuberosity and of the first metatarsal.

To correct the forefoot cavus deformity, a dorsal closing wedge osteotomy at the base of the first metatarsal osteotomy allows elevation of the metatarsal head and improves the talometatarsal angle. A Jones procedure was done, which consisted of the following steps: (1) release of the extensor hallucis longus from its insertion into the distal phalanx of the great toe, (2) fusion of the interphalangeal joint, (3) release of any dorsal contracture of the MTP joint capsule, and (4) routing of the extensor tendon into the dorsal aspect of the neck of the first metatarsal. The extensor tendon now acts to help dorsiflex the metatarsal rather than to hyperextend the MTP joint. This eliminates the clawing of the great toe as well as decreases the longitudinal arch. The clawing of the lesser toes was not severe enough to require correction. Surgical correction of lesser-toe deformities is discussed later in this chapter. These aspects of this patient's deformity were addressed: hindfoot varus, calcaneal dorsiflexion, plantar flexion of the first metatarsal, tethering of the plantar fascia, and cock-up of the great toe.

Not all of these procedures are required by every patient with cavus foot. The person whose hindfoot is in varus but whose forefoot is plantigrade may require only a calcaneal osteotomy. In another instance, the excessive plantar flexion of the first ray may be the only problem and may require only the dorsiflexion osteotomy of the first metatarsal.

If soft tissue imbalance is contributing to the deformity, appropriate tendon transfers and soft tissue procedures can be done in place of or in conjunction with bone procedures. In considering the surgical options, one should remember that the cavus

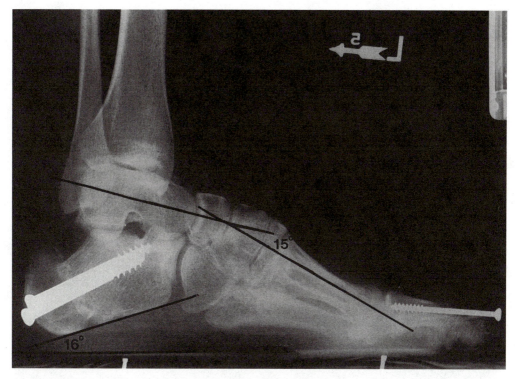

FIGURE 13–2. Postoperative radiograph of patient with heel varus and pes cavus following cal-caneal and first metatarsal osteotomies and a Jones procedure.

foot is already more rigid than normal. Therefore, every attempt should be made to preserve or increase existing flexibility. Conversely, if there is evidence of degenerative joint disease in the subtalar and transverse tarsal joints (Fig. 13–3), a triple arthrodesis may be indicated. In this case, the arthrodesis is performed to correct the hindfoot varus deformity and place the foot in a plantigrade position.

PES PLANUS

There are many causes of pes planus. An attempt must be made to establish the cause so that the appropriate surgical procedure can be selected. The following causes of pes planus and the surgical considerations of each are discussed: posterior tibial tendon rupture, tarsal coalition, Achilles tendon tightness, Charcot degeneration of the midfoot joints, hypermobile flatfoot of adulthood secondary to ligament laxity, calcaneal fracture, and rheumatoid arthritis.

Posterior Tibial Tendon Rupture

The insidious onset of unilateral, painful flatfoot in the adult is most common secondary to dysfunction of the posterior tibial tendon. The diagnosis is all too often

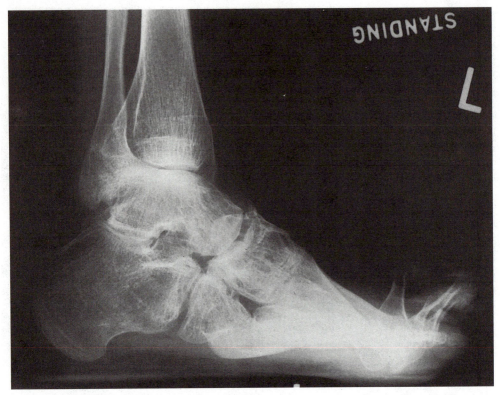

FIGURE 13–3. Radiograph of patient with degenerative joint changes requiring a triple arthodesis to correct the deformities.

missed. Delay in diagnosis can lead to chronic, irreversible changes in the foot. Posterior tibial tendon rupture is most frequently seen in women over the age of 40 years with no history of acute trauma.[1-3] During the early inflammatory phase of rupture, the primary complaint is pain over the posterior tibialis tendon, usually most pronounced on the posteromedial aspect of the ankle behind the medial malleolus or at the insertion on the navicular. Once the arch has collapsed, creating excessive pronation and abnormal heel valgus, subjective complaints may include pain over the lateral aspect of the hindfoot, which is caused by impingement of the calcaneus against the lateral malleolus. There is often also pain in the sinus tarsi as the subtalar joint is unevenly loaded with excessive forces laterally. Furthermore, the patient may complain of shoeing difficulties as the forefoot abducts from the hindfoot and pressure areas are created either over the navicular medially or over the head of the fifth metatarsal laterally.

If the problem is diagnosed early, before chronic changes develop in the bones and soft tissues, a tendon transfer can be performed using the flexor digitorum longus. The flexor digitorum longus is incised distally and rerouted through a drill hole into the navicular bone.[2] It then supplies motor function to supinate and adduct the foot. Considerable rehabilitation is required postoperatively to restore motion and strength in the transferred muscle-tendon unit, but good results of pain relief have been reported. Full function is generally not recovered because the flexor digitorum longus is weaker than the posterior tibialis. Also, if the ligaments have stretched without the support of the posterior tibialis, the foot does not regain the arch after the tendon transfers, even though pain may be relieved.

If treatment is delayed and the deformities of heel valgus and forefoot supination are no longer passively correctable, a soft tissue procedure is no longer an option. A triple arthrodesis is required to stabilize the calcaneus beneath the talus via a talocalcaneal fusion and to derotate and adduct the forefoot on the hindfoot by fusing the calcaneocuboid and talonavicular joints with the foot in a plantigrade position. Attempts should be made to maintain the normal function and flexibility of the foot; therefore, early diagnosis is desirable to avoid the necessity of arthrodesis.

Tarsal Coalition

Tarsal coalition is a congenital fusion of two or more tarsal bones, most commonly occurring between the talus and calcaneus or between the calcaneus and navicular. Symptoms usually occur when the patient reaches maturity, at which time the fibrous coalition ossifies, increasing the rigidity of the foot. If treatment is rendered before extensive degenerative changes occur in the surrounding joints, the coalition can be surgically excised with good results.[4] This intervention restores some motion and improves the biomechanics. Figure 13–4 is the radiograph of a 21-year-old college student who presented with symptoms of severe subtalar pain for only the last 2 years. He had flatfeet ever since childhood but had not had pain before this time. Because the radiographs demonstrated minimal degenerative joint changes, he was a candidate for surgical excision of the coalition, which united his calcaneus and navicular. Figure 13–5 is the radiograph after coalition excision.

If the condition goes untreated for many years or if the extent of coalition is such that the bones cannot be effectively separated with good results, a triple arthrodesis is required. The foot should be realigned and fused, with the heel in slight valgus and the forefoot plantigrade.

Charcot Joint Degeneration

A third cause of pes planus in adults is collapse and degeneration of joints of the hindfoot or midfoot secondary to neuropathy. This is most frequently secondary to diabetes. For reasons that are not yet clearly understood, the diabetic patient, who has some degree of loss of sensation to the foot, loses the structural integrity of the joints secondary to ligament and bone destruction. Occasionally the process can be initiated by an event as insignificant as twisting the foot or sustaining mild blunt trauma, but commonly there is no known history of trauma. The resulting arch undergoes collapse and disintegration, as seen in Figure 13–6. In the majority of cases, this condition is treated nonoperatively with compressive stockings, elevation, and non–weight bearing until the early inflammatory phase resolves and healing occurs. Surgery is required if the deformity causes repeated skin ulcerations over the bony prominences. Frequently, merely excising the prominences can suffice to prevent further problems, although the pes planus and abnormal biomechanics persist. Careful follow-up observation and fitting with custom-molded accommodative orthotic devices and shoe modifications are needed.

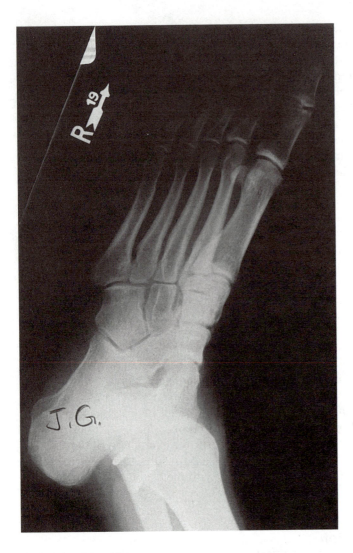

FIGURE 13–4. Preoperative radiograph of calcaneal-navicular coalition.

In rare instances, a patient with Charcot joint degeneration may be a candidate for arthrodesis of the affected joints to correct the deformity and stabilize the foot; however, the arthrodesis poses potential risks, such as infection and recurrence of the inflammatory phase of destruction. Arthrodesis requires extended periods of immobilization for healing to occur.

Hypermobile Flatfoot

As discussed in Chapter 2, flexible flatfoot is not necessarily a pathologic condition. During childhood, the ligaments of the feet are normally more flexible than in adulthood. As the child matures, the tensile strength of ligaments increases to prevent abnormal pronation and excessive pes planus. If abnormal excessive laxity persists into adulthood, however, abnormal stresses are placed on the hypermobile flatfoot.

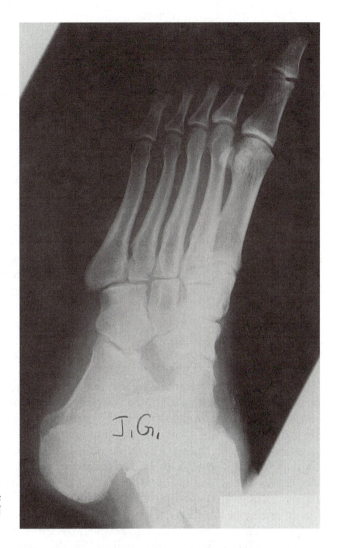

FIGURE 13–5. Postoperative radiograph after excision of C-N coalition.

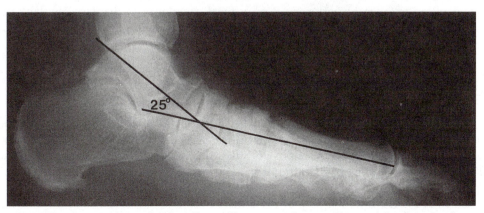

FIGURE 13–6. Radiograph of midfoot collapse secondary to Charcot joint degeneration.

The presence of excessive heel valgus is frequently accompanied by contracture of the Achilles tendon, which further worsens the biomechanical situation. If regular and faithful use of custom molded-plastic orthotic devices, as described by Bordelon,[6] and a properly administered program of Achilles tendon stretching are not successful in reducing the foot deformity, surgery can be considered.

Surgery in this case is also directed to the areas of most pronounced deformity. If the problem is primarily excessive heel valgus, a calcaneal osteotomy could reduce the valgus position of the calcaneus, and Achilles tendon lengthening may be all that is necessary. If the deformity is more severe and includes forefoot supination or abduction (or both), other surgical procedures may be performed to alleviate specific deformities. A plantar flexing osteotomy of the first metatarsal increases the arch and relatively pronates the forefoot. The forefoot abduction can be addressed by an opening wedge osteotomy of the cuboid or calcaneal neck or a closing wedge osteotomy of the cuneiform. The latter osteotomies can also pronate the forefoot, and in some instances, a calcaneocuboid arthrodesis is performed in association with the osteotomies.[7]

Calcaneus Fractures

Fracture of the calcaneus most frequently results from a fall from a height. The calcaneus is fractured as the talus is driven, like a wedge, into the body of the calcaneus, resulting in numerous fracture patterns. Commonly the fracture line goes through the posterior facet, leaving the medial portion of the calcaneus—the sustentaculum—relatively intact. The remainder of the body of the calcaneus is displaced laterally, which also effectively decreases the vertical height of the calcaneus. If the foot is allowed to heal in this position, the result is abnormal biomechanics owing to excessive heel valgus and pes planus.

In recent years, there has been an interest in primary operative intervention to openly reduce and internally fix calcaneal fractures. The goals of early surgery are to restore subtalar joint congruity, replace the displaced calcaneal tuberosity to its normal position, and begin early motion to decrease joint adhesions.

Patients with the sequelae of calcaneal fractures may develop arthritis as well as deformity. If there is a severe degree of deformity, the reconstructive procedure includes not only an arthrodesis of the subtalar joint or a triple arthrodesis, but also consideration is given to performing a calcaneal osteotomy to displace medially the heel and to increase the vertical height of the calcaneus to correct the pes planus deformity.[8]

Rheumatoid Arthritis

In rheumatoid arthritis, an inflammatory process attacks the joint surfaces and supporting ligaments and tendons. As the joints are eroded and bones sublux out of position, the foot collapses into a pes planus configuration. The joints may be unstable and painful when weight bearing. When orthoses and orthopedic shoes are inadequate, a triple arthrodesis, as discussed later in this chapter, restores the bony relationships and structural integrity of the foot.

HALLUX VALGUS

Adult acquired hallux valgus is associated with imbalance of the soft tissues and abnormal bony configuration of the first cuneiform/MTP joint complex. Components of hallux valgus pathology can include the painful "bump," or prominent exostosis, on the medial side of the foot; lateral deviation and pronation of the great toe; excessive metatarsus primus varus; subluxation or dislocation of the first metatarsal head from its sesamoid sling; attenuation of the medial MTP joint capsule; contracture of the adductor hallucis muscle and lateral MTP joint capsule; abnormal direction of pull of the intrinsic and extrinsic muscles of the great toe; degenerative joint disease; and associated second-toe deformities.

Adult acquired hallux valgus is found most often in women and is commonly associated with long-term wearing of fashionable, narrow box, pointed-toe shoes. Other associated findings, which may be implicated in the biomechanical cause of hallux valgus, include contracture of the Achilles tendon complex, pes planus, and hypermobility of the first metatarsal–medial cuneiform joint.

More than 100 different operations are described in the literature for correction of hallux valgus, and no single operation is perfect for all patients. Not every patient needs an operation, and careful patient selection is the byword. Patient personality, age, lifestyle, expectations, degree and type of deformity, presence of arthritis, and associated findings are just some of the factors to consider before surgical intervention is undertaken. There are, however, some basic principles when approaching this complex problem.

Figure 13–7 is a schematic representation of the normal tendons acting on the first MTP joint. The action of the long and short toe extensors is normally counteracted by the long and short toe flexors, just as the abductor hallucis is counterbalanced by the adductor hallucis. This counterbalance results in normal biplanar flexion and extension of the MTP joint. Figure 13–8 represents hallux valgus in which there is lateral displacement of the long flexors and extensors, overpull of the adductor, and plantar displacement of the abductor so that it no longer efficiently resists adduction of the great toe. A rotational component pronates the toe while the metatarsal head deviates medially, thus subluxing out of the sesamoid sling.

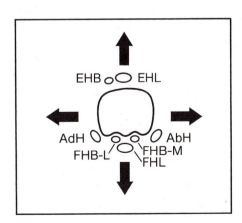

FIGURE 13–7. Schematic representation of forces acting across the normal first metatarsal phalangeal joint.

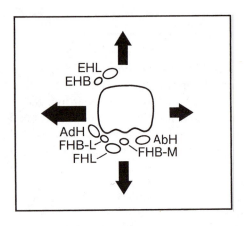

FIGURE 13–8. Forces acting across first MTP joint in hallus valgus.

If the primary complaint in hallux valgus deformity is a prominent medial eminence, the deformity is mild, and relatively rapid recovery is desirable, simple surgical removal of the medial eminence can be the answer. The disadvantages are that with removal of the medial eminence alone, realignment is not accomplished, and recurrence or progression of the deformity is likely.

For mild-to-moderate deformity in a young person with no degenerative joint disease, consideration can be given to performing a distal metatarsal osteotomy, such as a chevron osteotomy. This procedure affords limited realignment by lateral displacement of the head of the first metatarsal, removal of the medial prominence, and plication of the medial capsule. Healing is quick, and the procedure is technically less demanding than more extensive ones. A metatarsal osteotomy has other advantages, including shorter operating time, less pain in the immediate postoperative period, and earlier return to activities. Major shortcomings of this procedure are that it cannot adequately correct the deformity when the first and second intermetatarsal angle is greater than 15° or 16° and that the deforming force of the adductor muscle is retained.

Figure 13–9 is an illustration of the essential features of this procedure: (1) removal of the medial prominence, (2) lateral displacement of the metatarsal head after performing the osteotomy, and (3) removal of the residual medial prominence of the proximal metatarsal.[9] The lateral shift of the metatarsal realigns it over the sesamoid sling. As the medial capsule is plicated, the abductor tendon is realigned in its anatomic position medial to the metatarsal head. Thus, the tendon forces are realigned.

The procedure that has come to be known as the distal soft tissue procedure, which is a modification of the procedure originally described by McBride,[10] is used for a more extensive deformity. It was designed to provide more extensive correction of the abnormal biomechanics of the hallux valgus and is particularly useful in cases in which the deformity is more severe, that is, when the MTP joint angle is greater than 40° and the intermetatarsal angle is greater then 15°. In severe bunion deformities, the procedure is combined with a proximal metatarsal osteotomy to correct metatarsus primus varus.

The procedure as illustrated in Figure 13–10 has three major components: (1) An incision is made dorsally through the first web space, which releases the lateral MTP joint capsule, adductor hallucis tendon, and contractures about the lateral sesamoid.

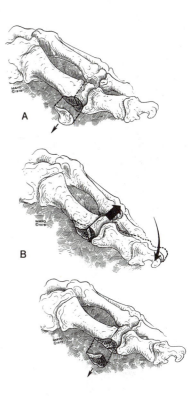

FIGURE 13–9. Schematic representation of Chevron osteotomy. (From Johnson, KA: Surgery of the Foot and Ankle. Raven Press, 1989, p 6, with permission.)

This allows reduction of the MTP joint, reduction of the sesamoid sling, and a correction of the hallux valgus. (2) The medial eminence of the metatarsal head is removed through a medial incision and the medial capsule is plicated and the abductor hallucis tendon is realigned to support the relocated sesamoid sling. (3) An osteotomy is performed at the base of the first metatarsal. Several osteotomies can be considered, including a lateral closing wedge osteotomy or a crescentic osteotomy performed through a separate dorsal incision at the proximal metaphyseal area.[13] Alternatively the medial incision could be extended more proximally, and a proximal Chevron procedure can be performed through the metaphyseal area, which displaces the entire metatarsal laterally.[14] Extreme care must be taken during the metatarsal osteotomy so that the metatarsal head is not dorsiflexed or the length excessively shortened, which would create a pressure transfer to the second metatarsal head. This procedure can be performed on patients of all ages, but it is better to avoid it in patients with degenerative arthritis of the first MTP joint.

Presence of severe degenerative joint disease limits the surgical procedures that can be used to correct the hallux valgus deformity. Arthrodesis is an excellent procedure for the deformity and elimination of pain secondary to arthritis. The disadvantages of this procedure include the elimination of joint motion and limitation of shoe selection to heel heights less than 1.5 inches. Resection arthroplasty involves removal of the proximal one third of the proximal phalanx, which allows correction of the angulation deformity of the toe while eliminating the opposing arthritic joint surfaces. The disadvantages include shortening of the toe; decreasing the weight-bearing function of the first toe, which can lead to lateral metatarsalgia; and failure to correct metatarsus primus varus. Replacement arthroplasty with a Silastic implant retains

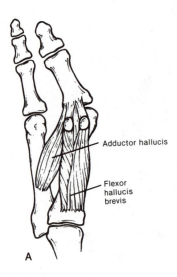

A

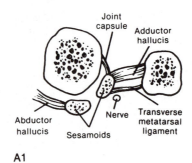

Joint
capsule

Adductor
hallucis

Abductor
hallucis

Sesamoids

Nerve

Transverse
metatarsal
ligament

A1

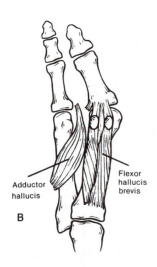

Adductor
hallucis

Flexor
hallucis
brevis

B

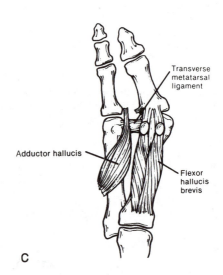

Transverse
metatarsal
ligament

Adductor hallucis

Flexor
hallucis
brevis

C

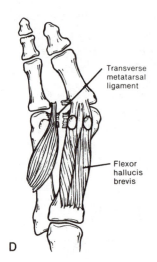

Transverse
metatarsal
ligament

Flexor
hallucis
brevis

D

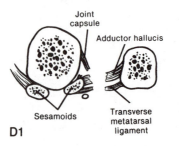

Joint
capsule

Adductor hallucis

Sesamoids

Transverse
metatarsal
ligament

D1

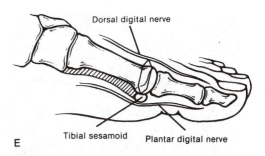

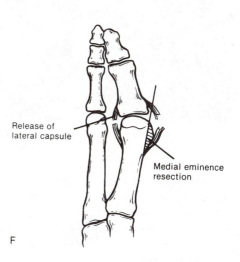

FIGURE 13–10. Schematic representation of distal soft tissue procedure. (*A*) The anatomy of hallus valgus. (*A1*) Subluxed sesamoids with contracted soft tissues. (*B*) Release deforming pull of the adductor hallucis. (*C*) The contracted intermetatarsal ligament is exposed. (*D*) Release contracted intermetatarsal ligament. (*D1*) The sesamoids and hallux valgus can now be reduced. (*E*) Medial incision. (*F*) Medial eminence is excised and the capsule plicated. (From Mann, RA and Coughlin, MJ: The Videotextbook of Foot and Ankle Surgery. Medical Video Production, St. Louis, 1991, pp 161–162, with permission.)

some joint function and can result in good cosmesis, but it continues to be fraught with numerous problems, including excessive tissue reaction by the body to foreign materials, breakage and loosening of the implant, necessity for removal if infection occurs, and increased expense.

HALLUX RIGIDUS

Hallux rigidus, or hallux limitus, is a degenerative joint disease of the first MTP joint that causes pain and limited motion. Roentgenographic findings include osteophyte formation on the dorsal aspects of the metatarsal head and at the base of the proximal phalanx (Fig. 13–11). Hallux rigidus seems to occur more frequently in people who demonstrate a relatively flat metatarsal head than in those whose MTP joint is more rounded (Fig. 13–12). One theory to account for this difference is that when stress of narrow pointed shoes is applied to the rounded MTP joint socket, lateral deviation of the toe occurs, causing hallux valgus. When similar stresses are applied to the flat metatarsal head, pressure is applied to the articular surface in an irregular manner, leading to traumatic arthritis.[10]

There are three primary procedures for the treatment of adult acquired hallux rigidus: cheilectomy, arthrodesis, and replacement arthroplasty with Silastic implant. Cheilectomy involves removal of excessive proliferative bone from around the metatarsal head and proximal phalanx. This procedure can be combined with a dorsi-

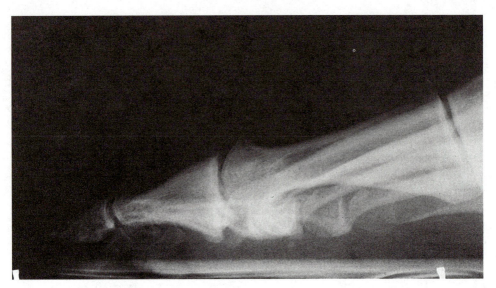

FIGURE 13–11. Preoperative lateral radiograph of hallux rigidus.

flexion osteotomy of the proximal phalanx to optimize the functional range of motion of the toe. If this procedure fails to resolve the symptoms or if the arthritis is too far advanced at the time of surgery, either arthrodesis or replacement arthroplasty can still be performed. Arthrodesis ensures relief of pain at the sacrifice of joint motion. Replacement arthroplasty, while maintaining joint motion, can be complicated by the problems listed under the previous discussion of the procedure for the treatment of hallux valgus.

MALLET TOES, HAMMER TOES, AND CLAW TOES

Occasionally, there is confusion regarding the definitions of the lesser toe deformities. For the purpose of this discussion, the following terms are used:

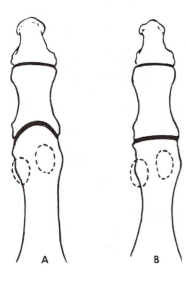

FIGURE 13–12. Schematic representation of the variations in the shape of the first metatarsal head. (*A*) Rounded or oval. (*B*) Flat. (From Mann, RA: Surgery of the Foot and Ankle, ed 6. CV Mosby, St. Louis, 1986, p 162, with permission.)

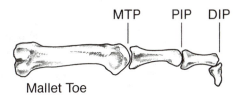

FIGURE 13–13. Mallet toe.   Mallet Toe

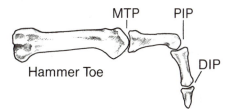

FIGURE 13–14. Hammer toe.

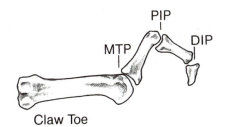

FIGURE 13–15. Claw toe.   Claw Toe

1. Mallet toe is a deformity of a lesser toe in which the distal interphalangeal joint (DIP) is flexed and the proximal interphalangeal (PIP) and MTP joints are normal (Fig. 13–13).
2. Hammer toe is a deformity consisting of abnormal flexion of the PIP joint with the DIP and MTP joints in neutral position (Fig. 13–14).
3. Claw toe is hyperflexion of both the PIP and DIP joints and hyperextension of the MTP joint (Fig. 13–15).

Which procedure is best for a given deformity varies from surgeon to surgeon and patient to patient. The following discussion includes approaches based on the authors' personal experience.

Mallet toe may be congenital or may develop in association with wearing ill-fitting shoes, which leads to contracture of the DIP joint. The symptomatic patient with a mallet toe usually has a painful callus on the tip of the toe, although a painful bursa may develop over the dorsum of the DIP joint. Detachment of the flexor digitorum longus from its insertion into the distal phalanx may be all that is necessary. If the volar plate is contracted, however, excision of a segment of the distal end of the distal phalanx may be necessary to allow the toe to rest in its normal extended position.

Hammer toe is most often seen in association with wearing ill-fitting shoes or hosiery, but it may also be caused by trauma when, for example, a sharp object cuts the extensor tendon over the PIP joint. Hammer toe can be classified into two categories: (1) flexible (or dynamic) and (2) fixed (or static). The categories can be distinguished by testing for contracture at the PIP joint. With the ankle in neutral position and the foot plantigrade, the PIP joint is passively manipulated into extension. If full

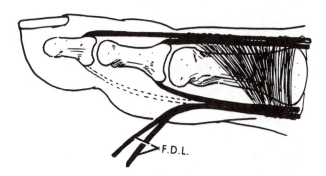

FIGURE 13–16. Detachment of the FDL from its insertion in this distal phalanx.

extension can be obtained, the hammer toe is flexible, and a soft tissue procedure such as a flexor-to-extensor tendon transfer can be performed. The procedure involves detaching the flexor digitorum longus from its insertion on the distal phalanx, splitting it along its median raphe (Fig. 13–16), and rerouting it to the dorsal aspect of the proximal phalanx (Fig. 13–17). It can now act to aid the extensor hood in flexing the MTP joint and extending the PIP joint. Some surgeons also detach the flexor digitorum brevis from its insertion at the base of the middle phalanx to remove its plantar flexing force at the PIP joint.

If the PIP joint cannot be fully extended, the hammer toe deformity is considered static or fixed. This deformity can be managed by excising the distal end of the proximal phalanx. Shortening the bone is usually sufficient to allow the toe to rest in a neutral position. If a neutral position cannot be achieved, more bone must be resected, or additional soft tissue releases must be performed. An excisional arthroplasty is accomplished at the PIP joint by retaining the joint surface of the middle phalanx and

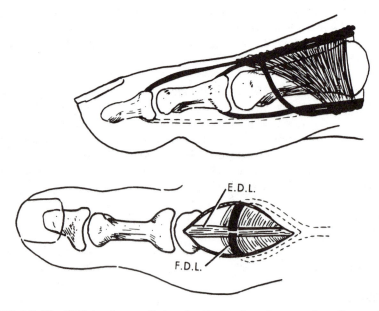

FIGURE 13–17. The FDL has been split longitudinally along its natural median raphe, each tail rerouted on either side of the proximal phalanx, and sutured to the dorsal extensor hood.

pinning the joint for 4 to 6 weeks. This maintains 10° to 20° of motion. Alternatively the PIP joint can be fused by removing the joint surface from the middle phalanx and fixing to the proximal phalanx.

Claw toes represent the simultaneous contracture of the long flexors and extensors of the lesser toes and a muscle imbalance between the extrinsic and intrinsic muscles.[10] A milder form of claw toes can develop as a natural progression of hammer toes, as the contracted PIP joint leads to a dorsiflexion contracture at the MTP joint. In the more severe form, claw toes develop in a disease in which there is neuromuscular dysfunction, such as Charcot-Marie-Tooth disease, Friedreich's ataxia, and diabetes, or when the joint or tendon is destroyed by an inflammatory condition, such as rheumatoid arthritis. In these more severe forms, multiple toes are involved. Claw toes may require release of the dorsal capsule of the MTP joints and lengthening of the extensor tendon, in addition to the procedures for treatment of hammer toes.

ANKLE INSTABILITY

Ankle instability generally occurs on the lateral rather than medial aspect. It is usually the result of a sprain of the anterior talofibular ligament, often combined with a sprain of the calcaneofibular ligament. In the acute injury, adequate healing usually occurs with 6 weeks of immobilization. In those instances, however, when the injury is untreated or when the ligament has, for unclear reasons, healed with laxity, the ankle or subtalar joint sublux when stressed into varus.

Often patients with ankle instability can be conservatively treated with orthoses or lateral heel wedges, taping or bracing the ankle during sports, and rehabilitating the strength and proprioception of the peroneal tendons. See Chapter 10 for further rehabilitation procedures. When rehabilitation of the ankle fails to reestablish joint stability and the patient suffers recurrent ankle sprains, surgery is considered.

Several reconstructions using one half or all of the peroneus brevis to substitute for the lateral ligament have been used with fairly good success over the years.[10] In the Evans procedure, for example, the peroneus brevis is divided proximally to the fibula, and the distal portion is anchored to the lateral malleolus (Fig. 13–18). Although this tethering effect is quite oblique to the line of the calcaneofibular ligament and anterior talofibular ligament, the operation actually works quite well in the clinical setting. The disadvantages are the difficulty in rehabilitating the compromised peroneal complex and the persisting potential for weakness of the peroneals in the high-demand individual.

In recent years, the modified Brostrom has gained acceptance. This operation involves a late repair with plication of the lax anterior talofibular and calcaneofibular ligaments with augmentation from the fascia of the extensor retinaculum (Fig. 13–19). This operation has the disadvantage that, in some instances, the quality of tissue is not as good as that of the tendons. It has the advantage of a more physiologic result and preservation of the peroneal tendons.

ARTHRITIS

From Chapter 1, the reader should recall that each joint works in concert with every other joint to ensure the dissipation of rotatory, angulatory, and compressive

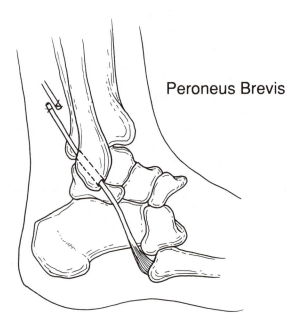

Peroneus Brevis

•FIGURE 13–18. Schematic representation of the Evans procedure. The peroneus brevis is transferred through the lateral malleolus to replace the anterior talofibular ligament and the calcaneofibular ligament. The ankle and subtalar joint are both stabilized with this transfer. (From Mann, RA and Coughlin, MJ: Surgery of the Foot and Ankle, ed 6. Mosby, St. Louis, 1993, p 1163, with permission.)

forces generated during gait. There are certain clinical conditions wherein the joint is so damaged, however, by trauma, infection, or inflammatory arthritis, that arthrodesis is the only viable solution.

Ankle

Although the ankle is primarily a biplanar joint for flexion and extension, it functions as a universal joint in conjunction with the subtalar joint. Elimination of ankle motion with an ankle arthrodesis places increased stress on the subtalar joint. Careful selection of the position for ankle arthrodesis becomes important. The degree of transverse rotation should approximate that of the contralateral ankle. Thus, the least amount of stress is placed on the subtalar joint. Too much internal rotation of the ankle holds the subtalar joint in a more rigid position, causing the patient to vault over a rather rigid, internally rotated forefoot unless compensatory external rotation of the hip and knee joint occurs. Too much external rotation forces the patient to roll off the medial side of the foot, which applies lateral stress to the great toe, causing hallux valgus.

Neutral is the most desirable position of flexion and extension, assuming that normal muscle strength and equal leg lengths exist. Some clinicians suggest that 10° of plantar flexion in women may be desirable, to allow for the wearing of a higher-heeled shoe. More compensatory plantar flexion than dorsiflexion, however, occurs at the midfoot joints. Thus, the patient is allowed more versatility if the ankle is fused in the neutral position. Too much dorsiflexion should be avoided because this causes concentration of forces on ground contact over a small area of the heel, which can cause pain. The optimal varus-valgus position of ankle arthrodesis is 5° to 7° of valgus in relation to the entire tibia. Too much varus places excessive stress on the fifth metatarsal and can cause pain and calluses.

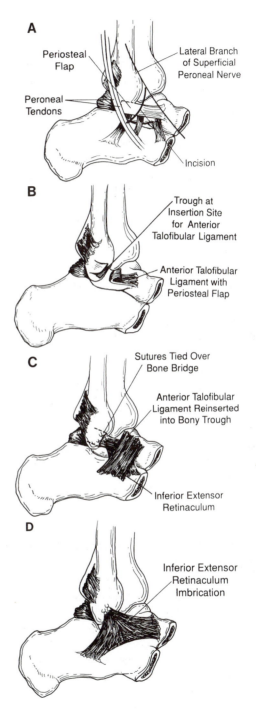

A
Periosteal Flap

Lateral Branch of Superficial Peroneal Nerve

Peroneal Tendons

Incision

B
Trough at Insertion Site for Anterior Talofibular Ligament

Anterior Talofibular Ligament with Periosteal Flap

C
Sutures Tied Over Bone Bridge

Anterior Talofibular Ligament Reinserted into Bony Trough

Inferior Extensor Retinaculum

D
Inferior Extensor Retinaculum Imbrication

FIGURE 13–19. The modified Brostrom procedure. (*A*) Incision over stretched anterior talofibular ligament. (*B*) Create trough to receive shortened ligament. (*C*) Suture ligament. Define inferior extensor retinaculum. (*D*) Imbricate inferior extensor retinaculum to lateral malleolus to reinforce repair. (From Mann, RA and Coughlin, MJ: Surgery of the Foot and Ankle, ed 6. Mosby, St. Louis, 1993, p 1163, with permission.)

Subtalar Joint

The subtalar joint uniquely translates the transverse rotation passing from the tibia into the foot. Proper alignment of this joint in fusion is critical. Slight valgus tilt of 5° to 7° allows the body weight to pass medially to the calcaneus, placing little stress on the lateral ankle ligament and maintaining some flexibility in the transverse tarsal joints. This allows even weight distribution across the foot. Too much valgus can result in excessive strain along the medial longitudinal arch, causing pain. Too much varus causes strain of the lateral collateral ankle ligament and excessive pressure under the lateral border of the foot and imparts rigidity to the transverse tarsal joints.

Transverse Tarsal Joints

The calcaneocuboid and talonavicular joints work in concert with the subtalar joint and with one another. If motion is eliminated in any one of these joints, motion in all three is essentially eliminated. When either or both of the transverse tarsal joints are fused, the subtalar joint should be held at a 5° of valgus position and the forefoot in a neutral plantigrade position. Too much supination results in pain under the lateral border of the foot. Too much pronation results in stresses under the first metatarsal head and sesamoids. Also, forefoot abduction or adduction must be avoided to prevent pressure areas on the medial or lateral borders when wearing shoes.

First Metatarsophalangeal Joint

Arthrodesis of the first MTP joint can result in minimal loss of function if done in the proper position of 10° to 15° valgus and 25° to 30° of dorsiflexion. The greater the degree of dorsiflexion, the higher the shoe heel that can be worn. Too much dorsiflexion, however, can result in rubbing in the top of the shoe at the interphalangeal joint when flatter shoes are worn. Insufficient dorsiflexion results in the need to vault over the great toe, resulting in hyperextension of the interphalangeal joint and in callus formation.

EXTRINSIC ABNORMALITIES OF THE LOWER EXTREMITY

As has been emphasized repeatedly in this book, each bone and joint in the kinematic chain works in concert with every other component. Extrinsic abnormalities of the hip, knee, femur, and tibia can exert a deleterious effect on the ankle and foot. The effect of each of these proximal components on the distal component must be considered in the patient evaluation and treatment. The surgical implications of four clinical problems are presented: femoral anteversion, tibial torsion, angular deformities of the tibia, and leg length discrepancy.

Femoral Anteversion

Femoral anteversion is exaggerated internal torsion of the femur affecting rotational alignment of the lower extremity. This common developmental deformity of children causes in-toeing and also may predispose to patellofemoral problems as the knee axis is internally rotated. Some rotational malalignment corrects spontaneously, independent of exercise and braces, as the child matures up to age 8. In rare cases, the deformity is severe enough to require surgery. Tachdjian recommends that surgery be reserved for the child 8 years and older whose hip cannot be externally rotated beyond neutral and whose functional disability and cosmetic appearance warrant correction.[12] An external rotation osteotomy may be performed at (1) the subtrochanteric region using a blade plate, (2) at the diaphysis using an intramedullary nail, or (3) at the distal metaphysis using pins or plate fixation. The bone is cut, and the foot is externally rotated so that approximately equal amounts of internal and external rotation of the foot can occur, and the knee axis is in a relatively physiologic position. The cut ends of the femur are then fixed in a stable configuration until healing occurs.

Tibial Torsion

Internal tibial torsion can occur alone or in conjunction with femoral anteversion and is another cause of in-toeing, which usually corrects spontaneously. In contrast to femoral anteversion, most cases correct with growth. In the rare child whose internal tibial torsion persists past 8 years of age, surgery can be performed. A derotation osteotomy of the tibia, similar to that for femoral anteversion, is performed to realign the transmalleolar axis at 25° of external torsion. Internal tibial torsion should be differentiated from Blount's tibia vara, which usually requires early bracing and surgical correction.

Angulatory Deformities of the Tibia

Two of the most frequently seen angulatory deformities of the tibia that cause clinical symptoms are genu varum and tibial shaft malunion.

Genu Varum

Genu varum or bowlegs is physiologic in a child below ages 2 to 3, probably as a result of the in utero position of the lower limbs. After age 3, the pendulum usually swings to genu valgus or knockknees, and finally there is a spontaneous correction by age 8 to 10 years. In those rare adolescents with severe persisting genu varum, tibia and fibula osteotomy may be necessary.

In the adult, genu varum can develop gradually as a result of asymmetric wearing away of the medial compartment of the knee secondary to osteoarthritis, rheumatoid arthritis, or tibial plateau fracture. If genu varum exists in conjunction with arthritis limited to the medial compartment of the knee, consideration can be given to a proximal tibial osteotomy. A tibial osteotomy surgery corrects the genu varum angular deformity, preserves the joint, and more evenly distributes weight-bearing stresses from the medial to the lateral compartment. If arthritis exists in the patellofemoral or lateral compartment, however, total knee arthroplasty should be considered. At the time of joint replacement, attention must be directed to correcting the varus malalignment with the appropriate soft tissue and bone techniques, to prevent failure of a malaligned prosthetic joint.

Tibial Malunion

Tibial malunions can occur at any level of the tibia. The more proximal the malunion, the greater the magnitude of angulatory deformity and the greater its effects on foot and ankle biomechanics. Because the subtalar joint has more motion into inversion than eversion, the arthrokinematic system of the foot and ankle is more effective in compensating for a valgus deformity of the tibia than for a varus deformity. Tibia varum can result in excessive compressive forces on the lateral aspect of the ankle, causing pain, and in callosities along the lateral border of the foot.

Surgical management includes corrective osteotomy, preferably at the level of greatest angular deformity, to bring the foot into correct alignment with the knee and hip. The osteotomy can be performed also to correct any rotational malalignment that might exist. The bone is fixed with an intramedullary rod, internal screws and plates, or external devices until healing occurs. Malunion may also include leg length inequality, which is discussed in the next section.

Leg Length Discrepancies

There are many causes of structural leg length inequality, including congenital anomalies, tumors, infection, trauma, and neuromuscular disease. The options for surgical management include retarding or permanently arresting the growth of the longer limb in the skeletally immature patient, shortening the longer limb, and lengthening the shorter limb. Some of the factors considered in the surgical evaluation include decisions about the skeletal site at which the leg length discrepancy occurs, the age of patient, the amount of discrepancy present and the total amount of discrepancy anticipated, the cause, the condition of the soft tissues, the predicted eventual total body height (if patient is skeletally immature), the presence of structural or functional compensation in the spine, the abnormality of gait, the degree of coordination, and the requirement for a lift.

If leg length discrepancy occurs in a child who has sufficient remaining growth potential in the shortened limb, the ideal solution would be selective and unilateral epiphyseal stimulation of the affected limb to allow growth of the short leg to "catch up" to the normal one. Unfortunately a safe, reliable technique of epiphyseal stimulation is not yet available.

Premature fusion of one or more of the physes of the limb that is longer allows the short extremity to equalize the disparate leg lengths as normal growth occurs. Using a complex system including serial limb measurements with orthoroentgenography, determination of skeletal maturity, relative size of the individual, and rate of growth, a growth prediction chart can be used to help determine at which anatomic site (femur or tibia) and at what age surgical growth arrest, or epiphysiodesis, can be most successfully employed. The surgical principles of epiphysiodesis include careful removal of the physis and packing of the space with bone graft to obliterate the growth plate.

The surgical options for the skeletally mature patient who has a leg length inequality are limited to lengthening the short leg or shortening the long leg. Once again, this decision is dependent on age; site and cause of discrepancy and the condition of the soft tissue; and the compensatory ability of the opposite leg, pelvis, and spine, among other factors.

Resecting a segment of the femur or the tibia and fibula provides a way to shorten the long limb. Leveling of the knees is an important cosmetic consideration as well as a biomechanical consideration. Ideally, if the loss of length of the short side has occurred at the tibial level, shortening the longer, contralateral tibia is preferable. Shortening of the tibia, however, is complicated by several factors. The muscles of the leg can become permanently weakened if more than 3 cm of bone is removed.[9] The surgery is more complex because resection of portions of both the tibia and the fibula is required and the leg is at risk for compartment syndrome.

Shortening of the femur offers fewer potential complications than the above-mentioned procedure and can be done in any number of ways. A current popular technique is the use of an intramedullary saw, which allows resection of the desired amount of the shaft of the bone without requiring a separate incision on the thigh. Using the closed technique, an intramedullary rod is passed through the same incision through which the saw is inserted over the greater trochanter. Femoral bone healing is more rapid and predictable than tibial healing, and there are fewer complications of muscle weakness, infection, and malunion.

Theoretically, lengthening the short leg makes more sense from a cosmetic and biomechanical standpoint. Bone lengthening, especially of the tibia, however, has been fraught with complications, such as overstretching, interference with the blood supply, insufficient fixation of the fragments, and problems of operative technique.[12] One of the most exciting current developments in limb lengthening has been the introduction of the Ilizarov technique of corticotomy and gradual bone lengthening. This technique involves subcutaneous fracture of the cortex of the bone and gradual distraction of the fragments using an external fixation device. Lengthening of up to 12 cm of the femur and 15 cm of the tibia has been reported, with fewer complications than with previous techniques.[15]

A combination of lengthening the short limb and shortening the long limb can be used to enhance symmetry of both limbs, and this approach can reduce the potential complications of either technique used alone. Operating on two limbs, however, creates a great deal of immobility in the postoperative period, and that has significant social implications to the patient.

SUMMARY

I will prescribe regimen for the good of my patients according to my ability and my judgment and never do harm to anyone.

Hippocrates of Cos

Before intervening with surgery that alters the biomechanics of the foot and ankle, the wise surgeon may well ponder these words of Hippocrates. Surgery is undertaken only if nonoperative or conservative measures have failed or are considered inappropriate for a given condition. As with any invasive procedure, the risks associated with surgery must be weighed against the potential benefits. Only after careful and thorough evaluation of the clinical condition can the surgeon embark on surgery. Understanding of this aspect of medicine is far from complete, and as technology and research in biomechanics of the foot increase, so will knowledge and success.

This chapter allows the clinician to gain an appreciation for the circumstances under which surgical interventions are undertaken to ensure maximal biomechanical efficiency of the foot and ankle complex. Factors contributing to surgical treatment of pes cavus, pes planus, hallux valgus, hallux rigidus, and toe deformities and ankle instability were presented. Circumstances under which arthrodeses of the ankle, subtalar joint, transverse tarsal joint, and first MTP joint are performed were reviewed. Last, a surgeon's perspective on specific extrinsic abnormalities in the lower limb was presented.

REFERENCES

1. Johnson, KA: Tibialis posterior tendon rupture. Clin Orthop 177:143, 1983.
2. Mann, R and Specht, L: Posterior tibial tendon ruptures: Analysis of eight cases. Foot Ankle 2:350, 1981.
3. Mann, R and Thompson, F: Rupture of the posterior tibial tendon causing flat foot. J Bone Joint Surg 67A:556, 1985.
4. Scranton, P: Treatment of symptomatic talocalcaneal coalition. J Bone Joint Surg 69A:533, 1987.
5. Swiontkowski, MF, et al: Tarsal coalitions: Long term results of surgical treatment. Pediatr Orthop 3:287, 1983.
6. Bordelon, RL: Surgical and Conservative Footcare. Slack, Thorofare, NJ, 1988, pp 72–73.
7. Richardson, EG: Pes planus. In Crenshaw, AH (ed): Campbell's Operative Orthopaedics, ed 8. Mosby, St. Louis, 1992, p 2693.
8. Romash, MR: Calcaneal osteotomy and arthrodesis for malunited calcaneal fracture. In Johnson, KA (ed): The Foot and Ankle. Raven Press, New York, 1994, p 425.
9. Johnson, KA: Surgery of the Foot and Ankle. Raven Press, New York, 1989.
10. Mann, RA and Coughlin, MJ: Surgery of the Foot and Ankle, ed 6. Mosby, St Louis, 1993.
11. Mann, RA and Coughlin, MJ: The Video Textbook of Foot and Ankle Surgery. Medical Video Productions, St. Louis, 1991.
12. Tachdjian, MO: Pediatric Orthopaedics, vol 2. WB Saunders, Philadelphia, 1972.
13. Coughlin, MJ: Proximal First Metatarsal Osteotomy. In Johnson, KA (ed): The Foot and Ankle. Raven Press, New York, 1994, p 85.
14. Sammarco, GJ, Brainard, BJ, and Sammarco, VJ: Bunion correction using proximal chevron osteotomy. Foot Ankle 14:8, 1993.
15. Paley, D: Current techniques in limb lengthening. J Pediatr Orthop 8:73, 1988.

Index

Numbers followed by an *f* indicate figures; numbers followed by a *t* indicate tabular material.